PRIMARY CARE
OF THE
GLAUCOMAS

PRIMARY CARE OF THE GLAUCOMAS

Thomas L. Lewis, OD, PhD
President
Associate Professor
Pennsylvania College of Optometry
Philadelphia, Pennsylvania

Murray Fingeret, OD
Chief, Optometry Section
St. Albans Veterans Administration Extended Care Center
Brooklyn Veterans Administration Medical Center
Brooklyn, New York
Associate Clinical Professor of Optometry
State University of New York College of Optometry
New York, New York
Adjunct Assistant Professor
Pennsylvania College of Optometry
Philadelphia, Pennsylvania

Illustrations by
Stephanie P. Schilling
Lori A. Messenger

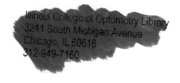

APPLETON & LANGE
Norwalk, Connecticut

Notice: The authors and the publisher of this volume have taken care to make certain that the doses of drugs and schedules of treatment are correct and compatible with the standards generally accepted at the time of publication. Nevertheless, as new information becomes available, changes in treatment and in the use of drugs become necessary. The reader is advised to carefully consult the instruction and information material included in the package insert of each drug or therapeutic agent before administration. This advice is especially important when using new or infrequently used drugs. The publisher disclaims any liability, loss, injury, or damage incurred as a consequence, directly or indirectly, of the use and application of any of the contents of this volume.

Copyright © 1993 by Appleton & Lange
Simon & Schuster Business and Professional Group

93 94 95 96 97 / 10 9 8 7 6 5 4 3 2 1

Prentice Hall International (UK) Limited, *London*
Prentice Hall of Australia Pty. Limited, *Sydney*
Prentice Hall Canada, Inc., *Toronto*
Prentice Hall Hispanoamericana, S.A., *Mexico*
Prentice Hall of India Private Limited, *New Delhi*
Prentice Hall of Japan, Inc., *Tokyo*
Simon & Schuster Asia Pte. Ltd., *Singapore*
Editora Prentice Hall do Brasil Ltda., *Rio de Janeiro*
Prentice Hall, *Englewood Cliffs, New Jersey*

Primary care of the glaucomas / [edited by] Thomas L. Lewis, Murray
    Fingeret.
        p.   cm.
    ISBN 0-8385-7998-1
    1. Glaucoma.   2. Optometrists.   I. Lewis, Thomas L.
    II. Fingeret, Murray.
    [DNLM: 1. Glaucoma—diagnosis.   2. Glaucoma—therapy.   WW 290
    P951]
    RE871.P75   1993
    617.7′41—dc20
    DNLM/DLC
    for Library of Congress   92-17702

Acquisitions Editor: Cheryl L. Mehalik
Senior Managing Editor: John Williams
Designer: Penny Kindzierski

ISBN   0-8385-7998-1

9 780838 579985   90000

This book is dedicated to
Harriet, Tracy, and Heather Lewis
and
Blanche Fingeret Pindus
for all their love and support

and to those with glaucoma who will benefit from the
knowledge gained by doctors from this book

Contents

Contributors

Larry J. Alexander, OD
Professor
Chief, Ocular Disease Clinic
University of Alabama in Birmingham
School of Optometry
Birmingham, Alabama

Connie L. Chronister, OD
Associate Professor
Pennsylvania College of Optometry
Philadelphia, Pennsylvania

John G. Classé, OD, JD
Associate Professor of Optometry
University of Alabama in Birmingham
School of Optometry
Birmingham, Alabama
Member of the Bar, State of Alabama

David M. Cockburn, DSc, MSc
Senior Academic Associate
University of Melbourne, Australia
Parkville, Victoria, Australia

Murray Fingeret, OD
Chief, Optometry Section
St. Albans Veterans Administration Extended Care
    Center/Brooklyn Veterans Administration Medical
    Center
Brooklyn, New York
Associate Clinical Professor of Optometry
State University of New York College of Optometry
New York, New York
Adjunct Assistant Professor
Pennsylvania College of Optometry
Philadelphia, Pennsylvania

Thomas F. Freddo, OD, PhD
Associate Professor of Ophthalmology, Pathology,
    and Anatomy
Director of the Eye Pathology Laboratory

Boston University School of Medicine
Associate in Ophthalmology (Optometry)
The University Hospital
Adjunct Associate Professor of Optometry
New England College of Optometry
Boston, Massachusetts

Ian F. Gutteridge, MSc Optom
Academic Associate
University of Melbourne, Australia
Parkville, Victoria, Australia

Cheryl Berger Israeloff, OD
New York, New York

Joanne Klopfer, OD, MPH
Associate Professor of Optometry and
    Community Health
Pennsylvania College of Optometry
Philadelphia, Pennsylvania

David Kowal, OD
Tallahassee, Florida

Peter A. Lalle, OD
Chief, Optometry Section
Ft. Howard/Baltimore Veterans Administration
    Medical Center
Baltimore, Maryland
Adjunct Assistant Professor
Pennsylvania College of Optometry
Philadelphia, Pennsylvania
Adjunct Assistant Clinical Professor
State University of New York
College of Optometry
New York, New York

Thomas L. Lewis, OD, PhD
President
Associate Professor
Pennsylvania College of Optometry
Philadelphia, Pennsylvania

Anthony B. Litwak, OD
Ft. Howard Veterans Administration
   Medical Center
Ft. Howard, Maryland

Adjunct Assistant Professor
Pennsylvania College of Optometry
Philadelphia, Pennsylvania
Adjunct Assistant Clinical Professor
State University of New York
College of Optometry
New York, New York

Linda Casser Locke, OD
Director, Indianapolis Clinics
Indiana University School of Optometry
Indianapolis, Indiana
Associate Professor of Optometry
Indiana University School of Optometry
Bloomington, Indiana

Sarah J. Paikowsky, OD, MS
Associate Center Director
Omni Eye Services of Baltimore
Baltimore, Maryland
Adjunct Assistant Clinical Professor
State University of New York
College of Optometry
New York, New York
Adjunct Clinical Professor of Optometry
New England College of Optometry
Boston, Massachusetts

Susan P. Schuettenberg, OD
Chief, Eye Service
East New York Neighborhood Family Care Center
Brooklyn, New York
Assistant Clinical Professor
State University of New York
College of Optometry
New York, New York

Thomas Stelmack, OD
Chief, Optometry Section
Westside Veterans Administration Medical Center
Associate Professor
Illinois College of Optometry
Assistant Professor
University of Illinois School of Medicine
Department of Ophthalmology
Chicago, Illinois

J. James Thimons, OD
Associate Professor
Chairman, Department of Clinical Science
Director of Professional Services
State University of New York
College of Optometry
New York, New York

Carla U. Vogel, RPh
Staff Pharmacist
Cooper Medical Center
Camden, New Jersey

Wolfgang H. Vogel, PhD
Professor of Pharmacology
Professor of Psychiatry and Human Behavior
Jefferson Medical College of Thomas
   Jefferson University
Philadelphia, Pennsylvania

Elliot B. Werner, MD
Associate Professor of Ophthalmology
Hahnemann University
Philadelphia, Pennsylvania

Joan Tanabe Wing, OD
Instructor
Pennsylvania College of Optometry
Philadelphia, Pennsylvania

Introduction

Optometry, as a profession, has grown and evolved over the time many of us have been in practice. Indeed a few years ago it would not have been imaginable that optometrists would write a book on glaucoma. Diagnostic pharmaceutical agents are now available for all optometrists to use and give us the ability to fully and completely differentially diagnose glaucoma. In addition the scope of practice has broadened so that many optometrists are able to treat and manage, or at least co-manage, their glaucoma patients. With this as a background, it appears timely that *Primary Care of the Glaucomas* is published.

The driving force behind this book since its inception was to create a text for the practicing optometrist. The book is intended to be clinical in nature, getting to the heart of the matter quickly and succinctly. As such we have enlisted many of the optometric experts in glaucoma to contribute to this text, asking them to keep their chapters practical and useful. *Primary Care of the Glaucomas* is not meant to be an all-inclusive textbook on glaucoma. Rather, we have attempted to stress relevant material without including rare, esoteric information. The artwork interspersed throughout the book is designed to illustrate the anatomic and pathologic correlations of glaucoma. The layouts often include photographs so that the optometrist has a clinical feel for what is being illustrated.

This book is composed of several sections: basic understanding of glaucoma, diagnosis of the glaucomas, and treatment and management of the glaucomas. We build a foundation in the early chapters, starting with the normal anatomy and physiology of the anterior segment and optic nerve so that the clinical significance of the pathophysiology, pharmacology, diagnosis, and treatment and management are fully appreciated by the reader.

It is our hope that this text will serve as a silent "colleague" for optometrists in the examination room, helping to guide them in the diagnosis, management, and treatment of their patients with glaucoma.

Thomas L. Lewis
Murray Fingeret

Acknowledgments

In a text such as this, many individuals play a role in either the research, writing, typing, copying, or in many of the other tasks involved. For all those individuals who have helped in some way, we thank you.

In particular we would like to especially thank several individuals: first, Craig Percy, who was the initial visionary and started us on this endeavor, and also Lou Catania, for always being "Lou."

We would also like to thank Jimmy Bartlett, Tony Cavallerano, Ron Davidoff, Gina Gladstein, Anita Goldstein, Rodney Gutner, Lisa Lonie, Esther Marks, Taryn Mathews, and Ruby Singleton for all their help.

Color Plates

Illustrations on the color plates are also reproduced in black and white with their relevant discussions in each chapter. The list below gives the page within the text where the black and white illustration occurs.

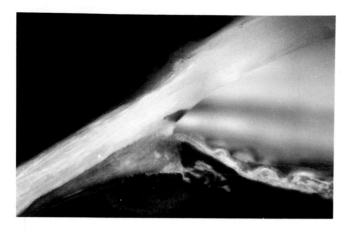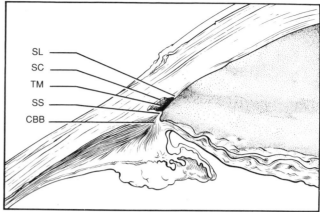

Figure 3–17. Macroscopic photograph and corresponding sketch identifying structures visible in a sagittal section of the normal anterior chamber angle. The anterior chamber is artifactually deepened due to posterior sagging of the iris following removal of the crystalline lens. SL = Schwalbe's line; SC = Schlemm's canal; TM = trabecular meshwork; SS = scleral spur; CBB = ciliary body band.

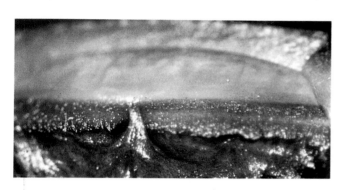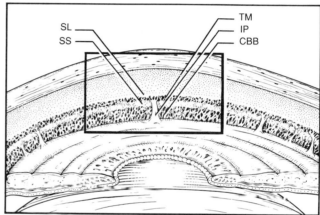

Figure 3–18. Macroscopic photograph and corresponding sketch of angle structures viewed from the perspective shown in the adjacent sketch. Schlemm's canal is filled with blood in this specimen, demonstrating its relationship to the other angle structures. An iris process is also shown. Compare the view of the angle structures in this figure with the corresponding sagittal view shown in Figure 3–17. SL = Schwalbe's line; SS = scleral spur; TM = trabecular meshwork; IP = iris process; CBB = ciliary body band.

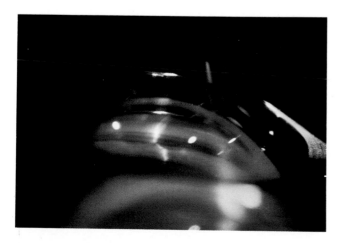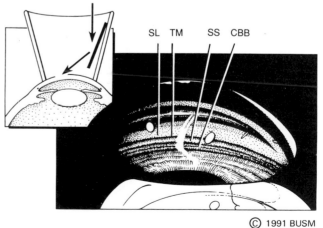

© 1991 BUSM

Figure 3–19. Goniophotograph of a normal open angle, and corresponding sketch representing a view analogous to that shown in Figure 3–18. *Inset* in sketch depicts the placement of the gonioscope onto the cornea and the manner in which the angle structures are viewed. SL = Schwalbe's line; TM = trabecular meshwork; SS = scleral spur; CBB = ciliary body band. *(Photo courtesy of Rodney Gutner, OD.)*

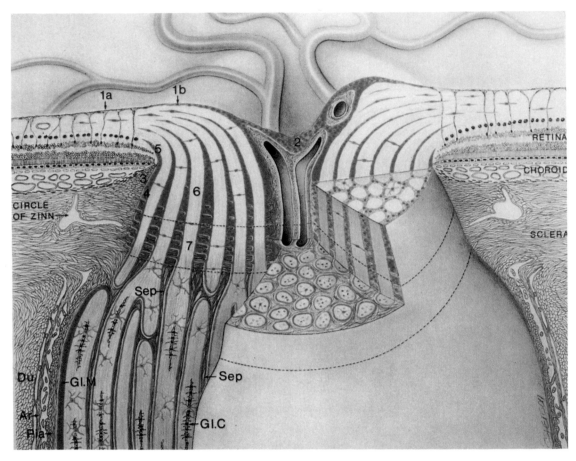

Figure 4–2. Three-dimensional drawing of the intraocular and part of the orbital optic nerve. The intraocular portion extends from the inner limiting membrane covering the optic nerve head to the back surface of the scleral lamina cribrosa. The nerve fibers of the retina (6) are separated into bundles by astrocytes. At the lamina cribrosa (upper dotted line), the nerve fascicles (7) and their surrounding astrocytes are separated from each other by the cribriform plate (drawn in blue). At the external part of the lamina cribrosa (lower dotted line), the nerve fibers become myelinated and the diameter of the nerve doubles. Columns of oligodendrocytes (black and white cells) and a few astrocytes (red cells) can be seen within the nerve fascicles. Other cells and regions include: Muller cells (1a), internal limiting membrane of Elschnig (1b), central meniscus of Kuhnt (2), and border tissue of Elschnig (3). Astrocytes line the optic nerve canal (4) and glial tissue is found at the termination of the retina (5). Septal tissue (Sep), glial mantle (Gl.M) and the dura (Du), arachnoid (Ar), and pia mater (Pia) are shown. *(Published courtesy of* Arch Ophthalmol, *1969; 82:506–530. Copyright, American Medical Association.)*

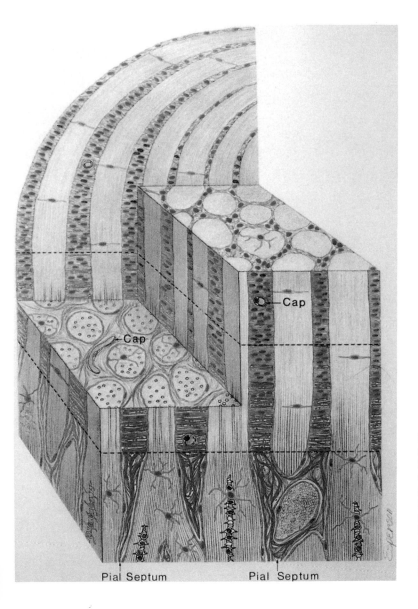

Figure 4–6. Detailed view of the prelaminar, laminar, and post laminar optic nerve. Astrocytes (red) separate the nerve fibers into bundles. Capillaries (Cap) are seen within these astrocytic columns. The lamina cribrosa is present between the dotted lines (drawn in blue). The connective tissue of the lamina cribrosa is continuous posteriorly with the pial septae. Nerve fibers become myelinated in the postlaminar region. *(Published courtesy of* Arch Ophthalmol. *1969; 82:800–814. Copyright, American Medical Association.)*

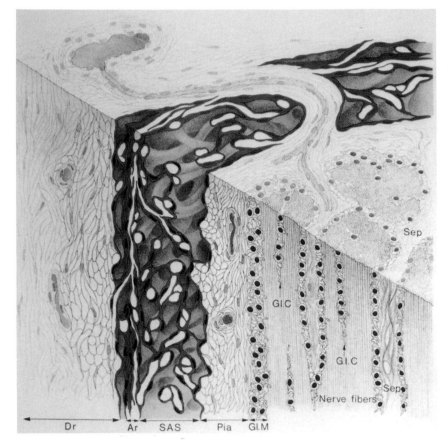

Figure 4–10. Photograph of vaginal sheaths of optic nerve, showing relationship between dura mater (Dr), arachnoid mater (Ar), subarachnoid space (SAS), and pia mater (Pia). Meningothelial cells contribute to the arachnoid mater and form linings for the dura mater, arachnoid trabeculae and pia mater. The inner surface of the pia mater is separated from the intraorbital portion of the optic nerve by a layer of fibrous astrocytes, forming the glial mantle (Gl.M) and glial columns (Gl.C). Elements from the pia mater form the pial septae (sep), which enclose the axonal bundles. The septae originate in the posterior lamina cribrosa, continue through the orbital and intracanalicular portions, and end in the intracranial portions of the optic nerve. *(Published courtesy of* Arch Ophthalmol. *1969; 82:659–674. Copyright, American Medical Association.)*

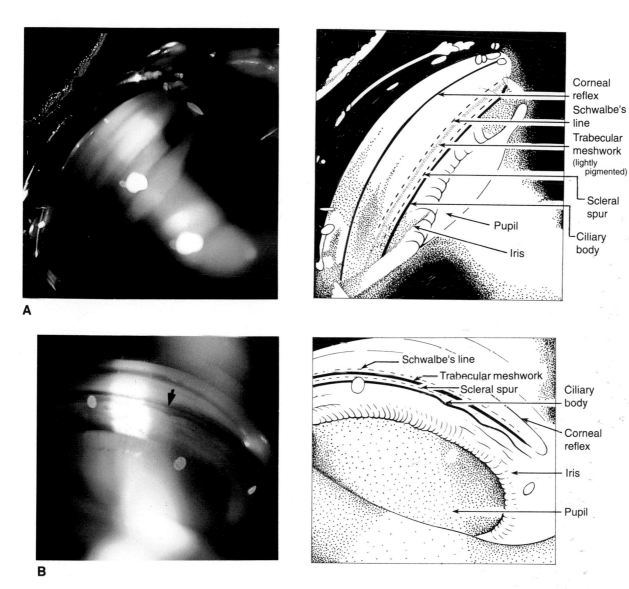

Figure 8–8. Normal angle anatomy. Note ciliary body, scleral spur, trabecular meshwork, and Schwalbe's line. The patient in (**A.**) has very little pigmentation in the trabecular meshwork. The patient in (**B.**) has a heavily pigmented trabecular meshwork. There may be considerable variation in the clinical appearance of the normal angle.

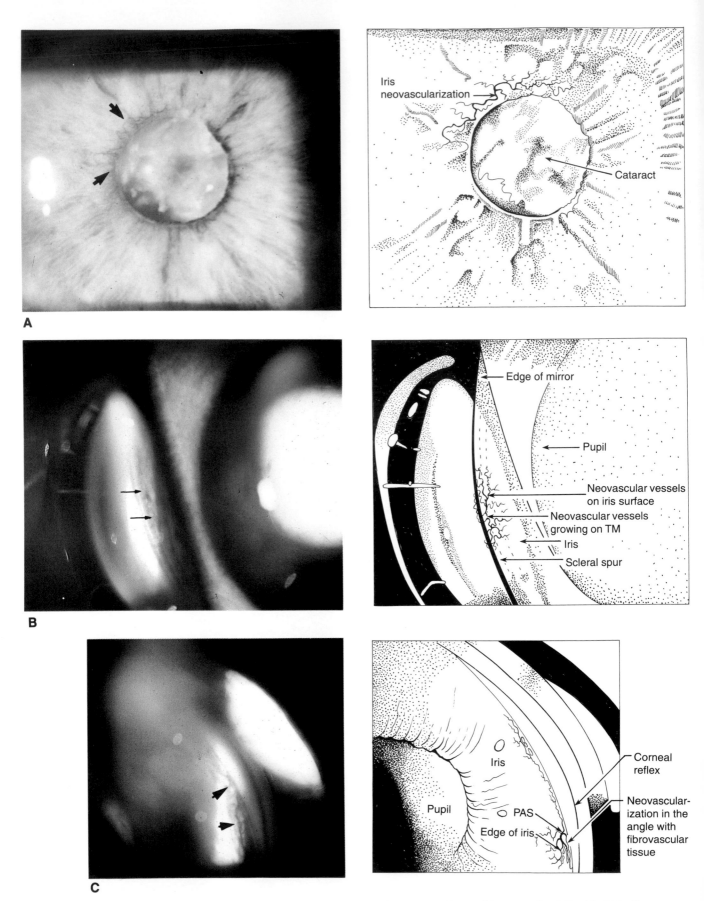

Figure 8–13. Iris neovascularization. Neovascular vessels typically occur at the pupillary margin of the iris **(A.)** after an ischemic event to the retina. These vessels may grow into the angle **(B.)** along with fibrovascular tissue forming PAS **(C.)** and neovascular glaucoma.

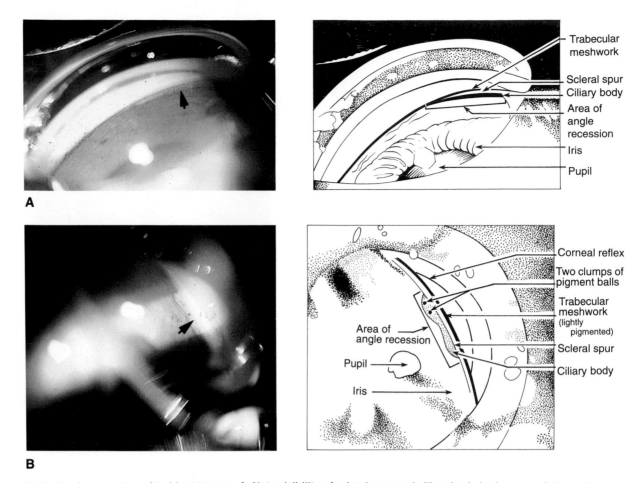

Trabecular meshwork

Scleral spur
Ciliary body

Area of angle recession

Iris

Pupil

A

Corneal reflex

Two clumps of pigment balls

Trabecular meshwork (lightly pigmented)

Scleral spur

Ciliary body

Area of angle recession

Pupil

Iris

B

Figure 8–14. Angle recession after blunt trauma. **A.** Note visibility of scleral spur and ciliary body in the area of the angle recess. **B.** Angle recession or clumps of pigment in the angle are indicators of possible damage to the trabecular meshwork and the risk of development of post-traumatic glaucoma.

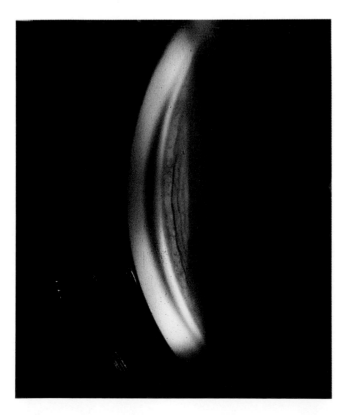

Figure 8–15. Blood in Schlemm's canal, a sign of elevated episcleral venous pressure. Schlemm's canal lies directly behind the trabecular meshwork and is not normally visible unless blood is present.

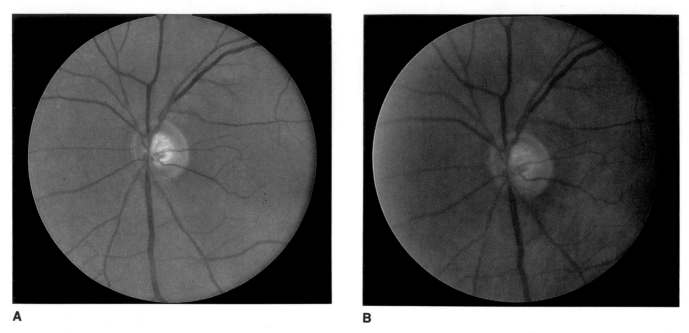

A

B

Figure 9–8. Serial disc photographs of a glaucoma suspect taken 4 years apart. Note progressive enlargement of the cup with localized deflection towards the inferior pole with shifting of the disc vessel at 4:30 o'clock **(B.)**.

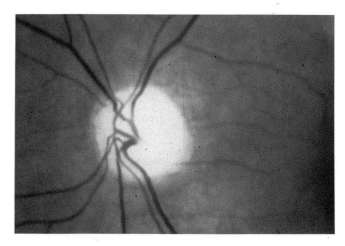

Figure 9–9. Optic cupping and diffuse pallor of the remaining neuroretinal rim tissue in an elderly patient with giant cell arteritis with anterior ischemic optic neuropathy. In glaucoma, the remaining neuroretinal rim tissue is a healthy orange-red color.

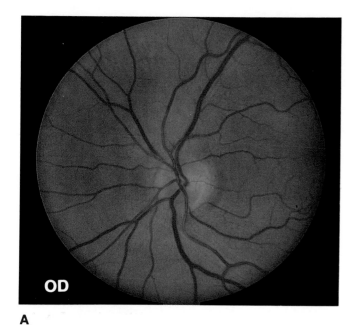

A

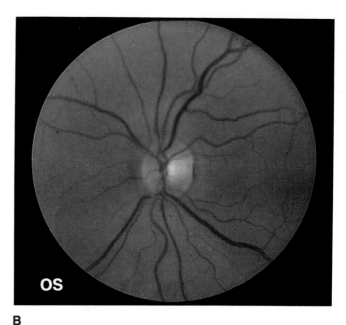

B

Figure 9–10. Cup-to-disc asymmetry secondary to unequal disc sizes. Photographs taken at same magnification with similar refractive errors, K readings, and axial lengths. Note larger cup and disc size in left eye compared to right eye. Cup-to-disc asymmetry of 0.2 or greater not due to unequal disc size should raise the suspicion of glaucoma.

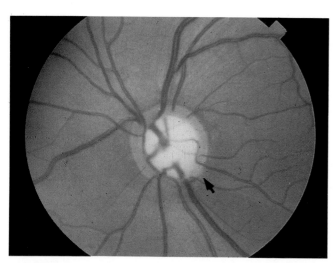

Figure 9–11. A. Notching of the inferior temporal pole of the optic disc in a glaucoma patient. Notches are usually associated with a wedge NFL defect and a corresponding visual field defect.

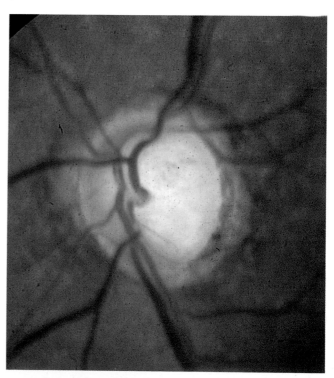

Figure 9–14. Peripapillary crescent associated with glaucoma. Note moth-eaten appearance of peripapillary crescent adjacent to thinning of the temporal rim in a normal-tension glaucoma patient. The specificity of this sign in glaucoma is unknown.

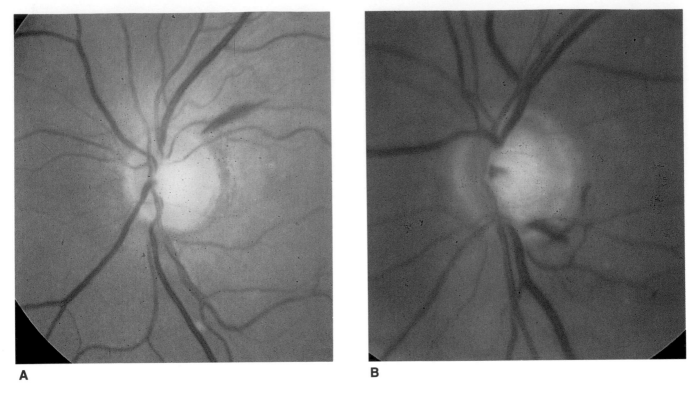

Figure 9–15. Disc hemorrhage (Drance hemorrhage) in glaucoma. Splinter hemorrhages on or adjacent to the optic nerve head usually in the inferior or superior temporal pole may be a sign of early glaucomatous damage **(A.)** or an indication of progressive glaucomatous damage **(B.)**. Disc hemorrhages are not pathognomonic for glaucoma.

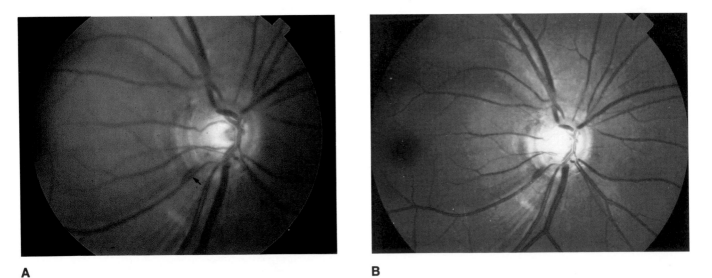

Figure 9–16. Drance hemorrhage with associated NFL defect. Note subtle disc hemorrhage at the 7 o'clock position **(A.)** with an accompanying slit NFL defect **(B.)**. Also note slit defects at 6:30 and 10:30 o'clock positions.

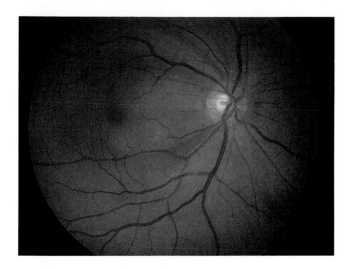

Figure 9–18. A. Glaucoma suspect with elevated IOP, non-glaucomatous cupping, and normal visual fields. NFL slit defects can be appreciated in the inferior and superior arcades with normal white light.

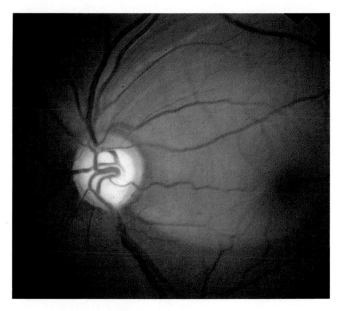

Figure 9–22. A. Advanced glaucoma patient with large cupping and an inferior notch of the optic disc. NFL loss inferiorly is visible.

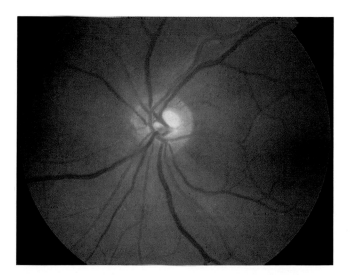

Figure 9–21. A. Glaucoma suspect with elevated intraocular pressure, non-glaucomatous cupping, and a normal visual field.

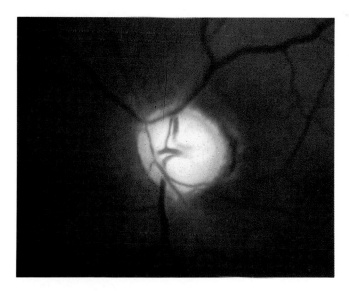

Figure 9–23. A. Endstage glaucomatous damage. Note complete cupping of the optic nerve.

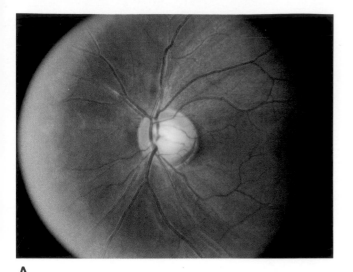

A

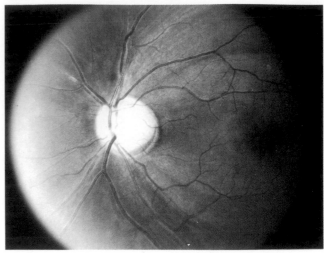

B

Figure 12–3. Focal nerve fiber layer dropout. Color and companion red-free photography of the left eye of a glaucoma patient with several slit-like defects in the nerve fiber layer between 12 and 2 o'clock and a large wedge defect between 5 and 7 o'clock.

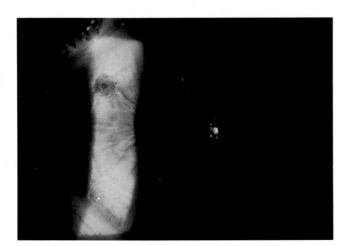

Figure 15–4. Postoperative photograph of a patent laser peripheral iridectomy. To be certain that the iridectomy is patent, the lens capsule should be seen through the iridectomy opening.

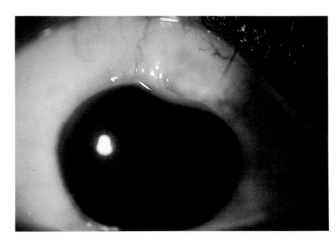

Figure 15–11. Photograph of a functioning filtering bleb. The bleb is translucent, avascular, and demonstrates microcysts at the anterior edge.

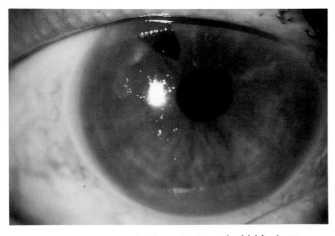

Figure 15–5. Photograph of a patent surgical iridectomy.

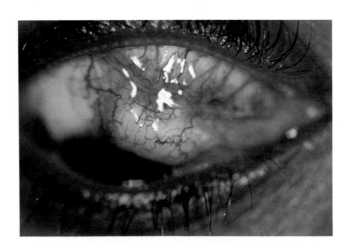

Figure 15–12. Photograph of an encapsulated bleb. The bleb is tense, opaque, elevated, and vascularized.

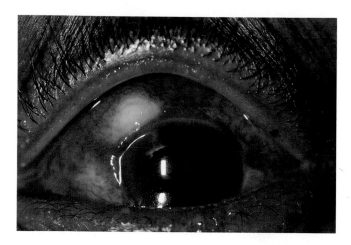

Figure 15–13. Photograph of an infected bleb. The eye is markedly hyperemic. The bleb is filled with pus and appears white.

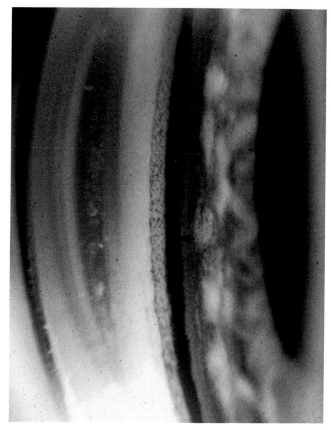

Figure 17–4. Dense trabecular meshwork pigmentation noted in an individual with pigmentary glaucoma.

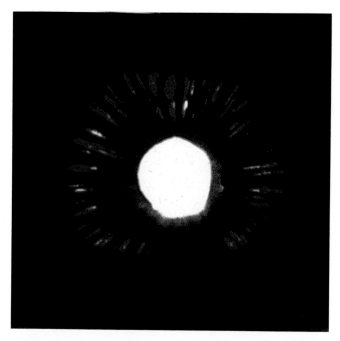

Figure 17–3. Iris transillumination defects, associated with pigment dispersion syndrome, occur in the mid-periphery and are circumferential in appearance.

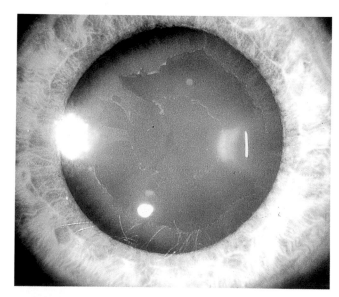

Figure 17–7. Classical pseudoexfoliative "bulls-eye" pattern on the anterior lens surface. *(Courtesy of Rodney Gutner, OD.)*

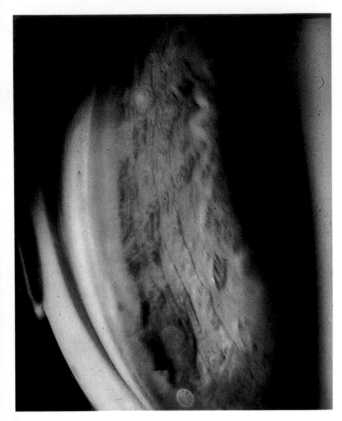

Figure 17–12. Severe angle recession. Note how wide open the angle appears.

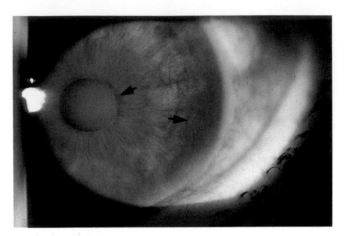

Figure 17–15. Early neovascular changes seen at the pupillary zone and mid-periphery of the iris.

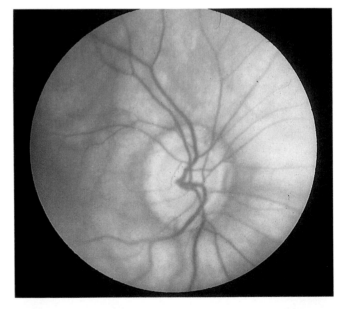

Figure 18–3. The pale atropic irregular annulus centered on the optic disc and bordered by a brown line is known as peripapillary halo or atrophy. Although common in normal eyes, peripapillary atrophy is over-represented in patients having glaucoma and particularly low-tension glaucoma.

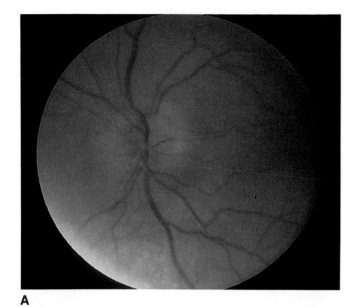

A

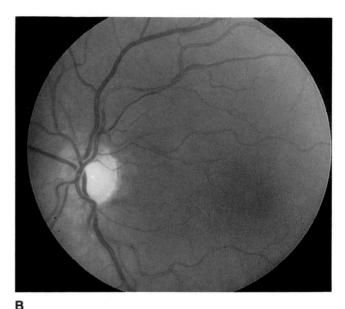

B

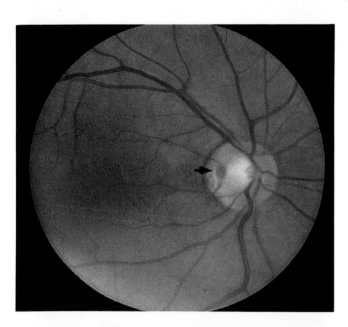

Figure 18–5 (above). **A.** Anterior ischemic optic atrophy (AION) presents acutely as a pale swelling of the disc, which may be localized to the area representing the watershed of one or more occluded short posterior cilliary arteries. **B.** Following resolution of the acute phase, the disc may assume the appearance of glaucomatous atrophy. Because IOP is within normal limits, a resolved case of AION may be mistaken for low-tension glaucoma.

Figure 18–6 (left). Optic nerve head pit. A congenital localized hiatus in the nerve head appears either as a hole or as a plug of glial tissue. This localized absence of axons gives rise to an arcuate scotoma, which could lead to an erroneous diagnosis of low-tension glaucoma in the presence of normal IOP.

Figure 18–7 (below). Optic disc drusen. These deposits within the optic nerve head may be visible as bubble-like excrescences on the surface of the disc (**A.**) or be partly buried and appear as a mildly raised nerve head (**B.**). In some instances the drusen may be totally hidden below the disc surface. Disc drusen are commonly associated with arcuate nerve fiber loss and, because IOP is usually normal, the condition could be mistaken for low-tension glaucoma.

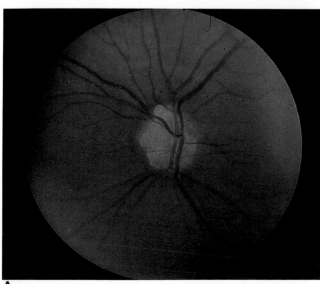

A

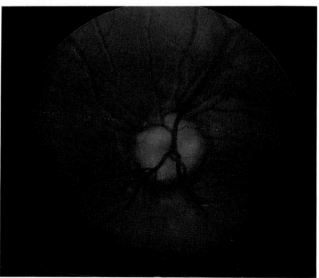

B

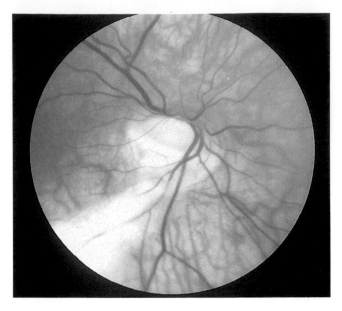

Figure 18–8. The tilted disc syndrome consists of crowding of axons at the superior portion of the disc and a relative deficiency at the inferior pole, which gives the disc the appearance of being tilted inferiorly. The remainder of the signs of tilted disc consist of a relative deficiency of pigment in the retinal pigment epithelium in the inferior ocular fundus, astigmatism, reduced visual acuity, and a relative visual field loss superiorly as a result of the deficiency of axons inferiorly. In the presence of normal IOP, this could be mistakenly diagnosed as low-tension glaucoma. In bilateral cases, the condition may mimic a bitemporal hemianopia. However, this mistake should be avoided because the field loss in an eye having tilted disc does not respect the vertical mid-line. This example of a tilted disc has incidental medulated nerve fibers.

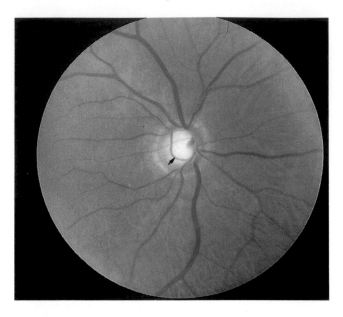

Figure 18–9. Baring of circumlinear vessels. On the normal disc, the surface vessels traverse and lie on the neuroretinal rim tissue, sometimes running for a short distance parallel with the rim. With progress of glaucomatous damage, the vessel may appear to be left suspended over the cup rather than resting on the rim tissue. Documentation of the location of such a vessel relative to the neuroretinal rim allows assessment of any progress of cupping.

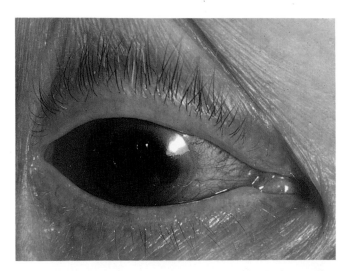

Figure 19–6. An angle closure attack typically presents with a red eye, cloudy cornea, and a mid-dilated pupil.

Section I

BASIC UNDERSTANDING OF GLAUCOMA

Chapter 1

DEFINITION AND CLASSIFICATION OF GLAUCOMAS

Thomas L. Lewis

DEFINITION

Glaucoma is not a single clinical entity. It represents a group of ocular diseases with various etiologies that ultimately result in a rather consistent optic neuropathy. Glaucomas are diseases in which intraocular pressure becomes "abnormal" for a given individual or in which that person's optic nerve becomes unusually susceptible to damage resulting in histopathological changes in this tissue. These changes eventually lead to a loss of visual function. Therefore, the classical triad of abnormal intraocular pressure, optic nerve damage, and visual function loss characterize most forms of glaucomas.

It is important to realize that various forms of glaucoma exist. From a clinical perspective, a generic diagnosis of glaucoma is inadequate to develop a proper management plan for the patient. A differential diagnosis, indicating the specific type of glaucoma, is necessary to predict the course and prognosis of the disease, and to assure appropriate and timely treatment.

CLASSIFICATION

Since glaucoma is a group of diseases with varying clinical presentations, prognoses, morbidity, treatment, and management, a system to properly classify these diseases is important. Various classifications have been proposed. These classification systems are either based on (1) etiology, i.e. the underlying cause of the change in aqueous dynamics, or (2) mechanics, i.e. the structural alteration in the anterior chamber angle, which results in an increase in intraocular pressure.

I have chosen a classification system with both an etiological and mechanical basis. This type of classification system seems to make the most sense clinically. The terminology used can assist the doctor in the proper diagnosis and management of glaucoma patients.

OPEN VERSUS CLOSED ANGLE

Glaucomas can be divided into *open angle* or *closed angle*. This relates to the gonioscopic appearance of the anterior chamber angle (Fig. 1–1). In open-angle glaucomas, the rise in intraocular pressure, if it occurs, is not due to a mechanical obstruction of the angle by the iris. In closed-angle glaucomas, the outflow of aqueous is obstructed by the root of the iris. This obstruction can be associated with *pupillary block* or can occur without pupillary block.

Both open-angle and closed-angle glaucomas can

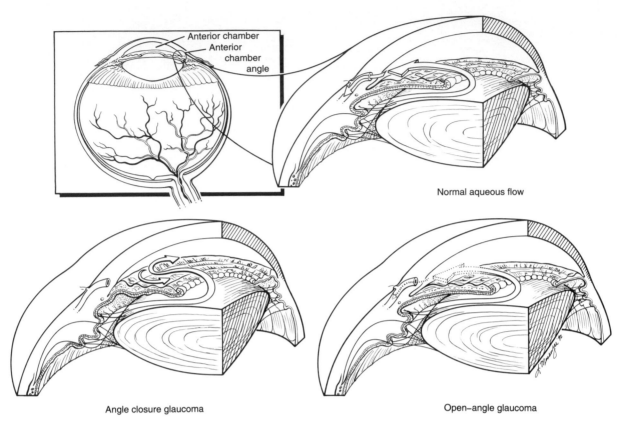

Figure 1–1. Representation of the differences in aqueous flow and the anterior chamber angle configuration between open-angle and closed-angle glaucomas.

result from underlying primary, secondary, or developmental etiologies. *Primary* glaucomas are not associated with any other apparent ocular or systemic disorder. In primary open-angle glaucoma, the obstruction to aqueous outflow is apparently occurring at a submicroscopic and/or biochemical level in the outflow pathways. These alterations are not visible on gonioscopic evaluation (Fig. 1–1). In primary closed-angle glaucoma, a pupillary block or *plateau iris* forces the iris into the anterior chamber angle, obstructing aqueous outflow (Table 1–1). Primary

glaucomas are usually genetically based and bilateral in their clinical presentation.

Secondary glaucomas are caused by a variety of ocular and/or systemic disorders, which, as a sequela of that condition, cause a decrease in aqueous outflow in either open-angle or closed-angle individuals. The obstruction of aqueous outflow in secondary open-angle glaucomas can occur by membrane formation over the anterior chamber angle; physical blockage of the trabecular meshwork by pigment, debris, or anatomical changes within the trabeculae; or

TABLE 1–1. PRIMARY GLAUCOMAS

Open-Angle
High tension
Normal (low tension)
Closed-Angle
With pupillary block
Prodromal
Subacute
Acute
Chronic
Without pupillary block
Plateau iris

TABLE 1–2. SECONDARY GLAUCOMAS: Open-Angle

Pigmentary	Inflammatory induced
Exfoliation	Tumor induced
syndrome	Lens induced
Neovascular	Intraocular hemorrhage
Post-traumatic	induced
Epithelial	Retinal detachment
downgrowth	Following intraocular surgery
Fibrous ingrowth	Following an increase in
Fuch's endothelial	episcleral venous pressure
dystrophy	

TABLE 1–3. SECONDARY GLAUCOMAS: Closed-Angle

With Pupillary Block
Miotic induced
Lens induced—swollen, ectopic
Synechiae to lens, vitreous, lens implant
Spherophakia

Without Pupillary Block

Anterior (Pulling)	*Posterior (Pushing)*
Neovascular	Central retinal vein
Fibrous ingrowth	occlusion
Iridocorneal endothelial	Iris or ciliary body cyst
syndrome	Ciliary block
Post-traumatic	Tumor induced
Inflammatory induced	Inflammatory induced
	Choroidal detachment
	Suprachoroidal hemorrhage
	Following panretinal
	photocoagulation
	Following scleral buckling

TABLE 1–4. DEVELOPMENTAL GLAUCOMAS

Primary	Secondary
Primary congenital (infantile)	Retinopathy of prematurity
	Post-traumatic
	Tumor related
	Inflammatory induced

Associated With Congenital Anomalies or Syndromes

Aniridia	Lowe's syndrome
Sturge-Weber syndrome	Microcornea
Neurofibromatosis	Microspherophakia
Marfan's syndrome	Rubella
Pierre Robin syndrome	Chromosome abnormalities
Homocystinuria	Persistent hyperplastic
Goniodysgenesis	primary vitreous

by changes in Schlemm's canal or the episcleral venous system (Table 1–2). Secondary closed-angle glaucomas are most easily divided into anterior forms, in which the iris is *pulled* into the angle by the contraction of structures in the angle, and posterior forms, in which the iris is *pushed* forward into the angle either from increased pressure caused by a pupillary block or from pressure building up behind the iris from a space-occupying change within the eye (Table 1–3). Secondary glaucomas can be inherited or acquired and be either unilateral or bilateral in their clinical presentation.

Developmental glaucomas are due to abnormalities in the anterior chamber angle, occurring during gestation, which result in a decrease in aqueous outflow. Most forms of developmental glaucomas are secondary; however, primary developmental glaucomas can occur (Table 1–4).

Whereas most forms of glaucoma are *chronic*, on rare occasions certain patients with closed-angle glaucoma can present with an *acute* form of the disease. A certain percentage of glaucoma patients will have a mixed-mechanism glaucoma, which is a combination of both open-angle and closed-angle glaucomas. Patients may show a change in their type of glaucoma over time. This is important to keep in mind since it influences the treatment plan for that patient.

Tables 1–1 through 1–4 presents a comprehensive but not exhaustive classification system for glaucoma. This textbook will concentrate on primary open-angle glaucoma, since it is the most common form of glaucoma seen in optometric practices. Primary closed-angle and secondary glaucomas will also be presented. Developmental glaucomas will not be discussed in detail because of the infrequency with which they are seen by optometrists.

All classification systems are arbitrary. Some cases do not fit neatly into one category. Remember, however, classification of glaucoma can be critical to the proper treatment of the patient. A specific diagnosis should differentiate open-angle from closed-angle, primary from secondary, and if possible, identify the specific disorder causing the secondary glaucoma.

Chapter 2

EPIDEMIOLOGY AND CLINICAL IMPACT OF THE GLAUCOMAS

Joanne Klopfer
Sarah J. Paikowsky

Epidemiology is the study of the occurrence of health-related states in populations and is concerned with patterns of disease as well as evaluation of factors thought to be responsible for the observed patterns.[1,2] Epidemiology can be viewed as an analytical tool to help the clinician make a judgment about disease and the relevance of risk factors in diagnostic decisions. The purpose of this chapter is to provide a synopsis of epidemiological principles that apply to understanding glaucoma in clinical practice. Emphasis will be on the epidemiology of primary open-angle glaucoma.

Two basic epidemiological principles are that disease and health are not randomly distributed in the population and there is usually a multicausal etiology involved in disease processes. Glaucoma follows along these principles. No single factor or measure has been isolated as responsible for the development of glaucoma.

Cataracts, primary open-angle glaucoma, and age-related macular degeneration are the leading causes of blindness in the United States.[3–5] For persons between the ages of 45 and 64 years, glaucoma is one of the leading causes of new cases of visual impairment.[6] Unlike cataracts, where vision can be restored, glaucomatous damage to the eye is irrepara-

ble. Each year in the United States, 95,000 patients lose some degree of sight from glaucoma.[7] National data from surveys conducted in the 1970s showed nearly 2 million persons over the age of 35 years were diagnosed as having glaucoma. More significantly, an estimated 1 million persons were reported to have undetected glaucoma.[6]

Blindness registries from selected states in the United States have reported glaucoma as the second leading cause of irreversible blindness.[8] In blindness registry statistics, a notable difference has been found between blindness rates in ethnic "white" and "nonwhite" populations. Glaucoma is the major cause of blindness among black Americans but only the fifth cause of blindness in persons of European descent or "white" American populations.[9] Other population-based or epidemiological studies also support glaucoma as a major cause of blindness in black populations.[4] Ethnicity, sometimes referred to as "race," has become a demographic factor of considerable interest in glaucoma.[10,11]

The treatment of glaucoma has been cited as the leading reason for office visits involving medical eye care. In the National Ambulatory Medical Care Sur-

A special thanks to Luanne M. Wislow for her technical support.

vey, there were approximately 2.6 million doctor visits for glaucoma in 1976.[6] This figure was based on a sample survey conducted of physician office services and specifically excluded ophthalmologists or optometrists practicing in eye clinics, hospitals, or nursing homes. The true number of doctor visits for the diagnosis and management of glaucoma is most likely greater. A recent estimation of the costs of treating glaucoma in the United States was $1.9 billion per year. This includes $903 million spent annually on visits to physicians, including diagnostic tests, $516 million on laser and incisional surgery, $351 million on prescription medications, and $94 million on blindness and low-vision rehabilitative services related to glaucoma.[12] An estimated $235 million of productive work time is lost annually because of glaucoma.[7] Since glaucoma is an age-related disease, implications for the future are significant given the aging of the population. Glaucoma is a disease that merits careful attention in order to prevent future blindness and visual impairment.

There is a wide variation in the presentation of glaucoma. Although the majority of glaucoma cases are primary in nature, genetic, developmental, and secondary conditions must be considered. This chapter will focus on the epidemiological information available on the prevalence, incidence, and risk factors for glaucoma. By definition, the *prevalence rate* is the number of individuals with a disease divided by the total population at risk of having the disease at one particular point in time.[2] Simply stated, prevalence represents the probability of having a disease. Most of the "statistics" quoted on glaucoma in populations are prevalence data. The *incidence rate* is a measure of the rate at which new cases of a disease develop in a specified period of time.[2] Disease incidence rates depict the number of new disease cases that develop in a disease-free population that has been followed for a defined period of time.[2] A *risk factor* can be defined as an attribute or exposure that increases the probability of developing a disease.[13] The challenge for the clinician is to identify the risk factors for a disease, to recognize these factors in the patient, and to be able to weigh the most important factors when establishing the diagnosis of glaucoma.

PRIMARY OPEN-ANGLE GLAUCOMA

Prevalence

Primary open-angle glaucoma (POAG) accounts for approximately 70% of all adult glaucoma cases.[14,15] Accurate figures on the prevalence of glaucoma are difficult to ascertain because diagnostic information is needed to define POAG. In addition, many statistics reported on the prevalence of glaucoma actually represent surveys of patients who sought care or committed to a vision screening program. These self-selected persons may be either healthier or sicker than the general population. Therefore, prevalence figures vary (Table 2–1). General estimates for the prevalence of POAG in the United States range from 0.27% in residents of Rochester, Minnesota over the age of 45 years[16] to as high as 5.6% for blacks over 40 years of age in the Baltimore Eye Survey.[4] Worldwide, the prevalence of POAG for populations over 40 years of age has been reported to be 0.86%[18] in Sweden and 0.64% in the United Kingdom.[19] The differences between these figures may be due to variation in the actual prevalences of glaucoma between countries or may reflect differences in how the prevalence rates were obtained.

Three population-based studies have provided the quintessential information on the prevalence of POAG. The Hollows and Graham study conducted in Ferndale, Wales collected data on residents 40 to 74 years of age in three Welsh villages during 1963. Ophthalmic examination included direct ophthalmoscopy, applanation tonometry, slit-lamp examination, and visual field testing on every third subject. A prevalence rate of 0.43% for POAG was reported.[20] In about one third of the cases, the glaucomatous visual field defects appeared in eyes with apparently "low" or normal intraocular pressures (IOPs). This altered the thinking of many clinicians, casting doubt on the effectiveness of determining glaucoma with tonometry alone.

The 1973 to 1975 Framingham Eye Study is a historical source of information on the prevalence of eye disease in the United States. In this study, 2675 residents of Framingham, Massachusetts, aged 52 to 85 years, were screened by history, tonometry, and ophthalmoscopy. The subjects were referred for Goldmann perimetry if they had one or more positive findings. A variety of prevalence rates for open-angle glaucoma in the Framingham population have been

TABLE 2–1. PREVALENCE[a] OF PRIMARY OPEN-ANGLE GLAUCOMA

	%
U.S.[4,15,16]	0.27–5.6
Sweden[17]	0.86
U.K.[18]	0.64
Wales[19]	0.43
Jamaica[22]	1.4
St. Lucia[23]	8.8–14.7

[a] Time period varies according to individual study.

reported, ranging from 1.2 to 2.1%.[5,21,22] For example, the POAG estimates were found to be at least 30% higher with subsequent analysis of the subgroup who had visual fields performed.[21] The Framingham Eye Study demonstrated the necessity of visual field examination to accurately define cases of POAG, and also clearly delineated increasing age as a strong risk factor for POAG.[21]

The Baltimore Eye Survey was conducted from 1985 to 1988 on noninstitutionalized persons over the age of 40 years who resided in east Baltimore. An eye screening examination consisting of refraction, visual acuity, tonometry, automated perimetry, ophthalmoscopy, detailed history, and stereo fundus photography of the optic disc and macula was administered to 5300 persons.[3] Unlike previous prevalence studies, the criteria for referral of diagnosis of POAG did not depend solely on tonometry or ophthalmoscopy. Evidence of glaucoma was based on the appearance of visual fields, optic disc, and/or nerve fiber layer atrophy. The results of this prevalence survey confirmed an increase of POAG with increasing age. More significantly, blacks were found to have a 4.7 times higher prevalence of POAG compared to whites.[4] Blacks were found to have higher rates of POAG in every age group, despite having lower IOPs. While the prevalence of glaucoma did not rise appreciably in the white population until 60 years of age or older, the black population had a linear trend beginning at 40 years of age (Fig. 2–1). These findings can be extrapolated to other multiracial urban populations in the United States because the Baltimore Eye Survey was a population-based investigation. The most significant finding of this study was the importance of evaluating the combined risk factors of age and race or ethnicity. The major public

health message derived from this study was that glaucoma evaluation should start early (no later than age 40) in the black population. Another striking finding was the amount of unrecognized disease and uncorrected refractive error found in the general population of an urban area.

Caribbean population-based studies provide prevalence data supportive of a higher rate of POAG in blacks. An ophthalmic survey in Jamaica, with a study design similar to that of the Wales study, reported a 1.4% prevalence rate for 574 persons age 35 years and older.[23] In St. Lucia, a more extensive study showed prevalence estimates to be 8.8 to 14.7%.[24]

A review of the POAG prevalence figures from various studies around the world (*see* Table 2–1) yields a disparate picture. Despite these differences, several conclusions can be derived. First, glaucoma has been diagnosed in significant numbers in persons with "normal" IOPs. Secondly, visual field testing improves the accuracy of detecting glaucoma. Finally, elevated IOP and age have been shown to increase the risk of POAG. More recent work has substantiated race or ethnicity as an added risk factor to consider.

Incidence

The incidence of glaucoma has not been clearly determined in population-based investigations. This is primarily because POAG occurs infrequently. Unlike prevalence studies where thousands of residents in a community are evaluated in order to find cases of glaucoma, it is much more difficult to follow the large number of disease-free individuals that are needed to diagnose the development of new cases of glaucoma.

Armaly conducted a 10-year longitudinal study on 3936 persons who were initially free of ocular disease in Des Moines, Iowa. Only four persons developed visual field loss during the first 5 years of the study and no patients developed visual field loss in the remaining 5 years.[25] The incidence rate could not be determined because of incomplete data on glaucoma patients lost to follow-up. An incidence rate of 0.1% over a 10-year period has been estimated from this study. The difficulties encountered by Armaly have been encountered in other incidence or longitudinal studies conducted in the United States.

In countries where there are centralized systems allowing greater access to health care for the entire population, data for glaucoma incidence rates are easier to obtain. In the Bedford Glaucoma Survey, 770 normal (non-ocular hypertensive) patients were followed. Four of the patients developed POAG resulting in a 5- to 7-year incidence rate of 0.52%.[26] Graham showed a similar incidence rate of 0.5% in a 4-year

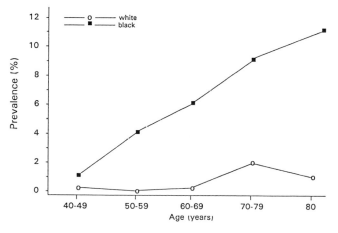

Figure 2–1. Primary open-angle glaucoma prevalence increases with age in East Baltimore, 1985–1988. Note the higher prevalence of POAG in the black population for each age group.

TABLE 2–2. INCIDENCE OF PRIMARY OPEN-ANGLE GLAUCOMA

U.S.[24]	0.1%/10 yrs
Sweden[26]	0.24%/1 yr
U.K.[25]	0.52%/5–7 yrs
Wales[19]	0.5%/4 yrs

study in Wales.[20] Bengtsson found a rate of 0.24% per year in Sweden.[27] Another 5-year Scandinavian study estimated POAG incidence to be between 0.25 and 1.0%.[28] Based on the Hospital Discharge Registry of Finland, Teikari found an age-adjusted cumulative incidence rate of 0.01% during a 10-year period.[29] This lower rate found by Teikari would be expected since not all patients would be treated for POAG in hospitals. Similar to prevalence studies reported, both Swedish and Finnish studies show an increasing incidence rate of POAG with increasing age.[27,29]

Since glaucoma is an infrequent, irreversible, and nonfatal disease, incidence rates can be calculated from population-based prevalence rates. Incidence rates of 0.19% per year for the 55- to 59-year group, increasing to 0.73% per year in the 75- to 79-year age group have been derived from the Framingham study.[30] It is important to note that these values have large standard errors and can only be regarded as approximate estimates. Furthermore, recall that this study was conducted on a predominantly white population and does not represent estimates of incidence of POAG for the entire United States.

In summary, due to difficulties in obtaining incidence data, reported POAG incidence rates are only approximations. The data in Table 2–2 show low POAG incidence rates throughout the world. New cases of POAG have been detected at a rate of 1 per 1000 to 1 per 100 per year.[31]

Evaluating Risk Factors: Non-Ocular

A basic premise of epidemiology is that causal relationships cannot be proven for either health or disease. The POAG studies we have described support this premise. In order to maximize available information, inferences can be made about the strength of association between risk factor(s) and a disease. In Tables 2–3 and 2–4, POAG risk factors have been summarized by supporting epidemiological studies. A large degree of confidence (noted as pluses in Tables 2–3 and 2–4) is shown where the risk factor has been substantiated by incidence studies. A prevalence study determines if the risk factor exists, but does not always provide information about whether the risk factor occurred before or after the disease.

Risk factors identified through case control studies should be evaluated based on the strength of each study. Clinical observations do not necessarily provide epidemiological risk factor data, but should be placed as evidence in the pool of risk factors to be considered.

The non-ocular risk factors for POAG are age, race or ethnicity, sex, family history of glaucoma, and systemic and environmental health factors (*see* Table 2–3). The strength of age as a POAG risk factor has been conclusively shown in a multicenter incidence study[32] and several prevalence studies.[4,5,18,20,24] The Collaborative Glaucoma Study showed a sevenfold increased risk for POAG when comparing the incidence rates in persons over the age of 60 compared to those under 40. Age, itself, is probably not directly related to POAG, but serves as a marker for degenerative metabolic or tissue changes that occur in the aging process, which contribute to the development of POAG.[33]

Data on race as a risk factor for POAG have been limited to specific ethnic groups. There are no published population-based rates for POAG in Hispanics, South Americans, or Mexicans. A lower prevalence of POAG has been reported in Alaskan Eskimos compared to other (non-Eskimo) Americans.[34] Zuni Indians in New Mexico were found to have a lower prevalence of POAG than non-Zuni Americans.[35] The prevalence of POAG in Shunyi County, Beijing, China was 0.11%.[36] Japanese have been reported to have lower rates of POAG and consistently lower IOP levels at all ages compared to Armaly's Iowa population.[37] The prevalence of POAG in Polynesians and Melanesians has also been found to be lower than in whites.[38,39] These studies have pointed to the ethnic Asian and Indian groups having lower rates of POAG compared to persons of European descent. In contrast, as previously discussed, there is significant population-based evidence showing blacks bearing a greater risk for POAG.[40]

The Baltimore Eye Survey not only found a 4.7-fold higher prevalence of POAG found in blacks compared to their white neighbors, but other significant information related to racial differences in the treatment and prognosis of the disease.[3] Blacks went "blind" (less than 20\400 in the better eye) from glaucoma an average of 10 years before whites. Other supportive evidence includes a case control study showing a 6.8-fold increased risk of POAG in the black population examined at the Massachusetts Eye and Ear Infirmary in Boston.[41] Clinicians have indicated that more aggressive medical and surgical treatment is necessary in black patients to control the disease.[42,43] Other observations point to blacks

TABLE 2–3. NON-OCULAR RISK FACTORS

Risk Factor	Risk Factor Strength	Description	Incidence Studies	Prevalence Studies	Other Supporting Studies
Age	++++	Increasing risk with increasing age	Collaborative Glaucoma Study, U.S.[32]	Ferndale, Wales[18] Framingham, U.S.[5,20] St. Lucia, West Indies[24] Baltimore, U.S.[4]	
Race					
Asians	+	Decreased risk with Eskimos, Zuni Indians	Eskimos[34]	Jamaica[23]	Wilson[41]
Eskimos			Zuni Indians[35]	St. Lucia, West Indies[24]	Katz[42]
Zuni Indians			Chinese[36]	Baltimore, U.S.[4]	Coulehan[43]
Whites	++		Japanese[37]		Wilson[44]
Blacks	+++	Increased risk with blacks	Polynesians[38] Melanesians[39]		
Sex					
Women > men	+/−	Not a strong risk factor	Finland Hospital Discharge[28] Dalby, Sweden[27]	Finland Medical Registry[28] St. Lucia, West Indies[24] Framingham, U.S.[21]	
Men > women					
Men = women			Ferndale, Wales[20] Baltimore, U.S.[4] Collaborative Glaucoma Study, U.S.[32]		
Family History of POAG	++	Increased risk with confirmed diagnosis of family members		Finnish Twin Cohort Study[52] Baltimore, U.S.[4] Collaborative Glaucoma Study, U.S.[32]	Miller[51] Wilson[41]
Systemic Health					
Diabetes	+	Increased risk with diagnosis of diabetes mellitus	Armstrong[53]	? Framingham, U.S.[21,22]	Wilson[41] Morgan[58] Reynolds[59] Katz[60]
Hypertension	?			? Framingham, U.S.[54]	Klein[45] Leske[61] Wilson[41] Leighton[62]
Cigarette Smoking	+/−				Katz[60] Morgan[58]
Alcohol Use	+/−			Framingham, U.S.[22]	Katz[60]
Working Indoors	+/−				Morgan[58]

presenting as younger POAG patients with a greater severity and more rapid progression compared to white POAG patients.[44] It is important to note that the risk factor of race is not thought to be causally related to POAG. As with age, race may serve as an important marker for possible underlying physiological factors related to POAG. Investigators have pointed to hypertension as a more prevalent condition in the black population[45] as well as higher IOP levels,[43,46] and larger cup-to-disc ratios.[47] Further studies are needed in order to elucidate the risk fac-

tors involved with the higher rates of POAG in blacks and the lower rates in Asian and Indian ethnic groups.

Data on gender as a risk factor for the development of POAG vary. In two Northern European countries, females had a higher incidence of POAG,[27,29] whereas, in the Framingham study males had a higher prevalence of POAG.[21] Other prevalence studies have reported no gender difference.[4,20,32] Little information can be derived from case control studies that generally match on gender for

TABLE 2–4. OCULAR RISK FACTORS

Risk Factor	Risk Factor Strength	Description	Incidence Studies	Prevalence Studies	Other Supporting Studies
IOP	++++	Increasing risk of POAG with increasing IOP	Collaborative Glaucoma Study, U.S.[25,32] Dalby Sweden[65] Norway[63]	Framingham, U.S.[5] Baltimore, U.S.[64]	Sommer[66] Quigley[67] Epstein[70] Kass[71] Katz[72]
Optic Nerve Head					
Vertical elongation	+	Good predictor of POAG			Weisman[78]
Neuroretinal tissue loss	+				Fazio[82] Airaksinen[80]
Increased volume or cup excavation	+				Fazio[82]
Asymmetrical cup-to-disc ratio	+		Yablonski[79]		Cartwright[68] Crichton[69]
Nerve Fiber Layer					
Loss or defect	+		Sommer[83]		Airaksinen[86]
Splinter hemorrhage	+		Diehl[84]	Bengtsson[85]	Bengtsson[87] Drance[88]
Myopia	+/−		Collaborative Study, U.S.[92]		David[89] Lotufo[91]

cases and controls. There may be a tendency to believe that females are at higher risk, because females outlive males and represent a greater proportion of the POAG patients. It is reasonable to conclude that gender is not a strong risk factor for POAG.

The role of family history of glaucoma as a risk factor for POAG has *not* been clearly demonstrated, despite information showing IOP,[48] cup-to-disc ratio,[49] and facility of outflow[50] to be genetically determined. Clinically based estimates have shown a four to eight times higher risk of POAG (based on reported history) for first-degree relatives of POAG patients.[51] Thus, it has been postulated that identical twin pairs would also show a high association for inheriting POAG. Surprisingly, a Finnish Twin Cohort study showed only 10.2% inheritance involved in POAG.[52] Follow-up studies on POAG have not been able to determine a genetic link between the risk of a family history of POAG and the disease. In the Collaborative Glaucoma Study in the United States, a much smaller than predicted incidence of POAG occurred among relatives of patients who had POAG.[32] Multiple factor case control comparison studies have shown only a "suggestive" association of family history of glaucoma to POAG.[41] Preliminary results from the Baltimore Eye Survey point to family history of glaucoma as a stronger risk factor for predicting POAG among the black population. In both white and black populations, the greatest association was found in sibling history compared to parent, children, or family history of POAG.[108] The mixed evidence for family history of glaucoma as a risk factor may actually reflect difficulties in obtaining accurate information on family history of POAG. It is also possible that a complex multigene process is involved in the development of POAG and historical documentation of family history alone cannot completely identify this risk factor.[14] We conclude that a family history of glaucoma is a risk factor and increases in strength when more information on confirmed diagnosis and treatment of family members for POAG is obtained.

There are only a few epidemiological studies linking systemic health and environmental risk factors to POAG. Diabetes mellitus is an important risk factor for POAG. The incidence of POAG has been documented to occur more frequently in diabetic patients compared to non-diabetic patients.[53] Case control studies that select POAG cases and then determine diabetic status point to a strong association of diabetes with POAG.[41,58–60] However, other population-based studies have not supported this association.[32,54,55] The Framingham data[21,22] and other studies have demonstrated only a relationship between elevated IOP and diabetes.[56,57] Some authors have hypothesized that systemic blood abnormalities such as in diabetes could affect vascular perfusion to the optic nerve in POAG.[33]

A positive association between increased IOP and high blood pressure has been found in several studies.[45,54,61] Whether the increase of IOP and concurrent increase in blood pressure are actually related to aging is not clear. The risk factor of systemic hypertension has not been tracked in longitudinal or cohort studies of visual field loss. One case control study showed a strong association between untreated high systolic hypertension and POAG. However, this association dissipated with treatment of the hypertension.[41] Another investigation has pointed to diastolic blood pressure as the risk factor of concern with POAG.[62] Analysis of Framingham prevalence data has shown no association of either systolic or diastolic blood pressure with POAG glaucomatous field defects.[54] Clinical studies have described sudden decreases in blood pressure, which cause vascular perfusion changes to the optic nerve, as resulting in subsequent glaucomatous visual field defects.[58,59] It is interesting to note that neither clinical nor case control studies have shown an association between a history of hypertension, or its treatment, and glaucomatous visual field loss.[58,60] Further population-based data are needed in order to assess the various features of blood pressure as risk factors for POAG. Since blood pressure is a dynamic process, it is reasonable to believe that more specific risk factors such as the level and control of systolic or diastolic pressures are involved in the relationship between blood pressure and POAG.

External risk factors cited for POAG include smoking, alcohol consumption, and some specific work environments. A relationship between smoking and increased IOP has been shown in a case control study. However, an association with glaucoma has not been determined.[58] In addition, smoking has been identified as a risk factor for POAG in only one of three other case control studies.[41,59,60] Two studies on predominantly white populations have shown a relationship between alcohol use and POAG in a small number of cases.[22,60] Larger population groups should be investigated in order to evaluate smoking and alcohol consumption as risk factors for POAG. An interesting case control study has shown indoor workers having a greater risk of POAG compared to outdoor workers.[58] Exposure to heavy metal, often by welding, has been reported to be related to an increased risk of POAG.[41] Whether working environment activities or other unrelated conditions of workers are actual risk factors for POAG should be examined in more robust epidemiological studies.

Evaluating Risk Factors: Ocular

Ocular risk factors for POAG include elevated IOP, optic nerve head appearance, cup-to-disc asymmetry, nerve fiber layer appearance, and myopic refractive error. Intraocular pressure has been most extensively evaluated in population-based studies. Other ocular risk factors have been studied more in clinical settings. The strength of epidemiological studies for these risk factors will be addressed in the following section, with supporting information from clinical observations.

Intraocular pressure has been shown to be one of the strongest ocular predictors of POAG. Although a causal relationship cannot be proven, deductions can be drawn from supporting evidence. An increase in prevalence and incidence of glaucoma occurs with increasing IOP.[25,63,64] The Framingham Eye Study showed the prevalence of POAG increased from 0.6% in eyes with IOPs less than 16 mm Hg to 7.1% among eyes with IOPs greater than 22 mm Hg.[5] The Collaborative Glaucoma Study showed a sixfold increase of POAG occurred in patients with a base-line IOP $\geq$ 24 mm Hg.[32] The Dalby Study showed a 5.4-fold increased risk with IOP > 21 mm Hg.[65] Sommer's review of incidence data on elevated IOP as a risk factor for POAG suggested that, even though the data are limited, higher IOP brings about a greater risk for developing glaucomatous damage.[66] The strong relationship between elevated IOP and glaucoma has also been supported by animal studies where artificially induced elevations in IOP were shown to result in glaucomatous cupping.[67] For patients with asymmetrical IOPs, visual field and optic nerve head damage correspond to the eye with increased IOP.[68,69] Clinical trials in a small number of ocular hypertensive patients have provided evidence that reducing IOP levels reduced the incidence of POAG damage.[70,71] Adult patients treated for glaucoma showed an improvement in visual field and optic nerve head appearance associated with the magnitude of IOP reduction.[71]

In contrast to the information supporting a dose-response relationship between IOP levels and POAG, another clinical investigation comparing three treatment modalities was unable to demonstrate that an intervention, which resulted in the lowest IOP level, was related to a decrease in visual field progression.[73] Further conflicting evidence on IOP as the leading ocular risk factor for POAG lies in those patients with pressures above 30 mm Hg who do not suffer visual field damage as well as patients with IOPs less than 20 mm Hg who do sustain significant glaucomatous visual field loss.[66,74] What is important to note is that the level of 21 mm Hg IOP is often selected as a cut-off point to delineate "normal" from "elevated" IOP was statistically derived as two standard deviations above the average or mean value in a normal population.[75] The sensitivity of using this arbitrary cut-off value is considerably less than 50%. Unfortunately, no other alternative IOP reading can be suggested that would provide a better balance between sensitivity and specificity.[5,66] Because of the misleading conclusions that could come about by relying on IOP readings alone, other ocular risk factors should be evaluated.

Screening Programs. The public is frequently exposed to the idea of glaucoma screenings. It is important to recognize that some aspects of glaucoma population-based screenings may be deceptive and impractical. Because the prevalence of glaucoma in any general population group is low, the positive yield of even a "perfect" glaucoma screening program would be small. The use of the IOP test as a single screening tool is not a good indicator of glaucoma. Follow-up of ocular hypertension cases have shown low yield for the diagnosis of glaucoma based only on IOP readings. It is also possible for patients with low IOPs to have undetected glaucomatous nerve damage. Thus, it is misleading to tell an individual that they have passed a glaucoma screening without first qualifying the sensitivity and specificity of the screening tools used, as well as making appropriate recommendations for further evaluation or treatment when needed.

Several optic nerve head findings have been associated with glaucomatous visual field loss. Whether these changes represent a risk factor for the development of POAG or result from the disease process has been debated. A common optic nerve head finding identified in POAG is the presence of an enlarged cup. Prevalence data show that a small proportion (7%) of the normal population have cup-to-disc ratios ≥0.5 while the majority (86%) are below 0.4.[76] In the glaucoma population, the majority (61%) of patients have cup-to-disc ratios ≥0.4.[77] As with IOP levels, no cut-off value for a cup-to-disc ratio can be recommended in order to provide an appropriate balance between sensitivity and specificity for detecting glaucoma.[5]

Vertical elongation of the cup has been reported to be a good predictor of glaucoma.[78] In the glaucoma population, 60% show a 0.1 difference in the vertical cup dimension compared to the horizontal dimension. The same difference exists in only 30% of the normal population. Asymmetrical cup-to-disc ratios between the two eyes have been shown to be particularly accurate predictor of glaucomatous visual field loss. A Washington University study found that 91% of patients with asymmetry of 0.2 or more developed visual field loss.[79] Observation of asymmetric cupping can be a useful prognostic ocular risk factor for POAG since a difference of ≥0.2 between the two eyes occurs in only 1% of the normal population. Neuroretinal rim loss in the optic nerve has been correlated with visual field loss.[80] In fact, loss of this rim tissue has a stronger association with POAG than does a large cup-to-disc ratio.

A significant consideration in evaluating the optic nerve is that the presence of multiple risk factors increases the likelihood of POAG. For example, in a 5-year study of patients with large cup-to-disc ratios combined with elevated IOPs, the eyes with a vertical cup-to-disc ratio less than 0.6 and an average IOP less than 28 mm Hg did not develop glaucomatous visual field loss. However, 91% of eyes with a vertical cup-to-disc ratio greater than 0.6 and an average IOP ≥28 mm Hg developed POAG.[79] The difficulty in relying on observations of optic nerve head risk factors in determining POAG is that large variation can be found in estimations even with experienced clinical observers using photographs.[81] New methods of computerized observations may provide more reliable data. Promising results have been shown with simultaneous optic disc topography measurements where large cup-to-disc ratios were found to be associated with decreased neuroretinal rim tissue area and increased disc volume.[82] Longitudinal follow-up studies that track these changes in large populations could provide more accurate criteria for evaluation of optic nerve head risk factors that could be used to predict POAG. Data from the Baltimore Eye Survey are being analyzed to provide this base-line information.

Loss of the nerve fiber layer has been championed as an excellent technique to identify patients with early glaucomatous nerve damage, since nerve fiber layer defects precede visual field loss. In a 10-year incidence study of an ethnically mixed population, 88% of nerve fiber layer defects were present when visual field loss first occurred. These same defects were infrequent in the normal subjects. Nerve fiber layer defects were noted in 60% of the POAG eyes approximately 6 years before visual field loss was found.[83] Unfortunately, the remarkable sensitivity of the nerve fiber layer technique is currently offset by a lack of training and expertise on the part of many clinicians.

Small hemorrhages occurring around the optic nerve head have been shown to be an important risk factor for the development of visual field defects due to glaucoma in both prevalence and incidence studies. These hemorrhages, termed "splinter" or "disc" hemorrhages, are associated with a substantially greater incidence of progression of visual field defects in patients with POAG.[84] Patients with elevated IOP and no visual field loss are also more likely to develop visual field changes after disc hemorrhages have been observed.[88] In a small group of 51 POAG eyes with recent glaucomatous visual field loss, a prevalence rate of 40% for disc hemorrhages was found.[85] The period between disc hemorrhage occurrence and visual field change has been documented to be 2 to 7 years.[87] Another study showed some subjects who were found to have disc hemorrhages that preceded nerve fiber layer damage from POAG.[86] It is important to note that, even though splinter hemorrhages are an early indicator of POAG or a sign of on-going glaucomatous damage, they may be missed because of their transient nature.

Myopia has been reported to be related to higher levels of IOP,[89] but there does not appear to be a direct relationship with an increased risk of developing POAG.[90] Clinical studies have shown that myopia over 3 diopters is associated with POAG in individuals under 35 years of age.[91] Selected records of POAG patients in the Collaborative Glaucoma Study showed four times as many myopic patients, over 1 diopter, compared to a similar age-matched sample of the U.S. population.[92] However, a case control study of patients in Boston showed only a weak relationship between myopia, greater than 1 diopter, and POAG.[41] Further studies are needed in order to understand whether myopia is in fact related to POAG. It is entirely possible that the reported association of myopic refractive error with POAG actually reflects the self-selected population of myopic patients who seek care because of visual complaints and are subsequently diagnosed as having glaucoma.

Other risk factors to be considered in deciding on the treatment and management of a glaucoma patient include the monocular patient, a patient who is unable to perform visual field testing, or a patient with a concurrent condition that may mask some of the signs or symptoms of glaucoma.

In conclusion, some ocular and non-ocular risk factors can be supported by epidemiological studies. It has been shown that use of multiple risk factor criteria can improve the probability of predicting POAG for an individual patient.[93] A "value" scheme is presented to portray an epidemiologically based profile for predicting POAG. In Tables 2–5 and 2–6, risk factors having epidemiologically based associations with POAG have been graded and assigned values. The factors have been designated with weighted, relative values of minimum risk (+), moderate risk (+ +), high risk (+ + +), and highest risk (+ + + +). Risk factors supported by sparse epidemiological data have not been included.

TABLE 2–6. RELATIVE VALUES OF OCULAR RISK FACTORS

	Noted
Cup-to-disc Asymmetry (≥0.2)	
Between the two eyes	+
Nerve Fiber Layer Appearance	
Defect or loss	+
Splinter hemorrhage	+
Optic Nerve Head Appearance	
Vertical elongation	+
Neuroretinal rim loss (thinning or notch)	+
Increased volume or excavation	+
Visual Fields	
Borderline threshold field	+
Suspicious nasal step or arcuate threshold defect	+ +
Repeated threshold defect	+ + +
Intraocular Pressure	
≤20 mm Hg	
21–23 mm Hg	+
24–26 mm Hg	+ +
27–29 mm Hg	+ + +
≥30 mm Hg	+ + + +

Scale: + minimum risk, + + moderate risk, + + + high risk, + + + + highest risk.

TABLE 2–5. RELATIVE VALUES OF NON-OCULAR RISK FACTORS

Risk Factor	Noted
Diabetes	
Confirmed diagnosis	+
Family History of Glaucoma	
Recalls family history	+
Reliable information about family member(s) diagnosed and treated for POAG	+ +
Race	
Hispanic, South American, mixed background	
Asian, Eskimo, American Indian	+
White	+ +
Black	+ + +
Age	
40–49 years	+
50–59 years	+ +
60–69 years	+ + +
>70 years	+ + + +

Scale: + minimum risk, + + moderate risk, + + + high risk, + + + + highest risk.

Building a Risk Profile: The Pyramid Concept

The *non-ocular risk factor profile* for POAG begins with the crucial factor of age. As the patient ages, the base of the POAG profile increases. Next, race or ethnicity is noted. In some instances, it may be difficult to categorize the patient in an ethnic group. Leaving this area blank is a reasonable alternative. It is important to probe the exact nature of a family history of glaucoma. Since family history related to glaucoma can be subject to considerable interpretation and recall bias, this question should be repeated at future office visits. Emphasis should be on specific details about how family members were diagnosed and treated for glaucoma. Similarly, the diabetes systemic health question needs to be repeated at subsequent examinations because patients may be diagnosed at later times.

To construct the *ocular risk factor profile,* clinical data are compiled by analyzing each eye separately, followed by a final comparison of cup-to-disc ratios between the two eyes. We suggest beginning with the IOP in the eye that is most suspicious for POAG. The relative risk values in Table 2–6 are based on data showing that eyes with IOPs over 30 mm Hg have a 15 times greater risk for developing glaucomatous visual field loss (41.2% developing field defects), which decreases to a fourfold relative risk (12% field defects) with IOPs in the 26 to 30 mm Hg range, and only 3% visual field loss occurring when IOPs are 21 to 25 mm Hg.[66] An additional plus mark should be added with subsequent increases in the IOP. Intraocular pressures below 20 mm Hg will not be marked; therefore, marks result in an inverse pyramid formation for low-tension glaucoma cases.

Visual field results are included at the next higher level of the ocular risk factor structure. Clinical decisions related to the diagnosis of glaucoma or the progression of visual field loss need to be based on accurate and repeated perimetry. In our relative value scheme, patients with a borderline threshold visual field are at a minimum risk level. Patients with a suspicious nasal step or arcuate field defect found during the first threshold visual field test are considered at "moderate" risk for further glaucomatous field loss. Three plus marks are given when a visual field defect is found on two repeated visual fields.

Evaluation of the optic nerve head and nerve fiber layer constitute the last two pieces of clinical information to be included in the POAG ocular risk factor profile. Large cup-to-disc ratios, when used alone, have been shown to be a poor prognostic factor for POAG. Thus, the clinician must use judgment to decide whether or not a large cup-to-disc ratio in a given patient should receive a mark on the ocular risk

factor profile. Additional plus marks should be added when vertical elongation, excavation, thinning or notching of the neuroretinal rim, optic disc hemorrhages, and nerve fiber layer loss are found. The final step involves comparing the cup-to-disc ratios between the two eyes to evaluate asymmetry. Mark one plus sign when asymmetries greater than 0.2 are found.

The concept of a clinical pyramid can be used to analyze the risk of developing POAG. An increase in the number of plus marks as you ascend the pyramid structure provides stronger epidemiological evidence supporting the diagnosis of POAG. Patients with a higher probability for developing POAG will have a triangular or pyramid shape in both the ocular and non-ocular risk factor profiles. Persons who are at low risk for POAG will have very few plus marks. Low-risk individuals can also be represented as having more of a linear or stick-like profile. The power of constructing these risk profiles lies with the clinician's ability to add plus marks after subsequent examinations in order to determine whether or not the risk of developing POAG is increasing over time. The best strategy is to examine the shape of the non-ocular profile first and then focus more attention on the ocular risk factor profile. Since age is such a strong predictor of disease, older patients would be expected to exhibit more of a pyramid shape in the non-ocular risk factor profile. Further evidence for determining the diagnosis of POAG will be based on an increase of plus marks resulting in a pyramid shape for the ocular risk factor profile. Expanding pyramid profiles should lead the clinician to modify treatment and/or refer for outside consultation. If no change in the size or shape of the pyramid is observed over time, it is reasonable to continue evaluating the patient at regular intervals.

CASE EXAMPLES OF SUSPECTED PRIMARY OPEN-ANGLE GLAUCOMA

The three case examples that follow are summarized in Table 2–7.

Case 1. 59-Year-Old Black Male

A 59-year-old black male presents to your office for a routine eye examination. He reports a vague history of glaucoma, believing that someone in his family went "blind" from glaucoma. He denies having diabetes. In the non-ocular risk factor profile, you mark two plus marks for age, since this individual is between the ages of 50 and 59 years. Being black gives him three plus marks in the race category. With an unsubstantiated family history of glaucoma, one plus

TABLE 2–7. PRIMARY OPEN-ANGLE GLAUCOMA PROFILE CASE EXAMPLES

	Case 1		Case 2		Case 3
	1995 Exam	*1996 Exam*	*1995 Exam*	*1997 Exam*	*1995 Exam*
Ocular Risk Factors					
Asymmetry					
NFL		+			?
Optic Disc	?	+ +			
Visual Fields	+	+ +			
IOPs	+	+ + +			+
Non-Ocular Risk Factors					
Diabetes		+			+
Family History POAG	+	+ +			+ +
Race	+ + +	+ + +	+	+	
Age	+ +	+ + +	+ + + +	+ + + +	
General Trends	Ocular risk factors identified. Beginning non-ocular pyramid shape (which will increase with age).	Increase in pyramid shape in 6 months.	No ocular pyramid. Age is the only non-ocular pyramid factor.	No pyramid shape growth.	Ocular factors involved. Beginning non-ocular pyramid shape (which will increase with age).
Plan	Monitor closely.	Referral/treatment warranted.	Routine care.	Routine care.	Monitor closely.

NFL = nerve fiber layer; IOP = intraocular pressure; POAG = primary open-angle glaucoma.

mark should be put in the family history of glaucoma slot. No mark is made in the diabetes category.

Your examination reveals presbyopia, a normal slit-lamp examination and IOPs of 23 mm Hg in each eye. There is a question in your mind as to whether the patient has a large physiological cup or acquired cupping from glaucoma. When you evaluate the optic disc more closely, no vertical elongation of the cup in the optic nerve head is found and there is no neuroretinal rim loss or notching in either eye. The nerve fiber layer in each eye appears plush without signs of drop-out. The results of the visual field are "borderline." There may be a paracentral nasal defect, but the reliability of this visual field is questionable.

Based on your examination, the ocular profile begins with a plus mark in the IOP section, since the IOP falls in the lower limits between 21 and 23. The borderline questionable visual field gets one plus mark. Excavation of the optic nerve head is a questionable sign that merits further attention. Since the nerve fiber layers are intact and there is no asymmetry between the cup-to-disc ratios, no further plus marks are included in the ocular profile. You advise the patient that he is at risk for POAG, explain your concerns based on the risk factors observed, and inform him that he needs to be monitored closely and re-examined in 4 to 6 months.

The patient returns for a follow-up evaluation in 6 months. At that time, the patient is 60 years of age.

Since your last examination, he has discovered that two of his brothers have been diagnosed and treated for glaucoma. The patient has also begun treatment for diabetes. Your examination reveals IOPs of 27 mm Hg in each eye, with what now appears to be definite cup excavation in the optic nerves and some neuroretinal rim loss. You suspect a slight inferior temporal slit defect in the nerve fiber layer of one eye. The visual field test confirms a small scotoma located in the area of question from the first visual field 6 months earlier.

In the non-ocular profile, three plus marks should now be included for age since the patient is 60 years old. Three plus marks remain in the race category. Two plus marks are now placed in the family history slot since open-angle glaucoma cases have been verified in this patient's immediate family. A plus mark should also be included in the diabetes section. For the ocular risk factor profile, three plus marks need to be included in the IOP slot because the IOP is between 27 and 29 mm Hg. Indicate two plus marks in the visual field slot to represent the definite glaucomatous defect found in the patient's second threshold visual field test. Two plus marks are now included in the optic disc appearance slot because of the presence of cup excavation and neuroretinal rim notching. One plus mark corresponds to the nerve fiber layer slit defect. Since no asymmetry between the cup-to-disc ratio of the two eyes has been noted, this slot should remain blank.

year period in a Swedish population over 65 years of age.[107]

With the exception of elevated IOP, migraine headaches, and local vasospasms, risk factors associated with LTG have been reported to be similar to those of POAG. Age appears to be a major risk factor.

CONCLUSION

Descriptive and population-based statistical information for several types of glaucoma have been presented. The main conclusion that can be drawn is that risk factors increase the probability of glaucoma disease occurring. For the clinician, building profiles based on observed risk factors can increase the probability for accurate diagnosis of glaucoma.

REFERENCES

1. Rothman KJ. *Modern Epidemiology.* Boston/Toronto: Little, Brown and Company; 1986.
2. Lilienfeld AM, Lilienfeld DE. *Foundations of Epidemiology.* 2nd ed. New York/Oxford: Oxford University Press; 1980.
3. Tielsch JM, Sommer A, Witt K, et al. Blindness and visual impairment in an American urban population: The Baltimore Eye Survey. *Arch Ophthalmol.* 1990;108:286–290.
4. Tielsch JM, Sommer A, Katz J, et al. Racial variations in the prevalence of primary open angle glaucoma: The Baltimore Eye Survey. *JAMA.* 1991;266(3):369–374.
5. Leibowitz HM, Krueger DE, Maunder LR, et al. The Framingham Eye Study Monograph: An ophthalmological and epidemiological study of cataract, glaucoma, diabetic retinopathy, macular degeneration, and visual acuity in a general population of 2,631 adults, 1973–1975. *Surv Ophthalmol.* 1980; 24(suppl):335–610.
6. National Society to Prevent Blindness. *Vision Problems in the U.S.* Data analysis, 1980.
7. Thomas JV. General considerations. In: Thomas JV, ed. *Glaucoma Surgery.* St. Louis: C.V. Mosby; 1992:1–2.
8. U.S. Department of Health, Education and Welfare. *Statistics on Blindness in the Model Reporting Area 1969–1970.* DHEW Publication No. NIH 73-427. Washington, DC: US GPO, 1973.
9. Hiller R, Kahn HA. Blindness from glaucoma. *Am J Ophthalmol.* 1975;80:62–69.
10. Javitt JC, McBean AM, Nicholson GA, et al. Undertreatment of glaucoma among black Americans. *N Engl J Med.* 1991;325:1418–1422.
11. Seddon JM. The differential burden of blindness in the United States. *N Engl J Med.* 1991;325:1440–1442.
12. Guzman G, Javitt J, Glick H, et al. Glaucoma in the United States population: The economic garden of illness. *Invest Ophthalmol Vis Sci.* 1992;33:759.
13. Last JM, ed. *A Dictionary of Epidemiology.* New York/Oxford/Toronto: Oxford University Press; 1983.
14. Leske MC, Rosenthal J. The epidemiologic aspects of open-angle glaucoma. *Am J Epidemiol.* 1979;109:250–272.
15. Eskridge JB, Bartlett JD. The glaucomas. In: Barlett JD, ed. *Clinical Ocular Pharmacology.* Stoneham, Massachusetts: Butterworth; 1989;733–798.
16. Kurkland LT, Taub RG. The frequency of glaucoma in a small urban community. *Am J Ophthalmol.* 1957;43:539–544.
17. Kini MM, Leibowitz HM, Colton T, et al. Prevalence of senile cataract, diabetic retinopathy, senile macular degeneration, and open-angle glaucoma in the Framingham Eye Study. *Am J Ophthalmol.* 1978;85:28–34.
18. Bengtsson B. The prevalence of glaucoma. *Br J Ophthalmol.* 1981;65:46–49.
19. Graham PA. Prevalence of glaucoma. Population surveys. *Trans Ophthalmol Soc UK.* 1978;98:288–289.
20. Hollows FC, Graham PA. Intra-ocular pressure, glaucoma, and glaucoma suspects in a defined population. *Br J Ophthalmol.* 1966;50:570–586.
21. Kahn HA, Milton RC. Revised Framingham Eye Study: Prevalence of glaucoma and diabetic retinopathy. *Am J Epidemiol.* 1989;111:769–776.
22. Kahn HA, Milton RC. Alternative definitions of open-angle glaucoma. Effect on prevalence and associations in the Framingham Eye Study. *Arch Ophthalmol.* 1980;98:2172–2177.
23. Wallace J, Lovell HG. Glaucoma and intraocular pressure in Jamaica. *AM J Ophthalmol.* 1969;67:93–100.
24. Mason RP, Kosoko O, Wilson MR, et al. National survey of the prevalence and risk factors of glaucoma in St. Lucia, West Indies. Part I. Prevalence findings. *Ophthalmology.* 1989;96:1363–1368.
25. Armaly MF. Ocular pressure and visual fields: A ten-year follow-up study. *Arch Ophthalmol.* 1969;81:25–40.
26. Perkins ES. The Bedford Glaucoma Survey. II. Rescreening of normal population. *Br J Ophthalmol.* 1973;57:86–92.
27. Bengtsson B. Incidence of manifest glaucoma. *Br J Ophthalmol.* 1989;73:483–487.
28. Jensen JE. Glaucoma screening. A 16 year follow-up of ocular normotensives. *Acta Ophthalmol (Copenh).* 1984;62:203–209.
29. Teikari JM, O'Donnell J. Epidemiologic data on adult glaucomas. Data from the Hospital Discharge Registry and Registry of Right to Free Medication. *Acta Ophthalmol (Copenh).* 1989;67:184–191.
30. Leske MC, Ederer F, Podgor MJ. Estimating incidence from age-specific prevalence in glaucoma. *Am J Epidemiol.* 1981;113:606–612.
31. Teilsch JM. The epidemiology of primary open angle glaucoma. *Ophthalmol Clin North Am.* 1991;4:649–657.
32. Armaly MF, Krueger DE, Maundir L, et al. Biostatisti-

cal analysis of the collaborative glaucoma study. I. Summary report of the risk factors for glaucomatous visual field defects. *Arch Ophthalmol.* 1980;98:2163–2171.

33. Wilson MR. Epidemiologic features of glaucoma. *Int Ophthalmol Clin.* 1990;30:153–160.
34. Arkell SM, Lightman DA, Sommer A, et al. The prevalence of glaucoma among Eskimos of Northwest Alaska. *Arch Ophthalmol.* 1987;105:482–485.
35. Kass MA, Zimmerman TJ, Alton E, et al. Intraocular pressure and glaucoma in the Zuni Indians. *Arch Ophthalmol.* 1978;96:2212–2213.
36. Hu CN. [An epidemiologic study of glaucoma in Shunyi County Beijing]. *Chung Hua Yen Ko Tsa Chih.* 1989;25:115–119.
37. Shiose Y. Intraocular pressure: New perspectives. *Surv Ophthalmol.* 1990;34:413–435.
38. Holmes WJ. Glaucoma in Central and South Pacific. *Am J Ophthalmol.* 1964;51:253–261.
39. Mann I. World distribution of certain eye diseases. Culture, race, climate, and eye disease. Springfield: Charles C Thomas; 1966:530–559.
40. Wilson MR. Glaucoma in blacks: Where do we go from here? *JAMA.* 1989;261:281–282.
41. Wilson MR, Hertzmark E, Walker AM, et al. A case-control study of risk factors in open angle glaucoma. *Arch Ophthalmol.* 1987;105:1066–1071.
42. Katz IM, Berger ET. Effects of iris pigmentation on response of ocular pressure to timolol. *Surv Ophthalmol.* 1979;23:395–398.
43. Coulehan JL, Helzlsouer KJ, Rodgers KD, et al. Racial difference in intraocular tension and glaucoma surgery. *Am J Epidemiol.* 1980;111:759–768.
44. Wilson R, Richardson TM, Hertzmark E, et al. Race as a risk factor for progressive glaucomatous damage. *Ann Ophthalmol.* 1985;17:653–659.
45. Klein BE, Klein R. Intraocular pressure and cardiovascular risk variables. *Arch Ophthalmol.* 1981;99:837–839.
46. Hiller R, Sperduto RD, Krueger DE. Race, iris pigmentation, and intraocular pressure. *Am J Epidemiol.* 1982;115:674–683.
47. Beck RW, Messner DK, Musch DC, et al. Is there a racial difference in physiologic cup size? *Ophthalmology.* 1985;92:873–876.
48. Armaly MF. The genetic determinants of ocular pressure in the normal eye. *Arch Ophthalmol.* 1967;78:35–43.
49. Armaly MF. Genetic determination of cup/disc ratio of the optic nerve. *Arch Ophthalmol.* 1967;78:35–43.
50. Armaly MF, Monstavicius BF, Sayegh RE. Ocular pressure and aqueous outflow facility in siblings. *Arch Ophthalmol.* 1968;80:354–360.
51. Miller SJH. Genetics of glaucoma and family studies. *Trans Ophthalmol.* 1978;98:290–292.
52. Teikari JM. Genetic factors in open angle (simple and capsular) glaucoma. A population based twin study. *Acta Ophthalmol.* 1987;65:715–720.
53. Armstrong JR, Daily RK, Dobson HL, et al. The inci-

54. dence of glaucoma in diabetes mellitus. *Am J Ophthalmol.* 1960;50:55–63.
54. Kahn HA, Leibowitz HM, Ganley JP, et al. The Framingham Eye Study. II. Association of ophthalmic pathology with single variables previously measured in the Framingham Heart Study. *Am J Epidemiol.* 1977;106:33–41.
55. Bengtsson B. Aspects of the epidemiology of chronic glaucoma. *Acta Ophthalmol.* 1981;146(suppl):4–26.
56. Klein BEK, Klein R, Moss SE. Intraocular pressure in diabetic persons. *Ophthalmology.* 1984;91:1356–1360.
57. Becker B. Diabetes mellitus and primary open-angle glaucoma. *Am J Ophthalmol (Copenh).* 1987;65:715–720.
58. Morgan RW, Drance SM. Chronic open-angle glaucoma and ocular hypertension: An epidemiological study. *Br J Ophthalmol.* 1975;59:211–215.
59. Reynolds DC. Relative risk factors in chronic open angle glaucoma: An epidemiological study. *Am J Optom Physiol Optics.* 1977;54:116–120.
60. Katz J, Sommer A. Risk factors for primary open angle glaucoma. *Am J Prev Med.* 1988;4:110–114.
61. Leske MC, Podgor MJ. Intraocular pressure, cardiovascular risk variables, and visual field defects. *Am J Epidemiol.* 1983;118:280–287.
62. Leighton DA, Phillips CI. Systemic blood pressure in glaucoma. *Br J Ophthalmol.* 1972;52:447–453.
63. Hovding G, Aasved H. Prognostic factors in the development of manifest open angle glaucoma. A long-term follow-up study of hypertensive and normotensive ages. *Acta Ophthalmol (Copenh).* 1986;107:186–188.
64. Sommer A, Tielsch JM, Katz J, et al. Relationship between intraocular pressure and primary open angle glaucoma among white and black Americans: The Baltimore Eye Survey. *Arch Ophthalmol.* (In press).
65. Bengtsson B. Aspects of epidemiology of chronic glaucoma. *Acta Ophthalmol.* 1981;146(suppl):4–26.
66. Sommer A. Intraocular pressure and glaucoma. *Am J Ophthalmol.* 1989;107:186–188.
67. Quigley HA, Addicks EM. Chronic experimental glaucoma in primates. II. Effect of extended intraocular pressure elevation on optic nerve head and axonal transport. *Invest Ophthalmol Vis Sci.* 1980;19:137–152.
68. Cartwright MJ, Anderson DR. Correlation of asymmetric damage with asymmetric intraocular pressure in normal-tension glaucoma (low-tension glaucoma). *Arch Ophthalmol.* 1988;106:898–900.
69. Crichton A, Drance S, Douglas GR, Schulzer M. Unequal intraocular pressure and its relation to asymmetric visual field defects in low-tension glaucoma. *Ophthalmology.* 1989;96:1312–1314.
70. Epstein DL, Krug JH, Hertzmark E, et al. A long-term clinical trial of timolol therapy versus no treatment in the management of glaucoma suspects. *Ophthalmology.* 1989;96:1460–1467.
71. Kass MA, Gordon MO, Hoff MR, et al. Topical timolol administration reduces the incidence of glaucomatous damage in ocular hypertensive individuals. *Arch Ophthalmol.* 1989;107:1590–1598.
72. Katz LJ, Spaeth GL, Cantor LB, et al. Reversible optic

disk cupping and visual field improvement in adults with glaucoma. *Am J Ophthalmol.* 1989;107:485–492.

73. Midgal C, Hitchings R. Control of chronic simple glaucoma with primary medical, surgical and laser treatment. *Trans Ophthalmol Soc UK.* 1986;105:653–656.

74. Armaly MF. The visual field defect and ocular pressure level in open-angle glaucoma. *Invest Ophthalmol.* 1969;8:105–124.

75. Armaly MF. On the distribution of applanation pressure. I. Statistical features and the effect of age, sex, and the family history of glaucoma. *Arch Ophthalmol.* 1965;73:11–18.

76. Armaly MF. The optic cup in the normal eye. *Am J Ophthalmol.* 1969;68:401–407.

77. Armaly MF. Cup/disc ratio in early open-angle glaucoma. *Doc Ophthalmol.* 1969;26:526–533.

78. Weisman RL, Asseff CF, Phelps CD, et al. Clinically detectable nerve fiber atrophy precedes the onset of glaucomatous field loss. *Arch Ophthalmol.* 1991;109:77–83.

79. Yablonski ME, Zimmerman TJ, Kass MA, et al. Prognostic significance of optic disk cupping in ocular hypertensive patients. *Am J Ophthalmol.* 1980;89:585–592.

80. Airaksinen PJ, Drance SM, Douglas GR, et al. Neuroretinal rim areas and visual field indices in glaucoma. *Am J Ophthalmol.* 1985;99:107–110.

81. Lichter PR. Variability of expert observers in evaluating the optic disc. *Trans Am Ophthalmol Soc.* 1976;74:532–572.

82. Fazio P, Krupin T, Feitl ME, et al. Optic disc topography in patients with low-tension and primary open angle glaucoma. *Arch Ophthalmol.* 1990;108:705–708.

83. Sommer A, Katz J, Quigley HA, et al. Clinically detectable nerve fiber atrophy precedes the on-set of glaucomatous field loss. *Arch Ophthalmol.* 1991; 109:77–83.

84. Diehl DLC, Quigley HA, Miller NR, et al. Prevalence and significance of optic disc hemorrhage in a longitudinal study of glaucoma. *Arch Ophthalmol.* 1990;108:545–550.

85. Bengtsson B, Holmin C, Krakau CET. Disc haemorrhage and glaucoma. *Acta Ophthalmol.* 1981;59:1–14.

86. Airaksinen PJ, Mustonen E, Alanko HI. Optic disk haemorrhages precede retinal nerve fibre layer defects in ocular hypertension. *Acta Ophthalmol.* 1981;59:627–641.

87. Bengtsson B. Optic disc haemorrhages preceding manifest glaucoma. *Acta Ophthalmol.* 1990;68:450–454.

88. Drance SM, Fairclough M, Butler DM, et al. The importance of disc hemorrhage in the prognosis of chronic open angle glaucoma. *Arch Ophthalmol.* 1977;95:226–228.

89. David R, Zangwill L, Tessler Z, et al. The correlation between intraocular pressure and refractive status. *Arch Ophthalmol.* 1985;103:1812–1815.

90. Daubs JG, Crick RP. Effect of refractive error on the risk of ocular hypertension and open angle glaucoma. *Trans Ophthalmol Soc UK.* 1981;101:121–126.

91. Lotufo D, Ritch R, Szmyd L, et al. Juvenile glaucoma, race and refraction. *JAMA.* 1989;261:249–252.

92. Perkins ES, Phelps CD. Open angle glaucoma, ocular hypertension, low tension glaucoma and refraction. *Arch Ophthalmol.* 1982;100:1464–1467.

93. Wilensky JT, Podos SM, Becker B. Prognostic indicators in ocular hypertension. *Arch Ophthalmol.* 1974;91:200–202.

94. Bankes JLK, Perkins ES, Tsolakis S, et al. Bedford glaucoma survey. *Br Med J.* 1968;1:791–796.

95. Stromberg U. Ocular hypertension. *Acta Ophthalmol.* 1962;69(suppl):1–75.

96. David R, Zangwill L, Stone D, et al. Epidemiology of intraocular pressure in a population screened for glaucoma. *Br J Ophthalmol.* 1987;71:766–771.

97. Leske MC. The epidemiology of open-angle glaucoma: A review. *Am J Epidemiol.* 1983;118:166–191.

98. Linner E, Stromberg U. Ocular hypertension. A five year study of the total population in a Swedish town, Skovde. Tutzing Castle: Glaucoma Symposium; 1966:187–214.

99. Linner E. Ocular hypertension. I. The clinical course during ten years without therapy. Aqueous humor dynamics. *Acta Ophthalmol.* 1976;54:707–720.

100. Lundberg L, Wettrell K, Linner E. Ocular hypertension. A twenty-year follow-up at Skovde. *Acta Ophthalmol (Copenh).* 1985;63:473–474.

101. Perkins ES. The Bedford Glaucoma Survey. I. Long-term follow-up of borderline cases. *Br J Ophthalmol.* 1973;57:179–185.

102. Seddon JM, Schwartz B, Flowerdew G. Case-control study of ocular hypertension. *Arch Ophthalmol.* 1983;101:891–894.

103. Kass MA, Hart WM, Gordon M, et al. Risk factors favoring the development of glaucomatous visual field loss in ocular hypertension. *Surv Ophthalmol.* 1980;25:155–162.

104. Von Graefe A. Uber die Iridectomie bei glaucom und uber den glaucomatosen process. *Graefe Arch Ophthalmol.* 1857;3:456.

105. Drance SM. Low-tension glaucoma, enigma and opportunity. *Arch Ophthalmol.* 1985;103:1131.

106. Shiose Y. Prevalence and clinical aspects of low tension glaucoma. In: Henkind P, ed. *Acta XXIV International Congress of Ophthalmology.* Philadelphia: JB Lippincott; 1983:587–591.

107. Bengtsson B. Manifest glaucoma in the aged. I. Occurrence nine years after a population survey. *Acta Ophthalmol.* 1981;59:321–331.

108. Presented by Tielsch JM, before the Dana Center for Preventive Ophthalmology faculty, Wilmer Eye Institute, The Johns Hopkins University Schools of Medicine and Public Health, Baltimore, Maryland, November 19, 1991.

Chapter 3

OCULAR ANATOMY AND PHYSIOLOGY RELATED TO AQUEOUS PRODUCTION AND OUTFLOW

Thomas F. Freddo

Central to an understanding of the glaucomas is an appreciation of the anatomy and physiology of the ciliary body and the aqueous outflow pathways as they relate to aqueous humor dynamics.

ANATOMY OF THE CILIARY BODY

The ciliary body, a portion of the anterior uvea, extends from the root of the iris to the ora serrata and is grossly subdivided into two portions, the pars plicata and the pars plana. Viewed from the posterior chamber, the pars plicata appears as a series of approximately 75 radially-oriented, fin-like ciliary processes (Fig. 3–1). Most of these project approximately 1 mm into the posterior chamber and are termed major processes. The intervening minor processes are only one third as high. The convoluted surface produced by the major processes in the pars plicata region serves to increase the area over which secretion of aqueous humor can occur. The absence of these surface specializations in the more posterior pars plana region of the ciliary body is consistent with the generally accepted view that the pars plana plays little, if any, role in aqueous production.

In sagittal sections, the ciliary body appears as shown in Figure 3–2. Although not an obvious feature, the ciliary body is separated from the sclera, over most of its length, by a potential space, the supraciliary space that is continuous posteriorly with the suprachoroid. Having only minimal physical connections to the sclera, except at its anterior and posterior margins, the ciliary body is held against the outer wall of the eye primarily by the intraocular pressure.

Most of the volume of the ciliary body is occupied by the ciliary muscle, a smooth muscle that is subdivided into three portions, longitudinal, radial, and circumferential, based on fiber orientation (*see* Fig. 3–2). A loose connective tissue stroma is present between the muscle and the bilayered ciliary epithelium that lines the posterior chamber.

The two cell layers of the ciliary epithelium are named based on their relative content of pigment. The layer closest to the ciliary body stroma is called the pigmented ciliary epithelium and that closest to the posterior chamber is called the nonpigmented ciliary epithelium (*see* Fig. 3–2, inset). The pigmented

Original work cited in this chapter was funded by National Eye Institute Grant # EY-04567. Excellent technical assistance was provided by Rozanne Richman, MS.

ciliary epithelium is continuous with the anterior myoepithelium of the iris anteriorly and with the pigmented epithelium of the retina at the ora serrata. The nonpigmented layer is continuous with the posterior pigmented epithelium of the iris anteriorly and undergoes expansion at the ora serrata to become continuous with the neurosensory layers of the retina. All of the aforementioned layers are derived from the neuroectoderm of the optic vesicle that invaginates on itself during embryogenesis. As a consequence, the epithelia of the iris, and those of the ciliary body, are peculiarly arranged such that the two epithelial layers are attached to one another at their apical surfaces. Thus, the basal lamina of the pigmented ciliary epithelium fronts the ciliary body stroma and that of the nonpigmented layer faces the posterior chamber.

THE ROLE OF THE CILIARY BODY IN AQUEOUS HUMOR FORMATION

Aqueous humor is a clear fluid, derived from a filtrate of plasma and secreted by the ciliary epithelium into the posterior chamber of the eye at a rate of approximately 2.5 μL/minute. Under steady-state conditions, this rate of inflow, matched by an identical rate of outflow, will result in complete turnover of the aqueous humor approximately every 1 to 2 hours. From the posterior chamber, the aqueous enters the anterior chamber of the eye through the pupil (*see* Fig. 3–2) where it circulates in a convection current driven by the temperature difference between the warm iris and the cooler cornea. Rising posteriorly and falling anteriorly, the aqueous humor finally leaves the eye via one of various outflow pathways described later. Along its route, aqueous provides for the metabolic needs of the avascular tissues of the ocular anterior segment. As a result, the chemical composition of the aqueous humor is continuously modified. Additional, potentially toxic, modifications occur as a result of interaction with incoming light.[1]

Correlating the anatomy with the physiology of aqueous humor formation, it is most convenient to describe the process in two steps: (1) elaboration of a plasma filtrate from which aqueous humor is derived, and (2) formation of aqueous humor from this filtrate. Although these steps are not independent, the first is related primarily to the ciliary body microvasculature and the second, to the ciliary epithelium.

Elaboration of a Plasma Filtrate From the Microvasculature of the Ciliary Body

Filtration is a process in which fluid is forced across a membrane by pressure. The volume of filtrate that crosses the membrane depends on the pressure dif-

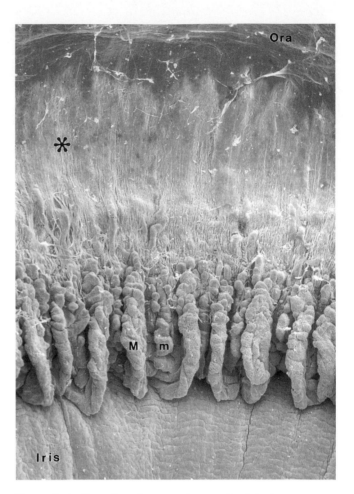

Figure 3–1. Scanning electron micrograph of the inner surface of the iris and ciliary body with the lens and zonules removed. The pars plicata region is distinguished from the more posterior pars plana region (*asterisk*) by the presence of major (M) and minor (m) ciliary processes. (×62) *(Modified from Morrison JC, Van Buskirk EM, Freddo T. Anatomy, microcirculation and ultrastructure of the ciliary body. In: Ritch R, Shields MB, Krupin T, eds. The Glaucomas. St. Louis, MO: C.V. Mosby; 1989.)*

ference across the membrane and the surface area over which filtration can occur. The composition of the filtrate (e.g., water, ions, proteins) is determined largely by the size of the pores in the membrane— that is, by the permeability of the blood vessel wall. In the ciliary body stroma, a filtrate of plasma is produced by filtration across the walls of its microvasculature.

The arterioles that serve the ciliary body stroma arise from the discontinuous major circle of the iris. Casts made of the ciliary body microvasculature of primate eyes have demonstrated that each major process is served by a set of anterior and posterior arterioles (Fig. 3–3).[2] The anterior arterioles supply the large diameter capillaries near the crests of the processes while the posterior arterioles supply the

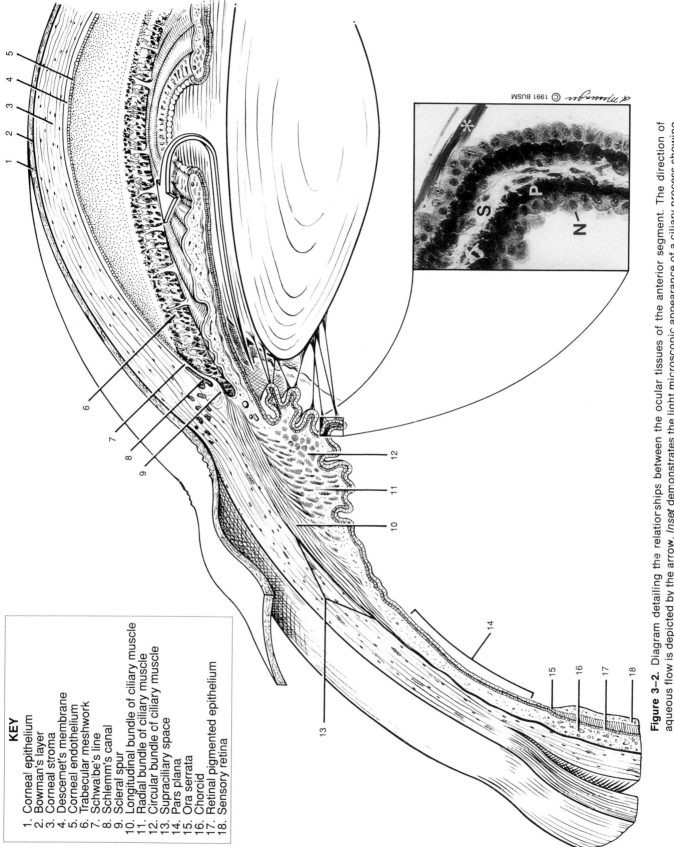

KEY

1. Corneal epithelium
2. Bowman's layer
3. Corneal stroma
4. Descemet's membrane
5. Corneal endothelium
6. Trabecular meshwork
7. Schwalbe's line
8. Schlemm's canal
9. Scleral spur
10. Longitudinal bundle of ciliary muscle
11. Radial bundle of ciliary muscle
12. Circular bundle of ciliary muscle
13. Supraciliary space
14. Pars plana
15. Ora serrata
16. Choroid
17. Retinal pigmented epithelium
18. Sensory retina

Figure 3–2. Diagram detailing the relationships between the ocular tissues of the anterior segment. The direction of aqueous flow is depicted by the arrow. *Inset* demonstrates the light microscopic appearance of a ciliary process showing the nonpigmented (N) and pigmented (P) ciliary epithelia, the ciliary body stroma (S) and a bundle of zonular fibers (*asterisk*). (×318)

25

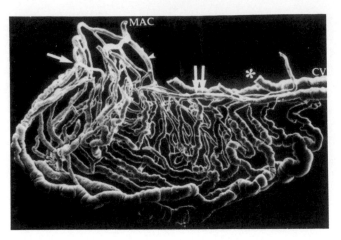

Figure 3–3. A cast of the vasculature within a single ciliary process. The major circle of the iris (MAC) gives rise to an anterior (*arrow*) and posterior (*arrowhead*) arteriole. Double arrow denotes choroidal vein (CV). Drainage from ciliary muscle to choroidal veins has been removed at asterisk. (×110) *(With permission from Morrison JC, Van Buskirk EM, Freddo T. Anatomy, microcirculation and ultrastructure of the ciliary body. In: Ritch R, Shields MB, Krupin T, eds. The Glaucomas. St Louis, MO: C.V. Mosby; 1989.)*

smaller caliber capillaries deep within each process. The direction of blood flow in both of these systems is from anterior to posterior, toward a network of choroidal veins (Fig. 3–4).

There is increasing anatomical and physiological evidence that blood flow in the ciliary body is regionalized and that these various regions respond differently to agents such as epinephrine.[3] Given the presence of adrenergic nerve endings associated with the ciliary body microvasculature, and the fact that blood flow in these vessels is reduced by sympathetic stimulation,[4,5] it is possible that controlled alterations in blood flow may occur that could, at various times, either enhance or reduce filtrate production.

The capillaries of the ciliary body stroma are lined by endothelial cells that are fenestrated and lack continuous tight junctions (Fig. 3–5). As can be demonstrated using tracers for plasma protein leakage such as horseradish peroxidase (HRP), the capillaries of the ciliary body stroma are very permeable to macromolecules as well as ions and fluid (Fig. 3–6). Not surprisingly, these vessels are limited in their capacity to serve as a selective permeability barrier. The proteins entering the plasma filtrate in this manner contribute to the oncotic pressure of the ciliary body stroma.

The ions, fluid, and small molecules of the plasma filtrate are driven into the ciliary body stroma by the hydrostatic pressure within the capillaries of the ciliary processes.[6] The magnitude of the hydro-

static pressure is, in part, dependent on neuroregulatory and/or humoral influences on the microvasculature.

Countering the hydrostatic pressure within the vasculature is the interstitial fluid pressure of the ciliary body stroma, which increases with increasing intraocular pressure (IOP).[6] Because of this relationship, moderate elevations of intraocular pressure give rise to reductions in aqueous inflow and, after a time delay, a decrease in intraocular pressure. The dynamics of this relationship are actually more complex, and the effect is insufficient to serve as a protective mechanism against the development of glaucoma.

There is nonetheless a clinical consequence of the relationship between intraocular pressure and inflow, but it has principally to do with measurements of aqueous *outflow*. Certain methods used to measure aqueous outflow facility, such as tonography and constant pressure perfusion techniques, rely on artificially elevating the intraocular pressure. Aqueous outflow facility is then calculated from the rate of decrease in the elevated pressure over time.[7,8] Since reduction in aqueous production contributes to the fall in intraocular pressure measured under these circumstances, the resulting outflow facility is proportionally increased. The proportion of total outflow facility resulting from the pressure-induced reduction in aqueous production is termed *pseudofacility*. Although early measurements suggested that pseudofacility might account for as much as 20% of total outflow facility,[9] improved methods suggest that pseudofacility probably accounts for only about 5 to 10% of the total.[10]

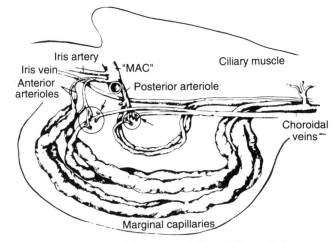

Figure 3–4. Diagrammatic representation of Figure 3–3 demonstrates the system of anterior and posterior arterioles that enter each process ultimately draining into a set of choroidal veins. *(With permission from Morrison JC, Van Buskirk EM, Freddo T. Anatomy, microcirculation and ultrastructure of the ciliary body. In: Ritch R, Shields MB, Krupin T, eds. The Glaucomas. St. Louis, MO: C.V. Mosby; 1989.)*

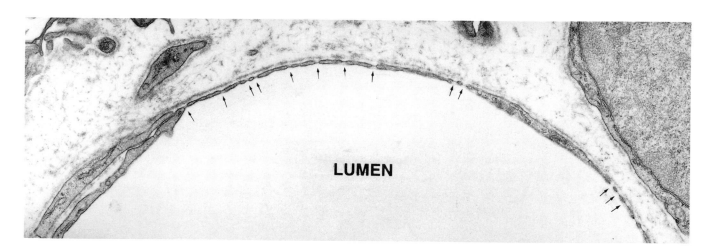

Figure 3–5. Transmission electron micrograph demonstrates the appearance of capillaries in the ciliary body stroma. Numerous fenestrations (*arrows*) are evident along the circumference of the vessel wall. (×34,800) *(Modified from Morrison JC, Van Buskirk EM, Freddo T. Anatomy, microcirculation and ultrastructure of the ciliary body. In: Ritch R, Shields MB, Krupin T, eds. The Glaucomas. St. Louis, MO: C.V. Mosby; 1989.)*

In summary, it appears that the dynamic equilibrium between the forces of the hydrostatic, interstitial, and intraocular pressures, combined with the vascular tone and permeability characteristics of the ciliary body microvasculature are the major factors determining the amount of filtrate available in the ciliary body stroma for aqueous production.

The Blood-Aqueous Barrier. In order for the aqueous humor secreted into the posterior chamber to have a composition different from that of the protein-laden filtrate in the ciliary body stroma, a selective permeability barrier must exist between the ciliary body stroma and the posterior chamber. And, because aqueous humor in the anterior chamber freely permeates the stroma of the iris, a barrier to plasma protein leakage must also exist within the walls of iris blood vessels. Several investigators have demonstrated that the morphologic equivalents of the blood aqueous barrier to macromolecules are the zonulae occludentes that join the cell membranes of adjacent iris vascular endothelial cells and those of the nonpigmented ciliary epithelial cells.[11–13]

Unlike the microvasculature of the ciliary body

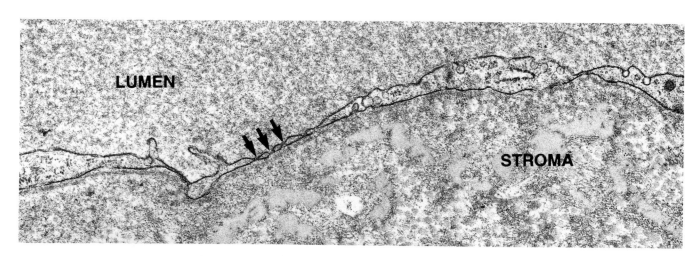

Figure 3–6. Transmission electron micrograph demonstrates that granular HRP reaction product leaks through fenestrations (*arrows*) into the surrounding ciliary body stroma. (×40,800) *(With permission from Morrison JC, Van Buskirk EM, Freddo T. Anatomy, microcirculation and ultrastructure of the ciliary body. In: Ritch R, Shields MB, Krupin T, eds. The Glaucomas. St. Louis, MO: C.V. Mosby; 1989.)*

stroma, the vessels of the iris do not leak plasma proteins or analogous macromolecular tracers such as HRP (Fig. 3–7). The reasons are twofold. The iris vessels are nonfenestrated and the endothelial cells of these vessels are joined by complex tight junctions. In cross-sections of iris vessels, zonulae occludentes (also commonly referred to as continuous tight junctions) are recognized as a series of contact points between the membranes of adjacent endothelial cells (Fig. 3–8). Using the technique of freeze-fracture electron microscopy, the membranes of these cells can be cleaved to reveal the three-dimensional organization of their tight junctions. In freeze-fracture electron micrographs, the series of contact points observed in cross-sections is revealed in actuality to be a complex network of branching and anastomosing lines of contact between strands of particles (probably proteins) embedded within the membranes of the adjacent cells (Fig. 3–9). The relationship between these two views of tight junctions is shown in Figure 3–10. This network of tight junctional strands serves to occlude the interendothelial cleft, preventing leakage of macromolecules from the bloodstream into the aqueous humor.

As mentioned, continuous tight junctions also constitute the morphologic equivalents of the blood-aqueous barrier in the ciliary body.[11,12] Following intravenous injection of HRP in primates, the tracer leaves the fenestrated capillaries of the ciliary processes, moving easily through the loose connective

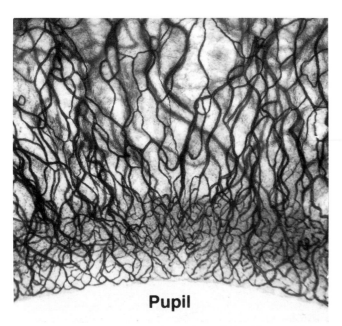

Pupil

Figure 3–7. Whole-mount preparation of the iris vasculature demonstrates that the macromolecular tracer HRP is confined within the vessels. (×38)

tissue of the ciliary body stroma to the bilayered ciliary epithelium. The tracer readily permeates the intercellular clefts between adjacent pigmented ciliary epithelial cells and between the adjoined apical surfaces of the pigmented and nonpigmented layers. However, further migration of the tracer toward the posterior chamber, between the cells of the nonpigmented layer, is blocked at their apicolateral surfaces by the presence of tight junctions (Fig. 3–11). The appearances of these junctions, in both sectioned material and freeze-fracture, are shown for comparison (see Fig. 3–11, inset and Fig. 3–12).

Despite these epithelial and endothelial barriers, a small amount of plasma protein does enter the aqueous humor. The protein concentration of aqueous humor equals approximately 1% of that in plasma,[6] but the route of entry of this protein has been uncertain. Examining the anterior segment of the eye, it is clear that no anatomical barrier exists between the protein-laden ciliary body stroma and the anterior chamber along the gonioscopically visible ciliary body band. Recently, it has been shown that most of the plasma-derived protein present in aqueous humor actually enters the anterior chamber directly, diffusing from the ciliary body stroma via the root of the iris.[14]

Formation of Aqueous Humor From the Plasma Filtrate by the Ciliary Epithelium

The formation of aqueous humor by the ciliary epithelium is dependent primarily on two forces: hydrostatic pressure and the magnitude of the oncotic pressure gradient across the ciliary epithelium.

One of the most widely accepted models for the process of aqueous secretion was reviewed by Cole[6] and represents a modification of the Diamond-Bossert model for standing gradient osmotic flow (Fig. 3–13).[15] A schematized representation of the factors involved is presented in Figure 3–13. The role of the pigmented ciliary epithelium is neglected since it is poorly understood. According to this model, sodium ions, bicarbonate ions, and possibly chloride ions as well are actively transported from the plasma filtrate into the intercellular clefts between adjacent nonpigmented ciliary epithelial cells. The presence of these solutes creates a standing osmotic gradient that draws water into the cleft. The tight junctions, joining the apicolateral surfaces of the nonpigmented cells, restrict aqueous flow at the apical end of the cleft, directing it toward the posterior chamber. Recently, it has been demonstrated that another type of intercellular junction, the gap junction, may coordinate the secretory activity of the ciliary epithelium by electrotonically and/or metabolically coupling the cells into a functional syncytium.[16]

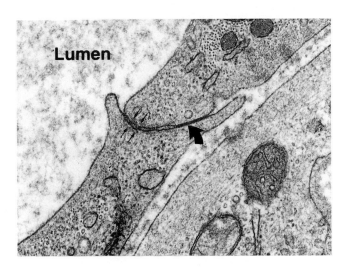

Figure 3–8. Transmission electron micrograph of an iris blood vessel demonstrates that the endothelial cells (E) are joined by tight junctions (*small arrows*) and gap junctions (*curved arrow*). (×40,000)

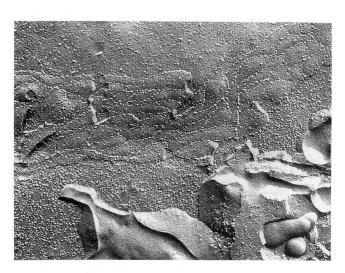

Figure 3–9. Freeze-fracture electron micrograph of iris vascular endothelial cells demonstrates the branching and anastomosing pattern of tight junctional strands that constitute the zonula occludens. (×38,000)

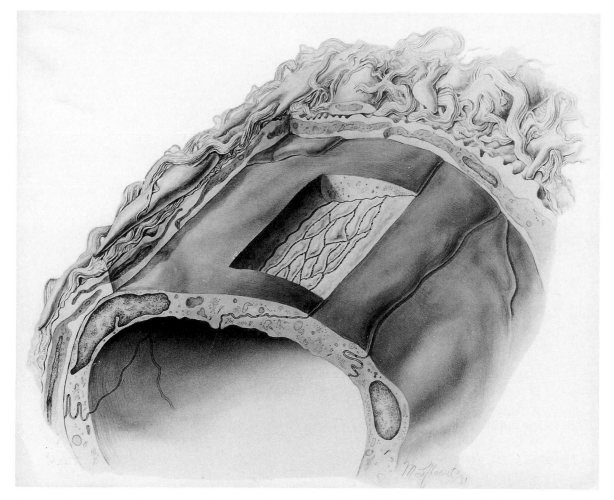

Figure 3–10. Diagrammatic representation of an iris blood vessel demonstrates the relationship between the sectioned and freeze-fracture appearances of the zonula occludens. *(With permission from Freddo T, Raviola G:* Invest Ophthalmol Vis Sci. *1982;23:154.)*

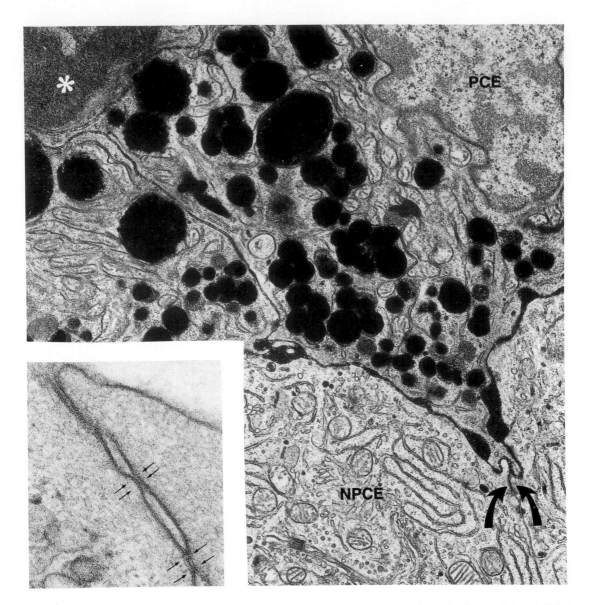

Figure 3–11. Black HRP reaction product fills the ciliary body stroma (*asterisk*), blackens the intercellular cleft between adjacent pigmented ciliary epithelial cells (PCE) and between the apical surfaces of the pigmented and nonpigmented layers (NPCE). Further diffusion of HRP toward the posterior chamber is blocked by tight junctions between adjacent nonpigmented epithelial cells (*curved arrows*). (×19,000) *Inset:* Higher magnification demonstrates the points of fusion (*arrows*) between membranes of adjacent nonpigmented ciliary epithelial cells that constitute the tight junction. (×131,000) *(With permission from Morrison JC, Van Buskirk EM, Freddo T. Anatomy, Microcirculation and ultrastructure of the ciliary body. In: Ritch R, Shields MB, Krupin T, eds. The Glaucomas. St. Louis, MO: C.V. Mosby; 1989.)*

Although the evidence for active transport of ions by the ciliary epithelium is quite substantial, there remains some evidence that the movement of ions into the intercellular cleft may be enhanced by ultrafiltration. Ultrafiltration is a process wherein dialysis (i.e., the separation of ions from an ion-protein mixture such as that existent in the ciliary body stroma) is augmented by application of a hydrostatic pressure. The relative contributions of these two components to the process of aqueous production continue to be debated but most authors now agree that secretion, in the form of metabolically-dependent active transport plays, by far, the greater role.[17]

Regardless of the mechanism used to move ions into the intercellular cleft, it is necessary that fluid in the apical part of the cleft remain hypertonic to assure a continuous flow of water.[6] It is thus important that the volume of the cleft remain small to avoid

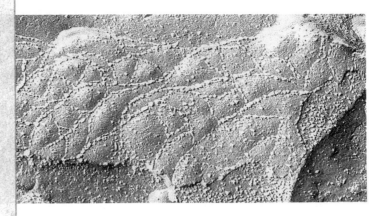

ograph demonstrates the branching and anastomosing tight junctional strands
npigmented ciliary epithelial cells. (×57,500) *(With permission from Morrison
icrocirculation and ultrastructure of the ciliary body. In: Ritch R, Shields MB,
O: C.V. Mosby; 1989.)*

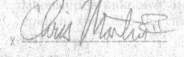

dhering in-
y epithelial
llular cleft
interfering
ns join the
f the inter-
e adhering
ciliary epi-
ith certain
bined (Fig.
e of this re-
ur only in
are secre-

nce for the
tive metab-
onstrating
xygen ten-
of aqueous

Na⁺/K⁺-ATPase. Evidence that ion transport is central to the process comes from studies that have localized sodium-potassium ATPase activity to the nonpigmented ciliary epithelium[21] and others documenting that inhibition of this enzyme with ouabain reduces aqueous secretion.[19]

Carbonic Anhydrase. Carbonic anhydrase also plays a significant role in the process of aqueous secretion by producing bicarbonate ions. This enzyme has also been histochemically localized to the pigmented and nonpigmented ciliary epithelium of the major ciliary processes.[22] Interestingly, this enzyme

was not found associated with the nonpigmented ciliary epithelium in the valleys between the major ciliary processes or in the pars plana, areas presumed not to be involved in aqueous production.

Carbonic anhydrase catalyzes the hydration of carbon dioxide to carbonic acid leading to the subsequent liberation of hydrogen and bicarbonate ions according to the following equation:

$$H_2O + CO_2 \leftrightarrow H_2CO_3 \leftrightarrow HCO_3^- + H^+$$

The roles of the ionic products of this reaction in the overall process of aqueous humor secretion remain uncertain. Inhibition of carbonic anhydrase decreases not only the entry of bicarbonate ions into the posterior chamber, but also the entry of sodium ions.[23] Whether a direct linkage between sodium and bicarbonate transport exists remains unclear, however. One theory regarding the role played by bicarbonate ions in aqueous humor production maintains that HCO_3^- is transported in parallel with Na^+, primarily to maintain electroneutrality. Another states that HCO_3^- movement may serve primarily to alter pH, optimizing sodium-potassium ATPase activity.[24]

Regardless of the mechanisms, the importance of this enzyme to aqueous secretion is amply attested to by the usefulness of carbonic anhydrase inhibitors (CAIs), such as acetazolamide, in the treatment of glaucoma. Currently, CAIs must be systemically administered, producing unwanted side effects that complicate therapy and can result in noncompliance. Efforts to develop a topically useful carbonic anhydrase inhibitor, thereby minimizing systemic side effects, have recently been reviewed by Podos.[25]

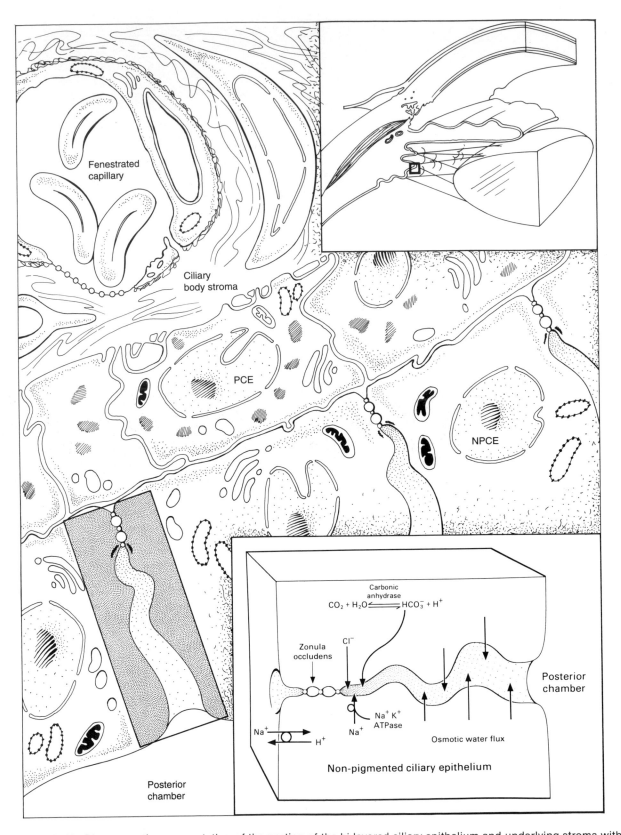

Labels within figure:

Fenestrated capillary

Ciliary body stroma

PCE

NPCE

Posterior chamber

Carbonic anhydrase

$$CO_2 + H_2O \rightleftharpoons HCO_3^- + H^+$$

Zonula occludens

Cl^-

$Na^+ K^+$ ATPase

Na^+

Na^+

H^+

Osmotic water flux

Posterior chamber

Non-pigmented ciliary epithelium

Figure 3–13. Diagrammatic representation of the portion of the bi-layered ciliary epithelium and underlying stroma with fenestrated capillaries that corresponds to the boxed area of the upper inset. The shaded area in the main figure corresponds to that shown in the lower inset depicting the major elements of the standing gradient model of aqueous flow. The role of the pigmented ciliary epithelium (PCE) has been neglected for simplicity. The gradient shown by stippling in the lower inset corresponds to the solute concentration along the intercellular cleft between adjacent non-pigmented ciliary epithelial (NPCE) cells. The normally narrow dimensions of the intercellular cleft ensure the hypertonicity required to maintain osmotic water flux and hence flow.

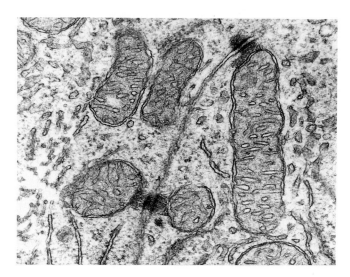

Figure 3–14. Mitochondria within adjacent nonpigmented ciliary epithelial cells are attached to desmosomal junctions that bridge the intercellular cleft. (×46,170) *(With permission from Freddo T, Cell Tiss Res. 1988;251:671.[18])*

Beta Adrenergic Receptors. Although a direct relationship with the model outlined above is unclear, there is convincing evidence that the secretory activity of the ciliary epithelium is influenced by β adrenergic activity, probably mediated by the adenyl cyclase enzyme-receptor complex.

Beta adrenergic receptors have been localized to the ciliary epithelium.[26] Stimulatory activation of these receptors initiates a signal transduction process (Fig. 3–15) beginning with activation of an intramembranous G protein. G proteins are regulators of certain enzymes and ionic channels (*see* Fig. 3–15). In the case of β adrenergic stimulation, the G protein activates the second messenger adenyl cyclase that has also been localized to the ciliary body.[27,28] Adenyl cyclase increases cytoplasmic levels of cyclic AMP leading to the phosphorylation of protein kinase-A. What is currently unclear is the mechanism through which these events lead to the ultimate effect on aqueous humor inflow. The literature in this area is remarkably contradictory, even disregarding the added complexities that arise in trying to compare data obtained from different species.[29] Regardless of the molecular mechanisms at work, it does seem clear that β antagonists such as timolol lead to reductions in both aqueous inflow and intraocular pressure.[30] Equally well established, if not well explained, is the belief that neither β agonists nor β antagonists demonstrate an outflow-mediated effect on intraocular pressure, despite the presence of β receptors on cells within the trabecular outflow pathways.[31]

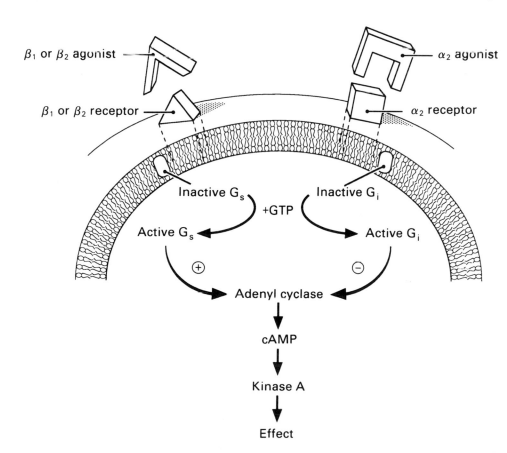

Figure 3–15. Diagrammatic representation of the signal transduction process that ensues following binding at β_1, β_2, and α_2 receptors. In each case, intramembranous G-protein activation occurs, which either increases or decreases cyclic AMP levels through alterations in adenyl cyclase activity.

Alpha Adrenergic Receptors. Alpha$_2$ adrenergic receptors are also present in the ciliary body.[32] They appear to be negatively coupled with adenyl cyclase, and can block the elevations of cAMP levels induced by β agonists (*see* Fig. 3–15).[31] A similar paradox to that described above for β receptors exists here as well, for *both* α adrenergic agonists and antagonists have been reported to lower intraocular pressure.[33] In the case of α_2 receptor-mediated agents, the sites of action appear to be different. Alpha$_2$ antagonists appear not to effect either inflow or trabecular outflow[34] suggesting a possible uveoscleral mechanism. Alpha$_2$ agonists, on the other hand, appear to act on aqueous inflow.[34] Currently, only one α_2 agent, the agonist p-aminoclonidine, is available in the United States and its principal use has been prophylactic, preventing elevations of intraocular pressure that may follow argon laser trabeculoplasty.

THE AQUEOUS OUTFLOW PATHWAYS

The major pathway for aqueous humor outflow is through the trabecular meshwork and the canal of Schlemm, into the venous system of the eye via a series of intrascleral collector channels and venous plexi. Three alternate pathways have also been identified that vary in their presumed importance to aqueous outflow from species to species. The most significant of these alternate routes is the uveoscleral pathway. Very minor additional contributions to outflow may occur via the vitreous body and the corneal stroma but an earlier assumption that iris vessels might participate in outflow has been refuted.[35] Of these pathways, only trabecular and uveoscleral outflow will be considered here.

ANATOMY OF THE TRABECULAR MESHWORK

The trabecular meshwork is a roughly triangular wedge of tissue encircling the anterior chamber and having as its apex the peripheral terminus of Descemet's membrane called Schwalbe's line. From this anterior boundary, the meshwork expands as it bridges the iridocorneal angle of the eye, ending posteriorly by blending with the stromas of the both the iris and ciliary body (Fig. 3–16). Projecting like a shelf into the meshwork near its posterior margin, is the scleral spur, which serves as a point of insertion for the longitudinal bundle of the ciliary muscle.

A portion of the meshwork lies wholly within a recess in the sclera termed the internal scleral sulcus.

The limits of this sulcus are defined by an imaginary line drawn on a sagittal section of the meshwork from Schwalbe's line to the anterior tip of the scleral spur (*see* Fig. 3–16). Within the confines of the sulcus are the corneoscleral and juxtacanalicular areas (also termed cribriform) of the meshwork and the canal of Schlemm. The portion of the meshwork that is not confined within the sulcus and that is most readily viewed gonioscopically is termed the uveal meshwork.

The importance of understanding the relationship between the views of the meshwork obtained from sagittal sections and those obtained gonioscopically cannot be overemphasized. In Figures 3–17 and 3–18, the macroscopic appearance of these structures and corresponding diagrammatic representations as seen from both perspectives can readily be compared. In addition, because the canal of Schlemm is filled with blood in Figure 3–17, the relationship between the canal and the other angle structures is also evident. These macroscopic views should be compared with the goniophotograph of a normal, open angle seen in Figure 3–19. The principal landmarks evident in such a view of an open anterior chamber angle include, from superior to inferior, (1) Schwalbe's line (i.e., the peripheral terminus of Descemet's membrane), (2) the trabecular meshwork, (3) the scleral spur, and (4) the ciliary body band.

The Uveal and Corneoscleral Portions of the Meshwork. The uveal and corneoscleral portions of the trabecular meshwork have an approximately analogous structure. Both are composed of series of trabeculae that delimit a system of aqueous flow channels. These channels become progressively smaller from the uveal to the corneoscleral meshwork.

The scanning electron microscopic appearance of the uveal face of the trabecular meshwork is seen in Figure 3–20. The cord-like trabecular beams seen in this view characterize only the innermost layers of the meshwork. The trabeculae of the corneoscleral meshwork have fewer, smaller openings that give them an appearance more aptly described as perforated sheets.

In microscopic sections, the uveal and corneoscleral trabeculae are each seen to be covered by a single layer of endothelial cells (Fig. 3–21). The cores of the beams and corneoscleral sheets are composed largely of various collagen subtypes and some elastic fibers, which have only recently been shown definitely to contain elastin.[36]

The intercellular junctions that join the trabecular endothelial cells include only gap junctions and

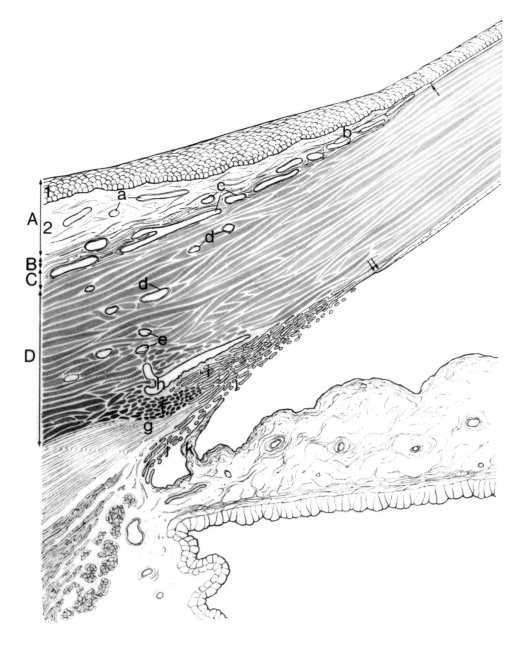

Figure 3–16. Drawing of the limbus to illustrate the structures evident by microscopic examination. The limbal conjunctiva (A) is formed by an epithelium (1) and an areolar connective tissue stroma (2). Tenon's capsule (B) forms an ill-defined connective tissue layer over the episclera (C). The limbal corneosclera occupies area (D). a = conjunctival vessels, b = corneal arcades, *single arrow* = terminus of Bowman's layer.

The triangular tissue wedge of the trabecular meshwork (i) originates at Schwalbe's line (*double arrows*) and broadens posteriorly to become continuous with the root of the iris and the ciliary body. An iris process (k) extends from the iris surface to the trabecular meshwork. Entering the posterior margin of the trabecular meshwork is the scleral spur (f) to which tendons of the longitudinal bundle of the ciliary muscle (g) are attached. Aqueous passing through the trabecular meshwork enters the canal of Schlemm (h), deep scleral plexus (e), intrascleral plexus (d), and, finally, the episcleral vessels (c). *(With permission from Hogan M, Alvarado J, Weddell J. Histology of the Human Eye. Philadelphia, PA: W.B. Saunders; 1971.)*

short, discontinuous tight junctional strands.[37] As such, aqueous humor readily permeates the cores of the trabecular beams and there is little evidence to suggest that the trabeculae are continually being deturgesced by their endothelial cells in any manner similar to that observed in the cornea. It is therefore unlikely that trabecular endothelial cells could operate to regulate outflow by varying the thickness of the trabeculae and, indirectly, the dimensions of the outflow channels.

The endothelial cells of the trabecular meshwork are known to be phagocytic.[38,39] They are capable of ingesting both endogenous materials such as pig-

ment[40,41] and exogenous particulates such as latex microspheres,[42] presumably for the purpose of keeping the trabecular outflow channels free of potentially obstructive debris. It appears that this phagocytic capacity may be at some long-term cost to the meshwork, however, for it is widely held that phagocytosis leads to detachment of endothelial cells from their beams and to their migration out of the eye.[38]

Given the limited capacity for cell division that is seen in the trabecular meshwork,[43] a progressive reduction in the number of trabecular endothelial cells is to be expected. These findings are consistent with the documented decrease in trabecular cell number

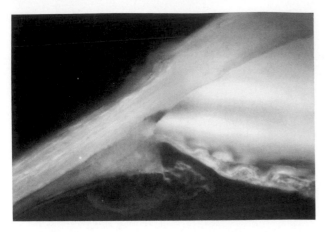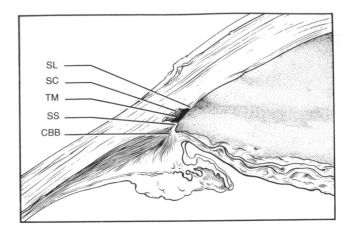

Figure 3–17. Macroscopic photograph and corresponding sketch identifying structures visible in a sagittal section of the normal anterior chamber angle. The anterior chamber is artifactually deepened due to posterior sagging of the iris following removal of the crystalline lens. SL = Schwalbe's line; SC = Schlemm's canal; TM = trabecular meshwork; SS = scleral spur; CBB = ciliary body band. (*See also* Color Plate 3–17.)

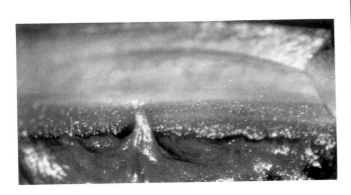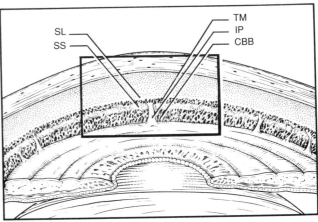

Figure 3–18. Macroscopic photograph and corresponding sketch of angle structures viewed from the perspective shown in the adjacent sketch. Schlemm's canal is filled with blood in this specimen, demonstrating its relationship to the other angle structures. An iris process is also shown. Compare the view of the angle structures in this figure with the corresponding sagittal view shown in Figure 3–17. SL = Schwalbe's line; SS = scleral spur; TM = trabecular meshwork; IP = iris process; CBB = ciliary body band. (*See also* Color Plate 3–18.)

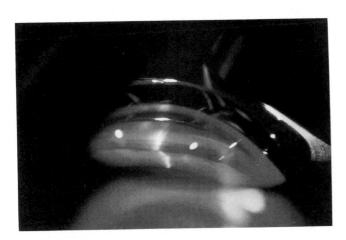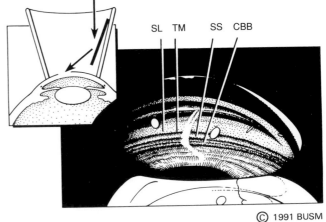

© 1991 BUSM

Figure 3–19. Goniophotograph of a normal open angle, and corresponding sketch representing a view analogous to that shown in Figure 3–18. *Inset* in sketch depicts the placement of the gonioscope onto the cornea and the manner in which the angle structures are viewed. SL = Schwalbe's line; TM = trabecular meshwork; SS = scleral spur; CBB = ciliary body band. (*See also* Color Plate 3–19.) *(Photo courtesy of Rodney Gutner, OD.)*

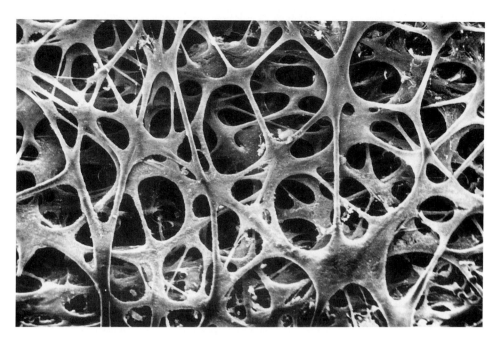

Figure 3–20. Scanning electron micrograph demonstrates the appearance of the uveal face of the trabecular meshwork as viewed from the anterior chamber. (×504). *(With permission from Freddo TF, et al,* Invest Ophthalmol Vis Sci. *1984;25:278.)*

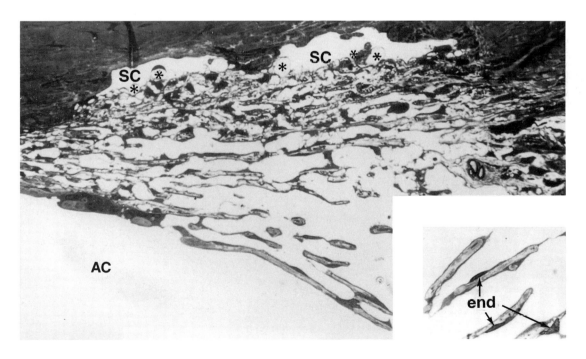

Figure 3–21. Light micrograph of the trabecular meshwork. Note that in this section Schlemm's canal (SC) is divided into two parallel channels. Outlines of giant vacuoles can be seen protruding into the lumen of the canal (*asterisks*). AC, anterior chamber. (×383) *Inset:* Higher magnification view of trabecular beams demonstrating the central connective tissue core surrounded by slender trabecular endothelial (end) cells. (×650).

seen with increasing age.[44,45] Whether this cell loss is a major factor leading to the development of glaucoma, however, remains to be established.[46]

The Cribriform or Juxtacanalicular Meshwork. The type of cell found in the region of the meshwork between the outermost corneoscleral trabecular beam and the inner wall of Schlemm's canal appears to be different from the endothelial cells that cover the trabeculae. They are more fibroblast-like and lack a basal lamina (Fig. 3–22).[47] The region of the meshwork occupied by these cells, and the extracellular matrix with which they are associated, represents the cribriform or juxtacanalicular region of the trabecular meshwork. Forming an integral part of the extracellular matrix in this region is a plexus of elastic-like fibers. These fibers are connected both to a subclass of tendons from the longitudinal bundle of the ciliary muscle (discussed below) and to the basal surface of the endothelial cells that line the inner wall of Schlemm's canal. This anatomical system, called the cribriform plexus,[48] has the potential to effect alterations in the permeability of this region. Such changes are likely of clinical importance, for it is the cribriform region of the aqueous outflow system that is generally held to represent the principal site of aqueous outflow resistance.[49,50]

The Role of the Ciliary Muscle in Trabecular Outflow. Three types of tendons have been reported to extend from the tips of the muscle fibers of the ciliary muscle either into or through the trabecular meshwork (Fig. 3–23).[51] One of these is responsible for attaching the longitudinal bundle of the ciliary muscle to the scleral spur. As a result, contraction of the ciliary muscle, whether it occurs naturally as a part of accommodation or is induced pharmacologically using miotics such as pilocarpine, pulls on the scleral spur and in this way serves to spread the trabecular sheets open, facilitating trabecular outflow.

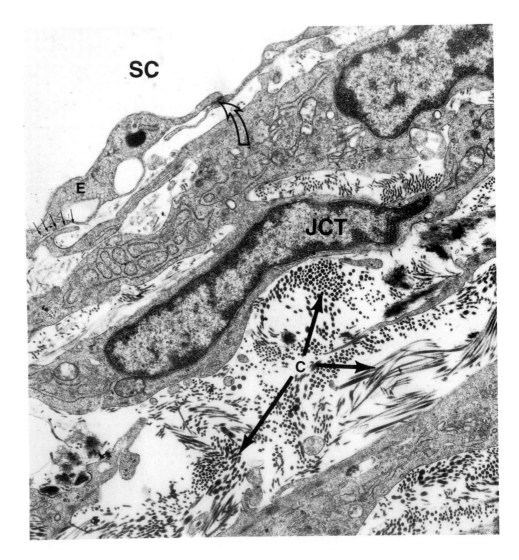

Figure 3–22. Transmission electron micrograph demonstrating the appearance of the cells predominant in the juxtacanalicular region of the trabecular meshwork (JCT). These cells lack a basal lamina and are enmeshed in a connective tissue matrix that includes fibrillar collagen (C). The relationship between these cells and the endothelial cells (E) lining the inner wall of Schlemm's canal (SC) is evident. Mushroom-like processes from JCT cells appear to contact the inner wall cells (*small arrows*). An interendothelial cell junction between two inner wall cells is also present (*curved arrow*). (×16,600) (*Courtesy of Haiyan Gong, MD, PhD.*)

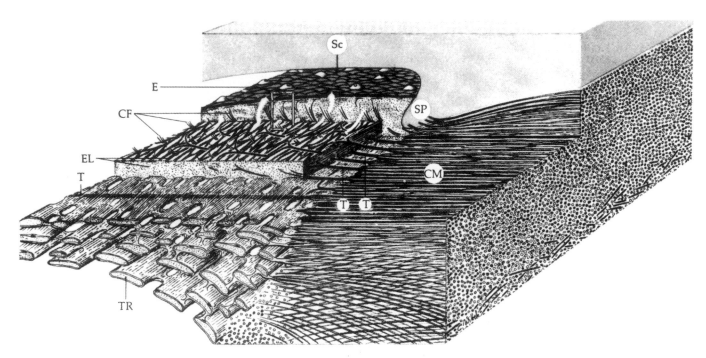

Figure 3–23. Anterior ciliary muscle tendons (T) and their connections with the trabecular meshwork. Tendons from the smooth muscle cells of the ciliary muscle (CM) extend to the scleral spur (SP), into the outermost corneoscleral trabeculae and into the juxtacanalicular region contributing to the cribriform plexus. Connecting fibrils (CF) extend from the plexus toward the endothelial cells (E) lining the inner wall of Schlemm's canal (Sc). *(Published courtesy of Rohen JW, Ophthalmology. 1983;90:758.)*

A second type of tendon extends through the trabeculae inserting into the peripheral corneal lamellae, having little apparent impact on outflow.

The third tendon type, extends into the outermost corneoscleral trabeculae and also inserts within the cribriform region of the meshwork. From these tendons, elastin-containing connecting fibrils (the cribriform plexus mentioned earlier) extend to the basal lamina of the endothelial cells lining the inner wall of Schlemm's canal (Fig. 3–24). Contraction of these fibers likely also contributes to increasing trabecular flow through the cribriform region of the meshwork.[51]

Underscoring the physiological importance of these various anatomical connections is the work of Kaufman and Bárány who first demonstrated that

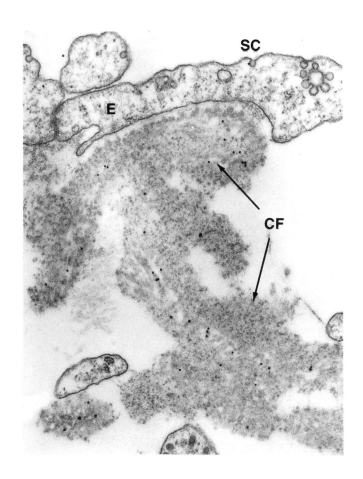

Figure 3–24. Transmission electron micrograph demonstrates the appearance of a connecting fibril (CF) corresponding to the area outlined in Figure 3–23. These fibrils extend from the cribriform plexus to endothelial cells (E) of the inner wall of Schlemm's canal (SC). Small black dots represent colloidal gold particles localizing sites of antielastin antibody binding, confirming the presence of elastin in these fibers. (×36,000) *(With permission of Oxford Press from Gong H, Trinkaus-Randall V, Freddo T, Curr Eye Res. 1989;8:1071.)*

surgical disinsertion of the ciliary muscle eliminates the outflow-enhancing effects of pilocarpine.[52] More recently, Kaufman and his co-workers have begun to question whether the progressive loss of ciliary muscle tone that contributes to presbyopia,[53] and the age-related loss of responsiveness to pilocarpine demonstrated in the monkey eye,[54] might also result in a diminished capacity to open up the meshwork, leading to a progressive accumulation of obstructive material and possibly glaucoma.[53,54]

The "Open" Spaces of the Trabecular Meshwork. It is always initially tempting to view the apparently ample "open" spaces seen in light or electron microscopic sections of the trabecular meshwork as though they represent an accurate depiction of the area available for aqueous flow. However, calculations of outflow resistance in the juxtacanalicular meshwork, using a mathematical model that assumed the "open" spaces to be real, have been shown to fall two orders of magnitude short of generally accepted values for outflow resistance.[55] From both biochemical and histochemical studies, it is evident that a substantial fraction of the space that appears empty in the trabecular meshwork is, in fact, filled by an extracellular matrix composed of proteoglycans, associated and unassociated glycosaminoglycans (GAGs), proteins, and other moieties.[56] Changes in the amount and distribution of these various constituents are known to influence, and may even regulate, the passage of aqueous humor out of the eye.[57–59] Indeed, recent studies of trabecular meshwork explants in organ culture[60] and earlier work in tissue culture[61] have demonstrated that dexamethasone increases GAG production, a process that may underlie the well-known phenomenon of steroid-induced elevation of intraocular pressure.

The Canal of Schlemm. The canal of Schlemm is a continuous circumferentially oriented channel situated deep within the internal scleral sulcus. The lumen of Schlemm's canal is in direct continuity with the venous system of the eye. Despite this connection, blood is not usually seen in the canal unless intraocular pressure falls below that of episcleral venous pressure.

Transected and viewed by scanning electron microscopy, the canal usually appears slit-like and, at several points around the circumference of the eye, can be seen to divide into two parallel channels that rejoin one another after a short distance (Figs. 3–21 and 3–25). One side of the canal directly abuts the sclera and is termed its outer wall. The opposite side, which faces the trabecular meshwork, is termed the

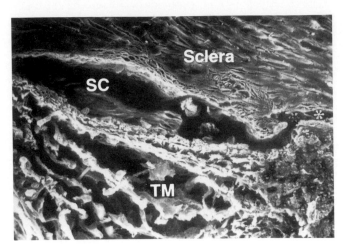

Figure 3–25. Scanning electron micrograph of transected trabecular meshwork (TM) and Schlemm's canal (SC) demonstrates the slit-like appearance of the canal, its relation to the sclera and its continuity with an external collector channel (*asterisks*). (×304).

inner wall of Schlemm's canal and it is the issue of how aqueous humor crosses this wall that has proven to be one of the most enigmatic in attempts to understand the dynamics of aqueous outflow.

There have traditionally been two schools of thought on the subject of how aqueous humor crosses the inner wall of Schlemm's canal. One argues that the aqueous passes between the endothelial cells that form the inner wall and the other argues that the aqueous passes through the cells via specialized structures commonly referred to as giant vacuoles.

Ultrastructural studies, using the technique of freeze-fracture electron microscopy, have demonstrated that the endothelial cells of the inner wall are joined by two types of intercellular junctions, gap junctions, and discontinuous tight junctions.[37] Unlike the *continuous* tight junctions of iris blood vessels, the *discontinuous* tight junctions between the endothelial cells of the inner wall do not form an uninterrupted system of branching and anastomosing strands (Fig. 3–26). Instead, maze-like pathways through the junctions exist that have been termed slit-pores (Fig. 3–27).[37] At first glance, these pores would seem to offer a potentially significant conduit for aqueous flow. In her manuscript reporting the existence of slit-pores, however, Raviola[37] went on to measure the dimensions of these pores and to calculate that they could not account for more than a small fraction of the aqueous humor that reaches the lumen of the canal. More recent studies, however, have demonstrated that under conditions of increased perfusion pressure, paracellular permeability increases, and a

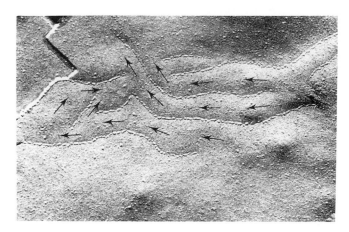

Figure 3–26. Freeze-fracture electron micrograph of the intercellular junctions between endothelial cells of the inner wall of Schlemm's canal. The tight junctional strands are discontinuous, providing a maze-like pathway through the junction as demonstrated by the arrows. (×62,300) *(With permission from Raviola G, Raviola E, Invest Ophthalmol Vis Sci. 1981;21:52.)*

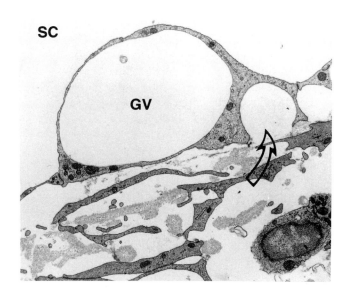

Figure 3–28. Transmission electron micrograph demonstrates a giant vacuole (GV) in the inner wall of Schlemm's canal (SC). Another vacuole is seen in the process of formation *(curved arrow)*. (×6,500)

reappraisal of the role of the paracellular pathway is in progress.[62]

Currently, most authors would continue to agree that the bulk of aqueous flow across the inner wall of Schlemm's canal is carried by giant vacuoles. Giant vacuoles in the wall of Schlemm's canal are demonstrated in Figure 3–28. These vacuoles appear to represent distentions within or between inner wall endothelial cells that are formed around an aliquot of aqueous humor.[63] This aliquot is then released into

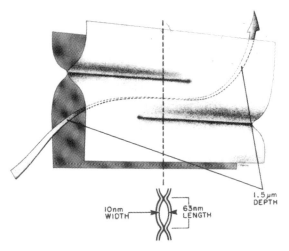

Figure 3–27. Diagrammatic representation of the freeze-fracture electron micrograph in Figure 3–26 demonstrates the nature of the "slit-pores" between adjacent endothelial cells forming the inner wall of Schlemm's canal. *(With permission from Raviola G, Raviola E, Invest Ophthalmol Vis Sci. 1981;21:52.)*

the lumen of Schlemm's canal through a small opening or pore that develops in the vacuole wall.[64] As odd as these vacuoles initially appear, there is precedent for the existence of such structures in other tissues. Specifically, it has been found that similar vacuoles are present in the arachnoid villi of the meninges, surrounding the brain, where they are felt to play a role in the resorption of cerebrospinal fluid.[64–66]

Giant vacuole formation is not energy dependent. The dynamics of this process are not fully understood but a relationship between these structures and outflow seems clear. Trabecular outflow, unlike uveoscleral outflow (described below) is pressure dependent.

As intraocular pressure is increased (within physiologically obtainable limits), the size of vacuoles in the inner wall of Schlemm's canal also increases.[65] Conversely, when intraocular pressure is reduced, as in paracentesis, vacuoles are also reduced.[67,68] Specimens of trabecular meshwork that are not under flow conditions while the tissue is being fixed for microscopic study commonly exhibit few, if any, vacuoles at all.

The Outflow Channels Beyond Schlemm's Canal.
From the canal of Schlemm, aqueous humor is conducted ultimately to the venous system. In this regard, it is important to appreciate that elevations of venous pressure can result in significant elevations of intraocular pressure. The pathways connecting the

canal of Schlemm to the venous system of the episcleral venous plexus are depicted in Figure 3–29. From the canal of Schlemm, aqueous passes into one of approximately 30 to 35 external collector channels (Figs. 3–25 and 3–29). These channels are unevenly distributed, with more on the nasal than on the temporal side of the eye. From the external collector channels, two separate pathways conduct the aqueous to the episcleral venous plexus. One pathway leads through an anastomotic system of deep and more superficial intrascleral plexi. The other is a more direct pathway to the venous system via a sparsely distributed set of aqueous veins. The aqueous veins, first described by Ascher, are identifiable clinically because there is a tendency for the aqueous and blood to resist immediate mixing and thus to be seen running in a laminar flow within these vessels.[69]

It appears that only about 20 to 25% of the normal resistance to aqueous outflow in the human or primate eye is attributable to the portions of the aqueous outflow system between Schlemm's canal and the venous system. Recently, there has been renewed interest in these channels, however, with identification of the contractile protein smooth muscle myosin

in cells adjacent to collector channels in human eyes. The presence of contractile elements in this distal portion of the outflow system raises the tempting possibility that they are capable of altering channel dimensions and, therefore, aqueous outflow.[70]

Fluid Mechanics of Trabecular Outflow

From the previous discussion, it is clear that a number of factors, influencing several anatomical sites and physiological processes, interrelate to account for aqueous flow and intraocular pressure. Although substantially oversimplified, a general appreciation of these interrelationships can be realized through an understanding of the equations developed by Goldmann in which:

$$\Delta P = P_i - P_e \text{ and } F = C_{tm} (P_i - P_e)$$

where

P_i = intraocular pressure in mm Hg
P_e = episcleral venous pressure in mm Hg
C_{tm} = facility of trabecular outflow
F = aqueous flow in μL/minute (at steady state, $F = F_{in} = F_{out}$)

This equation presumes that aqueous humor outflow represents an entirely passive, bulk flow down a pressure gradient from the anterior chamber to the venous system. It further assumes that *all* outflow is trabecular. Since, under steady-state conditions, the outflow facilities relating to pseudofacility and uveoscleral drainage are very low compared to trabecular flow, and the episcleral venous pressure is relatively stable, this equation represents a reasonable approximation of events affecting intraocular pressure in vivo. With addition of a flow component for uveoscleral outflow (F_{us}) and insertion of typical values for the various parameters as illustrated by Kaufman,[71] the Goldmann equation takes on additional clinical relevance.

Assuming
$F_{in} = F_{out} = 2.5 \mu$L/minute
$C_{tm} = 0.3 \mu$L/minute/mm Hg
$P_i = 16$ mm Hg
$P_e = 9$ mm Hg
$F_{us} = 0.4 \mu$L/minute

Then

$$F_{in} = F_{out} = C_{tm} (P_i - P_e) + F_{us}$$
$$2.5 = \quad 2.5 = \quad 0.3 (16 - 9) + 0.4$$

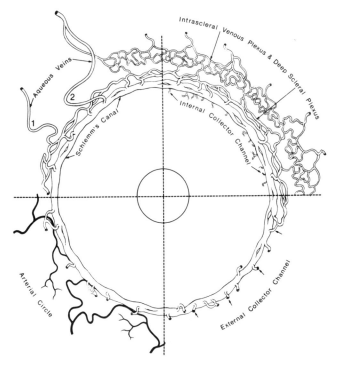

Figure 3–29. Diagrammatic representation of the distal portion of the aqueous outflow pathways from Schlemm's canal. External collector channels (*lower right*); deep and intrascleral plexi (*upper right*); aqueous veins (1 and 2) (*upper left*). *(With permission from Hogan M, Alvarado J, Weddell J. Histology of the Human Eye. Philadelphia, PA: W.B. Saunders; 1971.)*

A Role For Aqueous Humor in Aqueous Outflow Resistance. Until recently, little attention has been paid to the possibility that aqueous humor might be an active contributor to its own resistance. Interestingly, however, when aqueous humor is passed through microporous filters having pore dimensions of 0.2 μm, significantly greater resistance is produced than occurs using either saline or plasma diluted to the same protein concentration as aqueous.[72] This effect was shown to be mediated through hydrophobic interactions with the pore wall.[73] The fact that perfusion of obstructed filters with GAGases failed to relieve the obstruction, while perfusion with protease eliminated it, led to a presumption that proteins or glycoproteins were involved in the process.[72]

While the effects on nonphysiological filters described above have not been confirmed in vivo, several hydrophobic moieties (i.e., collagen and elastin) are present in the juxtacanalicular region. It may be the case that the outflow resistance in the juxtacanalicular region of the trabecular meshwork (JCT) results not simply from the nature of the extracellular matrix found here, but from the way in which these matrix components interact with constituents of the aqueous humor.

Uveoscleral Outflow

When particulate tracers such as thorotrast or fluoresceinated dextrans are perfused into primate eyes under appropriate conditions, some of the tracer can be demonstrated to enter the uvea through the tissues of the chamber angle, migrating through the interstices of the ciliary muscle to reach first the supraciliary and, finally, the suprachoroidal space (Fig. 3–30).[74,75] From the suprachoroidal space of the uvea, the aqueous passes either through the sclera or its emissaria, hence the choice of the term uveoscleral for this pathway.

Uveoscleral outflow appears to be pressure independent, representing a bulk flow rather than a diffusion-related phenomenon. The percentage of total aqueous outflow attributed to this pathway varies from species to species, but in human eyes, uveoscleral flow accounts for 10 to 20% of total outflow.[76]

Evidence of pressure independence comes directly from measurements in which uveoscleral flow rates were statistically unchanged at normal and elevated intraocular pressures.[76] One exception to this otherwise general rule was found for markedly lower intraocular pressure around 2 mm Hg. In this instance, uveoscleral outflow was demonstrated to decrease with decreasing pressure, although the mechanism remains unclear.[77]

Evidence that diffusion is not the primary driving force in uveoscleral outflow comes from several studies. It has been demonstrated that molecules having very different dimensions, and therefore presumably different diffusional characteristics, leave the anterior chamber at similar rates.[78] Furthermore, the rate of movement of macromolecular dextran from the suprachoroid to the anterior chamber is 200 times less than that in the opposite direction.[79] Clearly, if diffusion was the principal mechanism governing this movement, the rates would be essentially the same. Both of these results argue that another mechanism besides diffusion (i.e., bulk flow) underlies uveoscleral flow.

Because the uveoscleral outflow pathway involves the ciliary body, and specifically the intercellular spaces within the ciliary muscle, it should not be surprising that the state of contraction of the ciliary muscle can significantly alter the amount of uveoscleral flow. Although beneficial for trabecular flow, contraction of the ciliary muscle substantially reduces uveoscleral flow by compressing the intercellular spaces within the muscle that constitute the drainage pathway.[80]

Increasing effort is being directed at improving uveoscleral outflow as a means of reducing intraocular pressure in glaucoma. One of the most fruitful efforts has emerged from the studies of Bito[81] and others, on the ocular effects of prostaglandins (PGs). PGs are a family of compounds derived from arachidonic acid, which were examined originally for their role in mediating intraocular inflammation (cf review[81]). More recently, however, attention has been focused on certain subclasses of PGs that lower intraocular pressure. Most promising initially was prostaglandin $F_{2\alpha}$[82,83] and more recently, PGA_2, which

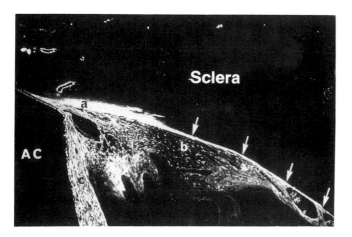

Figure 3–30. Light micrograph demonstrates the distribution of fluoresceinated dextran after intracameral perfusion into the anterior chamber (AC). The tracer has moved posteriorly into the angle tissues (a) including the ciliary muscle (b), ultimately to the supraciliary and suprachoroidal spaces (*arrows*). Tracer has also freely permeated the iris stroma (c). ($\times$38.5) *(With permission from Tripathi R, Exp Eye Res. 1977;25(suppl):305.)*

Schlemm's canal. *Invest Ophthalmol Vis Sci.* 1979;18:44.

64. Tripathi BJ, Tripathi RC. Vacuolar transcellular channels as a drainage pathway for cerebrospinal fluid. *J Physiol (Lond).* 1974;239:195.

65. Tripathi RC. The functional morphology of the outflow systems of ocular and cerebrospinal fluids. *Exp Eye Res.* 1977;25(suppl):65.

66. Gomez DG, Potts G. Effects of pressure on the arachnoid villus. *Exp Eye Res.* 1977;25(suppl);117.

67. Raviola G. Effects of paracentesis on the blood-aqueous barrier. An electron microscope study on *Macaca mulatta* using horseradish peroxidase as a tracer. *Invest Ophthalmol Vis Sci.* 1974;13:828.

68. Grierson I, Lee WR. Pressure-induced changes in the ultrastructure of the endothelium lining Schlemm's canal. *Am J Ophthalmol.* 1975;80:863.

69. Ascher KW. *The Aqueous Veins.* Springfield, IL: Charles C Thomas; 1961.

70. de Kater AW, Spurr-Michaud SJ, Gipson IK. Localization of smooth muscle myosin-containing cells in the aqueous outflow pathway. *Invest Ophthalmol Vis Sci.* 1990;31:347.

71. Kaufman PL. Pressure-dependent outflow. In: Ritch R, Shields MB, Krupin T, eds. *The Glaucomas.* Vol. 1. St. Louis, MO: C.V. Mosby; 1989:220.

72. Johnson M, Ethier CR, Kamm RD, et al. The flow of aqueous humor through microporous filters. *Invest Ophthalmol Vis Sci.* 1986;27:92.

73. Ethier CR, Kamm RD, Palaszewski BA, Johnson M, Richardson TM. Calculations of flow resistance in the juxtacanalicular meshwork. *Invest Ophthalmol Vis Sci.* 1986;27:1741.

74. Bill A. The aqueous humor drainage mechanism in the cynomolgus monkey (*Macaca irus*) with evidence for unconventional routes. *Invest Ophthalmol.* 1965;4:911.

75. Tripathi RC. Uveoscleral drainage of aqueous humor. *Exp Eye Res.* 1977;25(suppl):305.

76. Bill A. Further studies on the influence of the intraocular pressure on aqueous humor dynamics in cynomolgus monkeys. *Invest Ophthalmol.* 1967;6:364.

77. Toris CB, Pederson JE. Effect of intraocular pressure on uveoscleral outflow following cyclodialysis in the monkey eye using a fluorescent tracer. *Invest Ophthalmol Vis Sci.* 1985;26:1745.

78. Toris CB, Gregerson DS, Pederson JE. Uveoscleral outflow using different-sized fluorescent tracers in normal and inflamed eyes. *Exp Eye Res.* 1987;45:525.

79. Pederson JE, Toris CJ. Uveoscleral outflow: Diffusion or flow? *Invest Ophthalmol Vis Sci.* 1987;28:1022.

80. Bill A. Uveoscleral drainage of aqueous humor in human eyes. *Exp Eye Res.* 1971;12:275.

81. Bito LZ. Prostaglandins, other eicosanoids, and their derivatives as potential antiglaucoma agents. In: Drance SM, Neufeld AH, eds. *The Medical Treatment of Glaucomas.* New York: Grune and Stratton; 1984.

82. Giuffre G. The effects of prostaglandin $F_{2\alpha}$ in the human eye. *Graefe's Arch Clin Exp Ophthalmol.* 1985; 222:139.

83. Villumsen J, Alm A. The effect of prostaglandin $F_{2\alpha}$ eye drops in open angle glaucoma. *Invest Ophthalmol Vis Sci.* 1987;28:266.

84. Bito LZ, Baroody RA, Miranda OC. Eicosanoids as a new class of ocular hypotensive agents. 1. The apparent therapeutic advantages of derived prostaglandins of the A and B as compared with the primary prostaglandins of the E, F, and D type. *Exp Eye Res.* 1987;44:825.

85. Nilsson SFE, Stjernschantz J, Bill A. $PGF_{2\alpha}$ increases uveoscleral outflow. *Invest Ophthalmol Vis Sci.* 1987; 28(suppl):284.

86. Crawford K, Kaufman PL. Pilocarpine antagonizes prostaglandin $F_{2\alpha}$ induced ocular hypotension in monkeys. *Arch Ophthalmol.* 1987;105:1112.

Chapter 4

ANATOMY AND PHYSIOLOGY OF THE OPTIC NERVE

Thomas L. Lewis
Joan Tanabe Wing

An understanding of the normal anatomy and physiology of the optic nerve is necessary to fully comprehend the histopathological changes that occur in this tissue from abnormal levels of intraocular pressure. In addition, the clinician can better appreciate the clinical changes that appear in the optic nerve during the progression of glaucoma by having a strong foundation in the anatomy and physiology of this tissue. This chapter discusses the gross and microscopic anatomy and relevant physiology of the optic nerve, its blood supply, the process of axonal transport, and the clinical appearance and characteristics of the optic nerve and surrounding structures.

GROSS ANATOMY

The optic nerve is formed by ganglion cell axons and their accompanying glial cells. It extends from the retina through the posterior scleral foramen to the lateral geniculate body in the thalamus. The center of the optic nerve head is about 4 mm medial and 0.1 mm superior to the center of the macula. The optic nerve for descriptive purposes can be subdivided into various regions from its origin to the optic chiasm (Fig. 4–1). This chapter will concentrate on the intra-ocular and intraorbital portions since they are most important to an understanding of glaucoma.

Intraocular Portion
The anterior limit of the intraocular portion of the optic nerve is the inner limiting membrane covering the optic nerve head, while the posterior limit is the back surface of the scleral lamina cribrosa (Fig. 4–2). The intraocular portion is subdivided into the surface nerve fiber layer, the prelaminar and laminar regions. Its length can vary but it is usually about 1 mm. The width of this portion of the optic nerve often increases from anterior to posterior giving it a conical shape.

Intraorbital Portion
As the optic nerve extends beyond the posterior surface of the sclera and enters the orbit, several anatomical changes occur. The diameter of nerve doubles compared to the intraocular portion, primarily due to myelination of the ganglion cell axons, and the covering of the nerve by meningeal sheaths (Fig. 4–2). The central retinal artery and vein run along the inferior lateral aspect of the nerve and pierce the meningeal sheaths to enter the nerve about 12 mm behind the eye (Fig. 4–3).

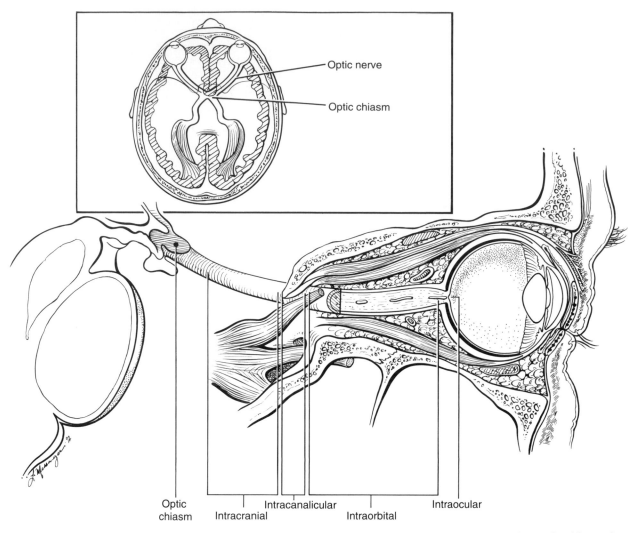

Figure 4–1. Schematic representation of the subdivisions of the optic nerve from its origin to the optic chiasm. *Inset* shows the intracranial course of the optic nerve to the lateral geniculate body.

MICROANATOMY

Intraocular Portion

Surface Nerve Fiber Layer. The nerve fiber layer of the retina is comprised of unmyelinated axons of retinal ganglion cells. It is supported by blood vessels and glial tissue that occupy about 5% of the volume of this layer.[1] The number of nerve fibers vary dramatically from individual to individual but is often estimated at about 1 million (700,000 to 1,250,000) per eye.[2–11] A possible reason for the great variability in the number of axons is the fact that, in mature adults, the number of axons results from an overproduction during the first half of gestation followed by elimina-

tion of approximately 70% of these fibers by the 16th through 30th week.[12] This type of developmental process can result in significant differences in the ultimate number of axons remaining in the adult eye.

There is debate whether or not a significant decrease in the number of axons occurs as a normal aging change. Studies have shown loss of axons ranging from approximately 500 to 5500 per year.[9–13] This becomes significant due to the fact that most people developing glaucoma are over the age of 60. If a larger number of axons are lost in the eyes of older individuals, they may be more susceptible to earlier visual field loss from glaucoma, and the differentiation of a normal from early glaucomatous nerve fiber layer and optic nerve may be more difficult.[11]

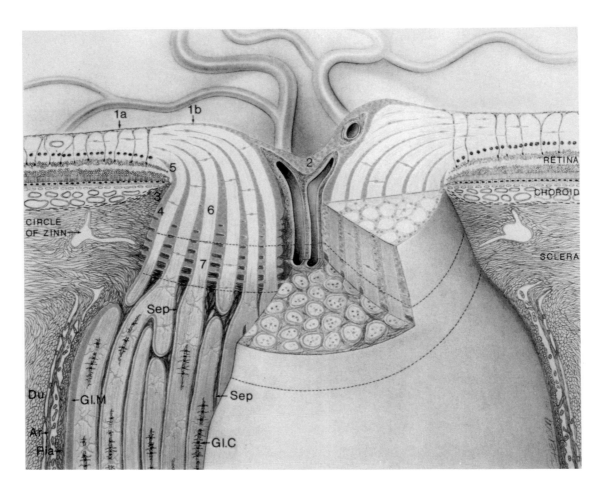

Figure 4–2. Three-dimensional drawing of the intraocular and part of the orbital optic nerve. The intraocular portion extends from the inner limiting membrane covering the optic nerve head to the back surface of the scleral lamina cribrosa. The nerve fibers of the retina (6) are separated into bundles by astrocytes. At the lamina cribrosa (upper dotted line), the nerve fascicles (7) and their surrounding astrocytes are separated from each other by the cribriform plate. At the external part of the lamina cribrosa (lower dotted line), the nerve fibers become myelinated and the diameter of the nerve doubles. Columns of oligodendrocytes (black and white cells) and a few astrocytes (red cells) can be seen within the nerve fascicles. Other cells and regions include: Muller cells (1a), internal limiting membrane of Elschnig (1b), central meniscus of Kuhnt (2), and border tissue of Elschnig (3). Astrocytes line the optic nerve canal (4) and glial tissue is found at the termination of the retina (5). Septal tissue (Sep), glial mantle (Gl.M) and the dura (Du), arachnoid (Ar) and pia mater (Pia) are shown. (*See also* Color Plate 4–2). (*Published courtesy of* Arch Ophthalmol. *1969; 82;506–530. Copyright, American Medical Association.*)

Ganglion cell axons converge on the optic nerve head in an organized pattern (Fig. 4–4). Axons from the nasal, superior, and inferior retina have a relatively straight course. Axons arising in the temporal retina arc above or below the macular region to enter the superior temporal and inferior temporal portions of the optic nerve, respectively. Axons arising in the macular region pass directly to the temporal edge of the optic nerve forming the papillomacular bundle.[14] Since the fovea is slightly inferior to the center of the optic nerve head, there are more axons entering the

temporal side of the disc inferiorly than superiorly, making the neuroretinal rim slightly thicker inferiorly.[15] The density of the axons is greatest in the papillomacular bundle; however, the greatest number of axons enter the superior and inferior poles of the optic nerve.

The ganglion cell axons arising in the temporal retina, arcing above or below the macular region, are known as arcuate nerve bundles. Ganglion cell axons, which are located in the temporal retina above an imaginary horizontal line passing through the

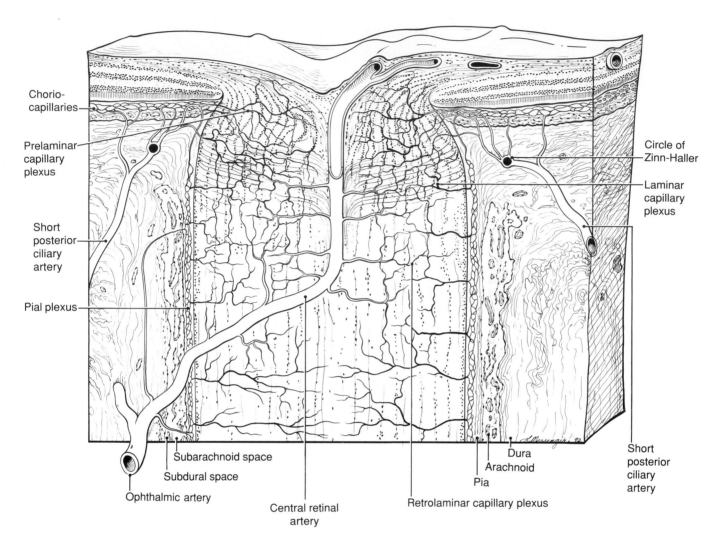

Choriocapillaries

Prelaminar capillary plexus

Short posterior ciliary artery

Pial plexus

Circle of Zinn-Haller

Laminar capillary plexus

Subarachnoid space

Subdural space

Ophthalmic artery

Central retinal artery

Dura

Arachnoid

Pia

Retrolaminar capillary plexus

Short posterior ciliary artery

Figure 4–3. Composite drawing of blood supply to the optic nerve. The central retinal artery, a branch of the ophthalmic artery, pierces the dura of the optic nerve. It sends branches to the central portion of the optic nerve and to the pial system of vessels. Transverse and longitudinal vessels emerge from the pia mater to supply the retrolaminar optic nerve. The laminar region receives its major centripetal blood supply from the circle of Zinn-Haller, which originates from the short posterior ciliary arteries. The prelaminar region is supplied by the short posterior ciliary arteries and by some centripetal branches from the peripapillary choroid. The nerve fiber layer receives its blood supply from branches of the central retinal artery and some choroidal vessels. Longitudinal capillary networks connect the laminar, prelaminar, and nerve fiber layer tissues.

macula, always enter the superior arcuate nerve fiber bundle; while axons located below this line always enter the inferior arcuate nerve fiber bundle. This creates the appearance of a horizontal raphe, temporal to the macula. This raphe is confined to temporal fibers comprising the posterior pole region of the retina and does not include fibers arising from the temporal peripheral retina. Knowledge of the pattern created by the direction of ganglion cell axons from all parts of the retina is important in understanding the

types of field defects seen in various types of retinal and optic nerve diseases, including glaucoma.

Not only is there a topographical pattern to the axons of ganglion cells but also an organization relating to their depth within the nerve fiber layer based on the original location of the ganglion cell nucleus (see Fig. 4–4). Axons from the peripheral retina tend to run deeper in the nerve fiber layer and enter the outer edge of the neuroretinal rim of the optic nerve. Axons from ganglion cells located closer to the poste-

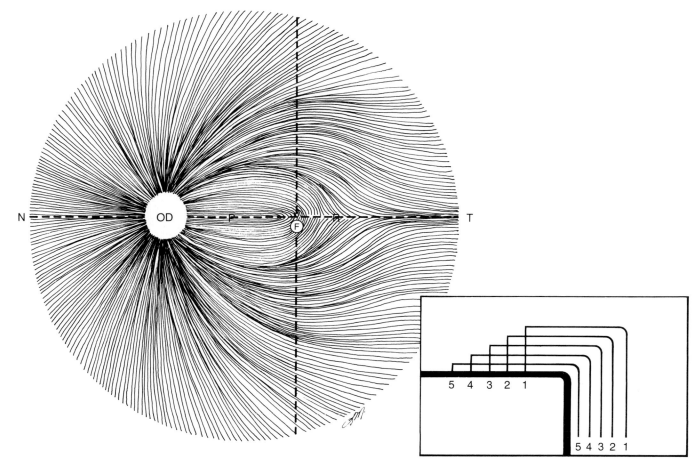

Figure 4–4. Drawing of the distribution of the retinal nerve fibers. Axons from the nasal, superior, and inferior retina have a relatively straight course. Axons arise in the temporal retina arc above or below the macular region. Axons from the macular region pass directly to the optic disc (OD) as the papillomacular bundle (P). Temporal to the fovea (F) is the horizontal raphe (R). N − nasal; T = temporal. *Inset:* Schematic drawing showing the relationship between ganglion cell axons in the retina and their position within the optic nerve. Axons from the peripheral retina run deeper in the nerve fiber layer and enter the outer edge of the neuroretinal rim. Axons originating closer to the posterior pole are more superficial in the nerve fiber layer and enter the optic nerve toward the inner edge of the neuroretinal rim. *(Adapted with permission from Hogan MJ, Alvarado JA, Weddell JE.* Histology of the Human Eye. *Philadelphia: W.B. Saunders, 1971.)*

rior pole are more superficial in the nerve fiber layer and enter the optic nerve toward the inner edge of the neuroretinal rim.[14,16,17]

Ganglion cell axons can vary in thickness but average about 1 micron.[10,11] There may be a decrease in the density of axons of the optic nerve with age,[13] possibly due to a selective loss of thicker axons.[10]

Prelaminar Region of the Optic Nerve

The prelaminar region of the optic nerve is comprised primarily of axons of ganglion cells along with their supporting glial tissue and blood vessels. It is located between the surface of the optic nerve head and the anterior border of the scleral lamina cribrosa (Fig. 4–5).

The surface of the optic nerve, next to the vitre-

ous, is covered by thin inner limiting membrane comprised of glial cells and their accompanying basement lamina (*see* Fig. 4–5). At the edge of the optic nerve, this inner limiting membrane merges with the much thicker internal limiting membrane covering the surface of the retina. The outer edge of the prelaminar portion of the optic nerve is covered by a mantle of glial cells that abut against the retina, retinal pigment epithelium, and the choroid (*see* Fig. 4–5).

As the approximately 1 million ganglion cell axons converge toward the optic nerve, they make a 90° turn to exit the eye through the posterior scleral foramen. As this turn is made, the axons become segregated into bundles or fasciculi by glial cells (Figs. 4–6 and 4–7; *see* Fig. 4–2). The exact number of fasciculi

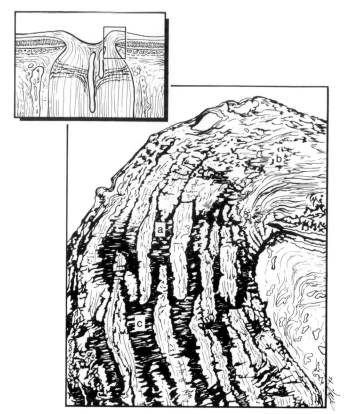

Figure 4–7. Drawing of the prelaminar portion of the optic nerve. Glial columns (a) arrange the ganglion cell axons (b) into bundles. The lamina cribrosa (c) is fenestrated to allow the nerve fiber bundles to exit the eye. *(Adapted with permission from Hogan MJ, Alvarado JA, Weddell JE.* Histology of the Human Eye. *Philadelphia: W.B. Saunders, 1971.)*

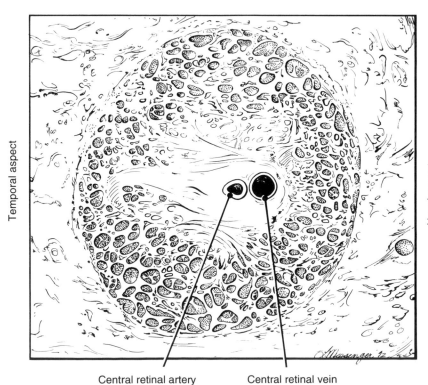

Temporal aspect

Nasal aspect

Central retinal artery   Central retinal vein

Figure 4–8. Drawing of the cross-sectional view of the lamina cribrosa shows the central retinal artery and vein. Pore size is larger in the superior and inferior region than in the nasal or temporal region.

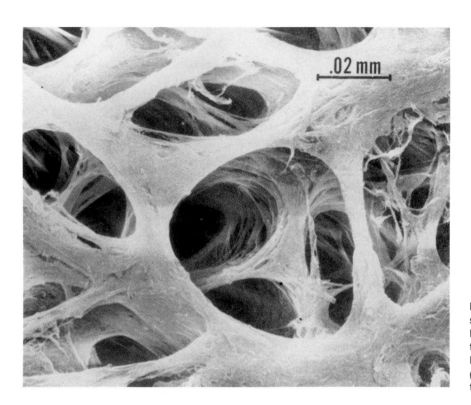

Figure 4–9. Scanning electron micrograph shows enlarged cross-sectional view of the lamina cribrosa. The lamellae of connective tissue contains fenestrations or pores to allow for the passage of nerve fiber bundles. *(Published courtesy of* Trans Am Acad Ophthalmol & Otolaryngol. *1974;78:290–297.)*

sels in the prelaminar region with a continuous endothelial cell lining with tight junctions and pericytes. The lamellae are coated on both sides with collagen, laminin, and fibrous astrocytes. The combination of elastin and collagen provides tensile strength and allows that region of the eye to resist distortion and potentially recover its original shape if compressed.[26,28]

The fenestra or pores in each lamella are lined by fibrous astrocytes. The approximately 200 to 600 pores[21] range in diameter from 10 to 250 microns (Fig. 4–9; *see* Fig. 4–8).[20,21,29] The pores are greater in number and larger in size in the lamellae located more anteriorly. Although some pores appear to branch and divide creating a labyrinth, in general, pores through which a specific bundle of ganglion cell axons pass are aligned in successive lamellae (*see* Figs. 4–8 and 4–9).

Pores in the superior and inferior poles of each lamella are larger and less supported by surrounding connective tissue than in the nasal or temporal regions[21,22] (*see* Fig. 4–8). Also, there is increased complexity of axonal channels superiorly and inferiorly. This may make these areas more susceptible to distortion from an increase in intraocular pressure.[21,23,25]

There does not appear to be a decrease in the number of pores with age. However, the proportion of the optic nerve occupied by pores does decrease with age, probably due to a loss of ganglion cell axons. The space created by a loss of axons is usually filled with connective tissue.[21,24,28]

Intraorbital (Postlaminar) Portion

Posterior to the scleral lamina cribrosa, the optic nerve leaves the eye and becomes intraorbital. The axons of the ganglion cells become myelineated, and meningeal sheaths cover the surface of the optic nerve (*see* Fig. 4–2). At the optic foramen, the meninges are continuous with the intracranial meningeal covering of the nerve. Anteriorly, the connective tissue components of the meninges blend with the outer layers of the sclera.

The outer meningeal coat, the dura mater, is composed of dense connective tissue and fibroblasts, with mesothelial cells (meningothelium) lining its inner surface (Fig. 4–10). Collagen and elastic tissue is prominent in the dura mater.[30] Beneath the dura is a potential subdural space separating the dura mater from the arachnoid (*see* Fig. 4–10).[30]

The arachnoid consists of several layers of meningothelial cells and a network of collagen bundles and some elastic fibers. The subarachnoid space is located between the inner surface of the arachnoid and the outer surface of the pia mater (*see* Fig. 4–10). Within the subarachnoid space is cerebrospinal fluid and trabeculae or columns of collagen that connect

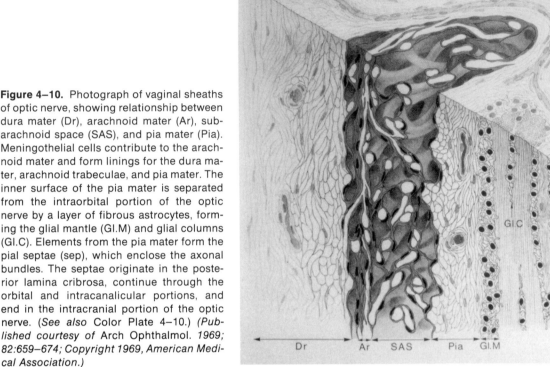

Figure 4–10. Photograph of vaginal sheaths of optic nerve, showing relationship between dura mater (Dr), arachnoid mater (Ar), subarachnoid space (SAS), and pia mater (Pia). Meningothelial cells contribute to the arachnoid mater and form linings for the dura mater, arachnoid trabeculae, and pia mater. The inner surface of the pia mater is separated from the intraorbital portion of the optic nerve by a layer of fibrous astrocytes, forming the glial mantle (Gl.M) and glial columns (Gl.C). Elements from the pia mater form the pial septae (sep), which enclose the axonal bundles. The septae originate in the posterior lamina cribrosa, continue through the orbital and intracanalicular portions, and end in the intracranial portion of the optic nerve. (*See also* Color Plate 4–10.) *(Published courtesy of* Arch Ophthalmol. *1969; 82:659–674; Copyright 1969, American Medical Association.)*

the pia mater to the arachnoid. These trabeculae contain blood vessels and are covered by meningothelium. In fact, the entire subarachnoid space is lined by meningothelial cells (Fig. 4–10).[30]

The innermost component of the meninges is the pia mater. It is mostly connective tissue with some elastic fibers, lined on its outer surface by meningothelium (*see* Fig. 4–10). The pia mater is highly vascularized containing capillaries with continuous, nonfenestrated endothelial cells. The inner surface of the pia mater is separated from the intraorbital portion of the optic nerve by a layer of fibrous astrocytes (*see* Fig. 4–10).

From the under surface of the pia mater, connective tissue extends inward to form longitudinal septa, which additionally separate ganglion cell axons into bundles (*see* Fig. 4–2). Each bundle is still surrounded by fibrous astrocytes as was true in the prelaminar and laminar regions (*see* Fig. 4–10). The pial septa, in addition to separating the nerve fiber bundles, also provide a pathway for vessels and nerves into the substance of the intraorbital portion of the optic nerve (*see* Figs. 4–2 and 4–10). The septa are attached to the

pia mater, to the connective tissue that surrounds the central retinal vessels located centrally within the optic nerve, and to the posterior surface of the scleral lamina cribrosa.

Meningothelial cells, which are so prominent within the meninges, resemble fibroblasts in their structure and function and are held together at many locations by desmosomes and some tight junctions.[30] A second type of glial cell, oligodendroglia, is also found in the intraorbital portion of the optic nerve and is responsible for the formation of myelin.

BLOOD SUPPLY

An understanding of the blood supply to the optic nerve is extremely important due to the fact that ischemia from vascular insufficiency is considered a likely contributing factor to the damage occurring from glaucoma.[23,31,32]

Tremendous interindividual variation exists in the blood supply to each specific portion of the optic nerve.[31,32] Not even the eyes of the same patient have similar vascular patterns. Therefore, it is difficult to draw precise conclusions regarding the anatomical pattern and the subsequent physiological impact that might occur from compression of a specific vessel in a given individual.

The blood supply to the optic nerve comes from one to five posterior ciliary arteries and the central retinal artery that arise from the ophthalmic artery (*see* Fig. 4–3). Usually, there are two to three posterior ciliary arteries distributed on the medial or lateral side of the optic nerve. The posterior ciliary arteries form both long and short posterior ciliary arteries. Each posterior ciliary artery is an end-artery system, supplying a specific territory of tissue with no anastomoses between vessels.[32,33] A watershed area is thus created at the outer edges of the territory supplied by adjacent posterior ciliary arteries and their major branches (Fig. 4–11). The watershed region for an individual with a medial and lateral posterior ciliary artery may be found anywhere between the nasal edge of the optic nerve and the fovea (*see* Fig. 4–11).[32,33] This individual variation may influence the relative susceptibility of the optic nerve to potential damage from an increase in intraocular pressure.

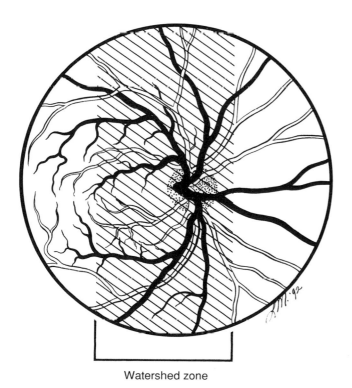

Watershed zone

Figure 4–11. Drawing of the vasculature of the posterior pole. The shaded region represents the potential water-shed area for an individual with a medial and lateral posterior ciliary artery.

Nerve Fiber Layer

The nerve fiber layer is supplied by branches of the central retinal artery (*see* Fig. 4–3) with venous drainage into the central retinal vein. There is a continuous capillary network from the level of the surface nerve fiber layer back through the postlaminar region of the optic nerve (*see* Fig. 4–3). Capillaries on the surface of the optic nerve are also continuous with those in the peripapillary retina.[34,35] Some choroidal vessels may contribute to the blood supply of the nerve fiber layer especially on the temporal side of the optic nerve head (*see* Fig. 4–3). If these are large in diameter, a cilioretinal vessel becomes apparent.[31]

Prelaminar

The prelaminar portion of the optic nerve receives its blood supply from centripetal branches from the peripapillary choroid (*see* Fig. 4–3). These branches arise from short posterior ciliary arteries and have a segmental (sectoral) distribution.[31] No anastomoses exist between vessels supplying the optic nerve and the choriocapillaris at this level. Longitudinal capillary networks connect the laminar, prelaminar, and nerve fiber layer tissues[35] (*see* Fig. 4–3). The temporal portion of the prelaminar region may be more vascularized than other areas.[31] Capillaries from the prelaminar region drain into the central retinal vein or through the choroid into vortex veins.

Laminar

The laminar region contains both a centripetal (transverse) system of vessels located within the lamellae and a longitudinal system of capillaries interconnecting the various regions of the optic nerve[31,35,36] (*see* Fig. 4–3). Although some centripetal vessels arise from pia mater arterioles, the major centripetal supply is from the circle of Zinn-Haller (*see* Figs. 4–2 and 4–3). This vascular complex is formed by an anastomosis within the sclera just outside the optic nerve of branches of adjacent short posterior ciliary arteries. In most individuals, this vascular circle is incomplete.

The central retinal artery does not contribute appreciably to the blood supply in the prelaminar or laminar regions. The venous drainage of the lamina cribrosa is primarily into the central retinal vein.

Intraorbital (Postlaminar)

Blood supply to the postlaminar region is more complex than in other portions of the optic nerve (*see* Fig. 4–3). It consists of one network of vessels supplying the periphery of the nerve and another supplying the central or axial portion.[35] The peripheral portion is supplied by branches from the pia mater vascular plexus. This plexus is formed by branches from muscular arteries, the ophthalmic artery, and recurrent branches from the peripapillary choroid and the circle of Zinn-Haller (*see* Fig. 4–3). These vessels enter the substance of the optic nerve through the pial septa. They anastomose freely within this portion of the optic nerve and extend forward as a continuous capillary network to more anterior regions of the optic nerve.

The central retinal artery contributes small branches to the central or axial portion of the postlaminar region of the optic nerve (*see* Fig. 4–3). Venous drainage from the postlaminar region is into the central retinal vein.

In summary, there are both centripetal (transverse) and longitudinal blood vessel systems in all portions of the optic nerve. Short posterior ciliary arteries contribute to some extent to the blood supply of all portions of the optic nerve, whereas the branches of the central retinal arteries supply only the nerve fiber layer and the axial portion of the postlaminar region. The longitudinal system of blood supply is continuous from the postlaminar region through to the nerve fiber layer.

PHYSIOLOGY OF THE OPTIC NERVE

Axonal Transport

An increase in intraocular pressure can ultimately damage the axons of the ganglion cells leading to clinically visible changes in the optic nerve and surrounding nerve fiber layer of the retina. As will be discussed in Chapter 5 on the pathology of glaucoma, damage to ganglion cell axons appears to occur at the level of the scleral lamina cribrosa by a blockage of axonal transport.[1,21,23] Therefore, in order to better understand glaucoma, the concept of axonal transport must be discussed.

Cells throughout the body must be able to transport material within their cytoplasm to all areas of the cell. This becomes especially important in cells, such as nerve cells, with long cytoplasmic extensions. The axon of a neuron is the cytoplasmic extension from the cell body that usually transmits impulses through synapses to other neurons or effector tissues (Fig. 4–12). Axons of neurons can be extremely long considering the fact that nerve cells located in the lumbar region of the spine send axons down as far as the foot. The difficulty in moving intracellular material along the axon is that the axonal extension does not contain many of the organelles found within the cytoplasm of the cell body. Axons of neurons, including those of the ganglion cell of the retina, contain only mitochondria, smooth endoplasmic reticulum, fine

filaments (6 to 7 nm), and microtubules (20 to 25 nm) (*see* Fig. 4–12).[14,19] Consequently, intracellular substances and material, which are necessary to sustain the axon and to supply the synapse of the axon, must be transported from the manufacturing source in the cell body down the axon to the synaptic junction. Conversely, byproducts of metabolism from the axon must be transported back to the nerve cell body for digestion and, in some cases, removal from the nerve cell.

The process of moving material back and forth is known as axonal transport. It is an energy-dependent process that is essential for the survival of the axon and, therefore, of the nerve cell. Material moving from the nerve cell to the synaptic end of the axon is considered axonal transport in an anterograde (orthograde) direction. Anterograde axonal transport can occur slow (0.5 to 3 mm per day)[37] or fast (200 to 1000 mm per day).[38] Slow anterograde axonal transport is believed to occur through peristaltic action of the axon cell membrane. It primarily serves the function of maintenance and assisting in growth of the axon. Fast anterograde axonal transport uses the microtubular elements within the axon as "railroad tracks" to move material from the cell body to supply the synaptic end.

Retrograde axonal transport moves material from the synapse back to the cell body at a rate of approximately 50 to 250 mm per day.[38] It also uses microtubules as a conduit.

Clearly, microtubules play an essential role in both orthograde and retrograde axonal transport. Compression of an axon resulting in a crushing, distortion, or bending of the microtubules could result in the blockage of axonal transport and ultimately death of the nerve cell. Since axonal transport is an energy-dependent process, an adequate supply of oxygen is also essential to maintain the transport systems. A reduction in blood supply to the nerve cell or any portion of the axon, to a level that results in ischemia, could also block axonal transport and lead to death of the nerve cell.

Therefore, blockage of axonal transport can occur through mechanical compression of the axon disrupting the microtubules or by a reduction in blood supply, which reduces the energy source necessary to maintain these transport systems. Glaucoma, ocular hypotony, and papilledema are some examples of ocular conditions that may have the blockage of axonal transport as their pathophysiological basis.

Ganglion Cell Types

There is an increasing use of electrodiagnostic testing including contrast sensitivity, pattern electroretino-

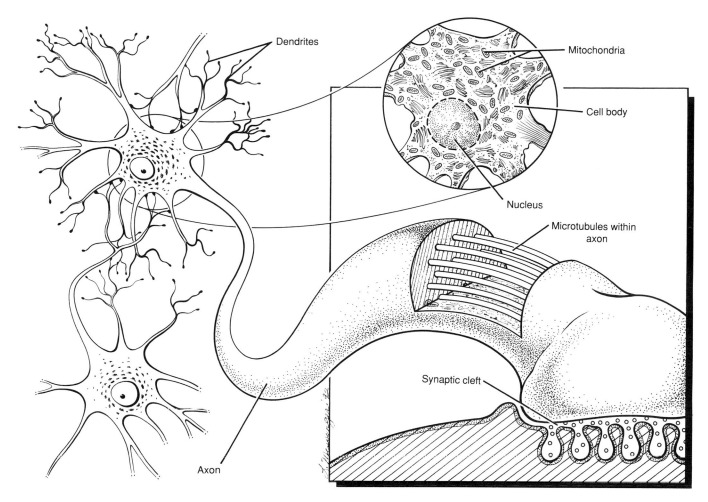

Figure 4–12. Schematic drawing showing the main components of a neuron. Axons contain microtubules and can synapse with effector tissues or other neurons. *Inset* shows the cell body of the neuron with its mitochondria and nucleus.

gram, and visual evoked potentials for the early diagnosis of glaucoma. To understand the psychophysical changes observed in glaucoma, it is necessary to appreciate how the visual system functions.

Retinal ganglion cells can be categorized into a variety of classes based on anatomical, physiological, or psychophysical criteria (Table 4–1). The different functional properties of these classes of ganglion cells are preserved throughout the visual pathway from the retina to the primary visual cortex and extrastriate regions. Although there is probably some overlap in functional characteristics and a mixing of the pathways at higher visual centers, parallel pathways do exist for visual processing.

P System. The P-ganglion cells comprise 80%[39] of the ganglion cells of the retina and are concentrated primarily in the fovea.[40] They are small in size, becoming larger toward the periphery of the retina.[41]

These cells project to the parvocellular layers (3, 4, 5, 6) of the dorsal lateral geniculate nucleus (dLGN).[42] Through thinly myelinated axons, the parvocellular layers of the dLGN project primarily to layer 4C beta of the visual cortex and on to layers II and III.[41,42] From here, connections are made with a variety of areas including the caudal portion of the inferior temporal cortex.

M System. The M-ganglion cells comprise 10% of the ganglion cells and are distributed evenly through the retina.[41] They have large cell bodies and axons, also increasing in size toward the periphery of the retina. These cells project to the magnocellular layers (1, 2) of the dLGN.[42] The magnocellular layers project through thickly myelinated axons primarily to layer 4C alpha and on to area 3 of the visual cortex.[41,42] From here, connections are made to a variety of extrastriate areas including the posterior parietal cortex.

to-disc ratio was 0.28 ± 0.17.[62] In a study of 475 normal eyes, Jonas and associates[53] found the mean horizontal cup-to-disc ratio to be 0.39 ± 0.28 and the mean vertical cup-to-disc ratio to be 0.34 ± 0.25. The clinician must know the size of the optic disc to evaluate properly the cup-to-disc ratio or neural rim area.[59]

The size of the cup area may be larger in blacks[57] and also in males.[61,62] There is debate whether or not the cup size changes with age[53,61,63–66] and also whether it is greater in high myopic patients.[53,64,65,67,68]

Peripapillary Tissue

The optic disc may be surrounded by peripapillary crescents or by hypopigmentation or hyperpigmentation. Crescents represent a misalignment of the edges of the neuroretina, retinal pigment epithelium, choroid, or sclera adjacent to the optic disc. Such misalignments occur developmentally or might be due to ocular stretching as in high myopia. Irregular pigment next to the optic disc may be caused by a lack of pigment or by hyperpigmentation of the retinal pigment epithelial cells. Hyperpigmentation may also be due to a double layer of retinal pigment epithelial cells.

Peripapillary crescents can change with time from aging processes in the retinal pigment epithelium, retinal diseases, or from acquired atrophy of the choroid or retinal pigment epithelium. In glaucoma, there may be changes in the peripapillary tissue such as marked atrophy of the retinal pigment epithelium and marked thinning of the chorioretinal tissue.[69–71]

Nerve Fiber Layer

The retinal nerve fiber layer is best observed clinically by using red-free light. The brightness of the red-free light reflected off the nerve fiber is directly proportional to the thickness of the layer. The nerve fiber layer adjacent to the optic nerve head is relatively thicker superiorly and inferiorly by as much as 150 to 200 microns compared to nasally and temporally.[72]

When observing the nerve fiber layer in the retina within two disc diameters of the optic disc, it will appear brightest and most visible in the inferior arcuate arcade, followed by the superior arcuate arcade, papillomacular bundle, and, finally, the nasal side of the optic nerve head.[73] There does not seem to be any difference normally between the appearance of the nerve fiber layer in the eyes of the same individual, nor a gender difference.[73]

Changes in the brightness of the nerve fiber layer adjacent to the optic disc may be one of the earliest signs of glaucomatous damage. As axons of the ganglion cells of the retina are destroyed in glaucoma, the nerve fiber layer thins and becomes less bright.

Large Discs

Large optic discs are defined clinically as those having an optic cup area greater than 2.1 mm².[53] Large discs tend to be associated with large neuroretinal rim areas and large cup areas. Physiological cupping greater than 0.6 was found in 91% of individuals with large optic discs but in only 25% of individuals with average or small discs.[74] Since the optic disc area, neuroretinal rim area, and optic cup area do not change proportionately, there is no constant ratio between these three clinical variables.

One of the greatest clinical challenges in glaucoma is the differential diagnosis of a large physiological cup from an optic disc that has acquired a large cup due to damage from glaucoma. In a comparison of normal-sized optic cups, large physiological cups and glaucomatous optic discs, Jonas and his colleagues[71] found that individuals with large physiological cups had large slightly vertical discs, normal neuroretinal rim area and configuration, a normal nerve fiber layer, no peripapillary chorioretinal atrophy, and slightly horizontal cups with a mean horizontal cup-to-disc ratio of 0.78. The glaucomatous group had a normal-sized disc area, a decreased neuroretinal rim area, an abnormal rim configuration (narrowing of the inferior and superior neuroretinal rim), defects in the retinal nerve fiber layer, a vertically oval optic cup, and a significant variation in the size of the cup-to-disc ratio.[71]

CONCLUSION

An understanding of the anatomy and physiology of the optic nerve helps to explain the clinical appearance of this tissue as well as the histopathological and clinical changes in this tissue in glaucoma. This allows the clinician to make an accurate and early differential diagnosis of the disease.

REFERENCES

1. Quigley HA. Early detection of glaucomatous damage. II. Changes in the appearance of the optic disc. *Surv Ophthalmol.* 1985;30:111–126.
2. Arey LB, Schaible AJ. The nerve-fiber composition of the optic nerve. *Anat Rec.* 1934;58(suppl):3.
3. Arey LB, Bickel WH. The number of nerve fibers in human optic nerve. *Anat Rec.* 1935;61(suppl):3.
4. Bruesch SR, Arey LB. An enumeration of myelinated and unmyelinated fibers in the optic nerve of vertebrates. *Anat Rec.* 1940;76(suppl):10.
5. Bruesch SR, Arey LB. The number of myelinated and unmyelinated fibers in the optic nerve of vertebrates. *J Comp Neurol.* 1942;77:631–65.

6. Kupfer C, Chumbley L, Downer JC. Quantitative histology of optic nerve, optic tract and lateral geniculate nucleus of man. *J Anat.* 1967:101:393–401.

7. Potts AM, Hodges D, Shelman CB, et al. Morphology of the primate optic nerve. I. Method and total fiber count. *Invest Ophthalmol.* 1972;11:980–988.

8. Quigley HA, Addicks EM, Green WR. Optic nerve damage in human glaucoma. III. Quantitative correlation of nerve fiber loss and visual field defect in glaucoma, ischemic neuropathy, papilledema and toxic neuropathy. *Arch Ophthalmol.* 1982;100:135–146.

9. Balazsi AG, Rootman J, Drance SM, et al. The effect of age on the nerve fiber population of the human optic nerve. *Am J Ophthalmol.* 1984;97:760–766.

10. Repka MX, Quigley HA. The effect of age on normal human optic nerve fiber number and diameter. *Ophthalmology.* 1989;96:26–32.

11. Jonas JB, Muller-Bergh JA, Schlotzer-Schrehardt UM, et al. Histomorphometry of the human optic nerve. *Invest Ophthalmol Vis Sci.* 1990;31:736–744.

12. Provis JM, van Driel D, Billson FA, et al. Human fetal optic nerve: Overproduction and elimination of retinal axons during development. *J Comp Neurol.* 1985;238: 92–100.

13. Dolman CL, McCormick AQ, Drance SM. Aging of the optic nerve. *Arch Ophthalmol.* 1980;98:2053–2058.

14. Hogan MJ, Alvarado JA, Weddell JE. Histology of the human eye. Philadelphia: W.B. Saunders; 1971:523–606.

15. Jonas JB, Nguyen NX, Naumann GOH. The retinal nerve fiber layer in normal eyes. *Ophthalmology.* 1989;96:627–632.

16. Radius RL, Anderson DR. The course of axons through the retina and optic nerve head. *Arch Ophthalmol.* 1979;97:1154–1158.

17. Minkler DS. The organization of nerve fiber bundles in the primate optic nerve head. *Arch Ophthalmol.* 1980;98:1630–1636.

18. Anderson DR. Ultrastructure of human and monkey lamina cribrosa and optic nerve head. *Arch Ophthalmol.* 1969;82:800–814.

19. Anderson DR, Hoyt WF. Ultrastructure of intraorbital portion of human and monkey optic nerve. *Arch Ophthalmol.* 1969;82:506–530.

20. Emery JM, Landis D, Paton D, et al. The lamina cribrosa in normal and glaucomatous human eyes. *Trans Am Acad Ophthalmol Otol.* 1974;78:OP-290–297.

21. Quigley HA, Addicks EM. Regional differences in the structure of the lamina cribrosa and their relation to glaucomatous optic nerve damage. *Arch Ophthalmol.* 1981;99:137–143.

22. Radius RL. Regional specificity in anatomy at the lamina cribrosa. *Arch Ophthalmol.* 1981;99:478–480.

23. Radius RL. Anatomy of the optic nerve head and glaucomatous optic neuropathy. *Surv Ophthalmol.* 1987;32: 35–44.

24. Ogden TE, Duggan J, Danley K, et al. Morphometry of nerve fiber bundle pores in the optic nerve head of the human. *Exp Eye Res.* 1988;46:559–568.

25. Jonas JB, Mardin CY, Schlotzer-Schrehardt U, et al. Morphometry of the human lamina cribrosa surface. *Ophthalmol Vis Sci.* 1991;32:401–405.

26. Hernandez MR, Luo XX, Igoe BS, et al. Extracellular matrix of the human lamina cribrosa. *Am J Ophthalmol.* 1987;104:567–576.

27. Tamura Y, Konomi H, Sawada H, et al. Tissue distribution of type VIII collagen in human adult and fetal eyes. *Invest Ophthalmol Vis Sci.* 1991;32:2636–2644.

28. Hernandez MR, Luo XX, Andrzejewska W, et al. Age-related changes in the extracellular matrix of the human optic nerve head. *Am J Ophthalmol.* 1989;107:476–484.

29. Elkington Ar, Inman CBE, Steart PV, et al. The structure of the lamina cribrosa of the human eye: An immunochemical and electron microscopical study. *Eye.* 1990;4:42–57.

30. Anderson DR. Ultrastructure of meningeal sheaths: Normal human and monkey optic nerves. *Arch Ophthalmol.* 1969;82:659–674.

31. Hayreh SS. Anatomy and physiology of the optic nerve head. *Trans Am Acad Ophthalmol Otol.* 1974;78:240–251.

32. Hayreh SS. Interindividual variation in blood supply of the optic nerve head. *Doc Ophthalmol.* 1985;59:217–246.

33. Hayreh SS. Segmental nature of the choroidal vasculature. *Br J Ophthalmol.* 1975;59:631–648.

34. Anderson DR, Braverman S. Reevaluation of the optic disk vasculature. *Am J Ophthalmol.* 1976;82:165–174.

35. Lieberman MF, Maumenee AE, Green WR. Histologic studies of the vasculature of the anterior optic nerve. *Am J Ophthalmol.* 1976;82:405–423.

36. Fryczkowski AW, Grimson BS, Peiffer Jr RL. Scanning electron microscopy of vascular casts of the human scleral lamina cribrosa. *Intern Ophthalmol.* 1984;7:95–100.

37. Griffin JW, Watson DF. Axonal transport in neurological disease. *Ann Neurol.* 1988;23:3–13.

38. Yanoff M, Fine BS. *Ocular Pathology.* Philadelphia: J.B. Lippincott; 1989:486.

39. Perry VH, Oehler R, Cowley A. Retinal ganglion cells that project to the dorsal lateral geniculate nucleus in the macaque monkey. *Neuroscience.* 1984;12:1101–1123.

40. DeMonasterio FM. Properties of concentrically organized X- and Y-ganglion cells of the macaque retina. *J Neurophysiol.* 1978;41:1435–1449.

41. Bassi CJ, Lehmkuhle S. Clinical implications of parallel visual pathways. *J Am Optom Assoc.* 1990;61:98–110.

42. Kulikowski JJ. Terminology of P and M pathways. In: *Seeing Contour and Colour.* Proceedings of the third international symposium of the Northern Eye Institute. Oxford: Pergamon Press; 1989:11–17.

43. Kaplan E. The role of P and M systems: (A) Introductory remarks. In: *Seeing Contour and Color.* Proceedings of the third international symposium of the Northern Eye Institute. Oxford: Pergamon Press; 1989:224–227.

44. Hubel DH, Livingstone MS. Segregation of form, colour, movement and depth processing: Anatomy and physiology. In: *Seeing Contour and Colour.* Proceedings of the third international symposium of the Northern Eye Institute. Oxford: Pergamon Press; 1989:116–119.

45. Kulikowski JJ. The role of P and M systems: (C) Psy-

chophysical aspects. In: *Seeing Contour and Colour*. Proceedings of the third international symposium of the Northern Eye Institute. Oxford: Pergamon Press; 1989:232–237.

46. Merigan WH. Assessing the role of parallel pathways in primates. In: *Seeing Contour and Colour*. Proceedings of the third international symposium of the Northern Eye Institute. Oxford: Pergamon Press; 1989:198–206.

47. Glovinsky Y, Quigley HA, Dunkelberger GR. Retinal ganglion cell loss is size dependent in experimental glaucoma. *Invest Ophthalmol Vis Sci*. 1991;32:484–491.

48. Quigley HA, Sanchez RM, Dunkelberger GR, et al. Chronic glaucoma selectively damages large optic nerve fibers. *Invest Ophthalmol Vis Sci*. 1987;28:913–920.

49. Johnson MA, Drum BA, Quigley HA, et al. Pattern-evoked potentials and optic nerve fiber loss in monocular laser-induced glaucomatous primate eyes. *Invest Ophthalmol Vis Sci*. 1989;30:897–907.

50. Marx MS, Podos SM, Bodis-Wollner I, et al. Flash and pattern electroretinograms in normal and laser-induced glaucomatous primate eyes. *Invest Ophthalmol Vis Sci*. 1989;27:378–386.

51. Airaksinen PJ, Lakowski R, Drance SM, et al. Color vision and retinal nerve fiber layer in early glaucoma. *Am J Ophthalmol*. 1986;101:208–213.

52. Jonas JB, Gusek GC, Guggenmoos-Holzmann I, et al. Size of the optic nerve scleral canal and comparison with intravital determination of optic disc dimensions. *Graefe's Arch Clin Exp Ophthalmol*. 1988;226:213–215.

53. Jonas JB, Gusek GC, Naumann GOH. Optic disc, cup and neuroretinal rim size, configuration and correlations in normal eyes. *Invest Ophthalmol Vis Sci*. 1988;29:1151–1158.

54. Jonas JB, Gusek GC, Guggenmoos-Holzmann I, et al. Variability of the real dimensions of normal human optic discs. *Graefe's Arch Clin Exp Ophthalmol*. 1988; 226:332–336.

55. Britton RJ, Drance SM, Schulzer M, et al. The area of the neuroretinal rim of the optic nerve in normal eyes. *Am J Ophthalmol*. 1987;103:497–504.

56. Caprioli J, Miller JM. Optic disc rim area is related to disc size in normal subjects. *Arch Ophthalmol*. 1987; 105;1683–1685.

57. Quigley HA, Brown AE, Morrison JD, et al. The size and shape of the optic disc in normal human eyes. *Arch Ophthalmol*. 1990;108:51–57.

58. Jonas JB, Fernandez MC, Naumann GOH. Correlation of the optic disc size to glaucoma susceptibility. *Ophthalmology*. 1991;98:675–680.

59. Quigley HA, Coleman AL, Dorman-Pease ME. Larger optic nerve heads have more nerve fibers in normal eyes. *Arch Ophthalmol*. 1991;109:1441–1443.

60. Bengtsson B. The variation and covariation of cup and disc diameters. *Acta Ophthalmol (Copenh)*. 1976;54:804–818.

61. Carpel EF, Engstrom PF. The normal cup-disc ratio. *Am J Ophthalmol*. 1981;91:588–597.

62. Liebowitz HM, Krueger DE, Maunder LR, et al. The Framingham Eye Study monograph. *Surv Ophthalmol*. 1980;24(suppl):335–610.

63. Pickard R. The alteration in size of the normal optic disc cup. *Br. J Opthalmol*. 1948;32:355–361.

64. Ford M, Sarwar M. Features of a clinically normal optic disc. *Br J Ophthalmol*. 1963;47:50–52.

65. Snydacker D. The normal optic disc: Ophthalmoscopic and photographic studies. *Am J Ophthalmol*. 1964;58: 958–964.

66. Schwartz JT, Reuling FH, Garrison RJ. Acquired cupping of the optic nervehead in normotensive eyes. *Br J Ophthalmol*. 1975;59:216–222.

67. Colenbrander MC. Measurement of the excavation. *Ophthalmologica*. 1960;139:491–493.

68. Perkins ES, Phelps CD. Open angle glaucoma, ocular hypertension, low-tension glaucoma, and refraction. *Arch Ophthalmol*. 1982;100:1464–1467.

69. Fantes FE, Anderson DR. Clinical histologic correlation of human peripapillary anatomy. *Ophthalmology*. 1989;96:20–25.

70. Jonas JB, Fernandez MC, Naumann GOH. Glaucomatous optic nerve atrophy in small discs with low cup-to-disc ratios. *Ophthalmology*. 1990;97:1211–1215.

71. Jonas JB, Zach FM, Gusek G, et al. Pseudoglaucomatous physiologic large cups. *Am J Ophthalmol*. 1989; 107:137–144.

72. Caprioli J. The contour of the juxtapapillary nerve fiber layer in glaucoma. *Ophthalmology*. 1990;97:358–366.

73. Jonas JB, Nguyen NX, Naumann GOH. The retinal nerve fiber layer in normal eyes. *Ophthalmology*. 1989;96:627–632.

74. Maisel JM, Pearlstein CS, Adams WH, et al. Large optic disks in the Marshallese population. *Am J Ophthalmol*. 1989;107:145–150.

Chapter 5

ETIOLOGY AND PATHOPHYSIOLOGY OF PRIMARY OPEN-ANGLE GLAUCOMA

Thomas L. Lewis
Connie L. Chronister

Understanding the causes for the increase in intraocular pressure and the damage to the optic nerve that occurs in glaucomas improves the ability to properly diagnose and treat these diseases. Unfortunately, definitive explanations of the etiology and histopathology of glaucoma are still not available. This chapter summarizes current research and clinical data and reviews the theories being proposed to explain the disease.

THE CAUSES OF ELEVATED INTRAOCULAR PRESSURE

With age, there is a progressive increase in the resistance to the outflow of aqueous humor along with a concurrent decrease in aqueous production. This can result in a slight increase in intraocular pressure. In a few individuals, an imbalance is created between the increased resistance to outflow and the decrease in aqueous production, resulting in a more significant rise in intraocular pressure. Of these individuals, those with susceptible optic nerves will develop an optic neuropathy from the elevated intraocular pressure, resulting in glaucoma.

In primary open-angle glaucoma, there is no apparent systemic or secondary condition contributing to the decrease in aqueous outflow. Although the exact etiology of the decreased outflow is not known, the most likely causes involve biochemical or histological changes in both the conventional outflow pathway (i.e., Schlemm's canal) and the uveoscleral pathway.[1–22]

The most direct method of uncovering the etiology of the glaucomatous changes in the anterior segment of the eye would be by comparing histological specimens from normal eyes with those from glaucomatous eyes of similar age.[2,4,5–9] Studies of tissue from glaucomatous eyes are hampered by changes that may result from treatment with drugs, lasers, or surgery, rather than from the disease itself. Furthermore, most available specimens reflect late rather than early stages of the disease. Attempts to overcome these problems have led to the use of animal models, cell culture, organ culture, and model systems. Human trabecular meshwork tissue has been grown in cell culture and organ culture and used as monolayer filters to create research models.[1,3,25–28]

The results of ultrastructural and biochemical studies of both normal and glaucomatous human tissue have led to the conclusion that many, if not all, of the pathological features associated with glaucoma

TABLE 5–1. ANTERIOR CHAMBER CHANGES SEEN WITH AGING AND PRIMARY OPEN-ANGLE GLAUCOMA

Loss of trabecular endothelial cells

Pigment accumulation within trabecular endothelial cells

Thickening of trabecular lamellae

Fusion of trabecular lamellae

Thickening of scleral spur

Increase in extracellular (plaque) material in juxtacanalicular zone

Decrease in giant vacuoles along inner wall of Schlemm's canal

are really exaggerated and accelerated changes that occur with age in all eyes[2,22,25,29] (Table 5–1). Therefore, in discussing the etiology of primary open-angle glaucoma, it makes more sense to first describe the normal aging changes in the anterior chamber angle. A detailed explanation of the normal anatomy of the anterior chamber is found in Chapter 3.

NORMAL AGING CHANGES

1. *A loss of trabecular endothelial cells.* In 1984, Alvarado and colleagues demonstrated that trabecular cellularity decreases rapidly during the first 2 years of life and continues to decline at a slower, linear rate for the next 98 years.[2] Between ages 20 and 80, there is an approximate 350,000 cell (47%) loss.[2] The loss of endothelial cells from the trabecular lamellae is greatest posteriorly and in the uveal meshwork and least in the juxtacanalicular zone.[2,22] This cell loss and the associated enlargement of remaining cells on the trabeculae is similar to the aging changes occurring in the corneal endothelium.[2,30]

    The continuous loss of endothelial cells is accompanied by an increase in abnormal lattice (curly) collagen within the trabeculae and by swelling and lamellation of the basement membrane.[13,22]

2. *An increase in pigmentation accumulation within the endothelial cells of the trabecular meshwork.* At age 20, approximately 3% of the cells covering the trabeculae contain melanin within their cytoplasm.[22] By age 80, 18% of the cells contain melanin.[22] The source of the melanin is most likely from the pigmented epithelia cells of the ciliary body and iris.[22]

3. *Thickening of the trabecular lamellae.* There is a 30% increase in the thickness of the trabeculae from ages 20 to 80.[22] This occurs primarily from an accumulation of material in the base-

ment membrane of the endothelial cells and also the addition of extracellular material within the core of the trabecular beam.[22] It is possible that this thickening is a result of loss of the endothelial cell covering.[22]

4. *Fusion of trabecular lamellae.* This most likely is a result of endothelial cell loss.[22,25]

5. *Thickening of the scleral spur.* This occurs as a result of hyalinization and/or atrophy of the ciliary muscle along with collapse and condensation of the uveal trabecular meshwork.[16,29]

6. *Increase in extracellular (plaque) material in the juxtacanalicular zone.* Some of the tendons of the longitudinal portion of the ciliary muscle are connected to a specific network of elastic-like fibers in the juxtacanalicular zone, which in turn are connected by fine fibrils to the basement membrane of the endothelial cells lining the inner wall of Schlemm's canal. These small "connecting fibrils" are oxytalan fibers.[1] Sheath material composed of fine fibrils embedded in a homogenous matrix cover the anterior ciliary muscle tendons and continue over the elastic-like fibers in the juxtacanalicular zone.[1] With age, proteoglycan deposits accumulate as plaques within the sheaths covering the elastic-like fibers.[7] Ultimately, these plaques may form broad interlacing plates of extracellular deposits.

    Sheath-derived plaques have also been observed to accumulate with age in the outer wall of Schlemm's canal and in the tips of the longitudinal ciliary muscle tendons.[7,8]

7. *A loss of the ability to form giant vacuoles along the inner wall of Schlemm's canal.*[22]

8. *A proliferation of connective tissue cells from the endothelial cell lining and juxtacanalicular tissue into the lumen of Schlemm's canal.*[16]

GLAUCOMATOUS CHANGES

The increase in intraocular pressure in glaucoma may occur from a variety of possible causes. In the late 1960s, it was proposed that the elevated intraocular pressure was due to an increase in intrascleral venous pressure.[1,31] By increasing intrascleral venous pressure, the pressure head for aqueous outflow would decrease, and intraocular pressure would rise.[1,31] Nesterov (1970) concluded that the greatest resistance to aqueous outflow in primary open-angle glaucoma was not in the intrascleral veins, but in the juxtacanalicular tissue of the anterior chamber angle.[1,32] Thus, although an increase in intrascleral venous pressure could cause a rise in intraocular pressure, this appears not to be the most likely cause for the chronic pressure elevation found in primary open-angle glaucoma.

Canalicular blockage from a direct collapse of Schlemm's canal along its inner wall was another early idea as a cause for decreased aqueous outflow in glaucoma.[1,32] Moses and colleagues suggested that the collapse of Schlemm's canal was not the primary cause of increased intraocular pressure, but secondary to a primary defect along the inner wall of the canal leading to an increase in resistance to the outflow of aqueous.[1,33]

Endothelial Cell Loss

The loss of endothelial cells from the trabecular meshwork, which occurs normally with age, may occur earlier and to a greater extent in individuals with primary open-angle glaucoma. The excessive loss of endothelial cells seen in glaucoma is not uniform but greatest in the inner (uveal) meshwork.[2] On the other hand, the juxtacanalicular zone has a similar number of cells as age-matched normal eyes.[2] Alvarado found fewer endothelial cells at a given age in glaucomatous eyes than in normal eyes, although the rate of decline in the two groups was similar.[2] Thus the age-cellularity curves for normal and glaucoma individuals are parallel.[2] Those that develop primary open-angle glaucoma seem to reach their "critical" level of cell loss sooner than normal people.[2]

The rapid and excessive decrease in cellularity seen in primary open-angle glaucoma may be due to a congenital defect resulting in the person being born with fewer endothelial cells.[2] An alternative explanation is that a critical depletion of trabecular endothelial cells occurs rapidly in adulthood as a result of a "glaucoma factor."[22] Grierson believed that excessive wear-and-tear on endothelial cells could be the glaucoma factor for certain individuals.[22] Grierson and other investigators found that prolonged phagocytic activity of these cells can cause injury and necrosis.[22,23,34] Other causes of cell loss could be nutritional insufficiencies or toxins in the aqueous or excessive intracellular pigment accumulation.[22]

The loss of certain endothelial cells results in a reparative response from the remaining cells similar to that which occurs as a result of aging changes in the corneal endothelium.[2] The innermost trabeculae respond to the endothelial cell loss by marked enlargement (hypertrophy) of the remaining cells in order to cover over the denuded areas.[2,25,29] These activated cells may extend across trabecular beams, partially covering the usually opened "aqueous channels" creating a new and abnormal cellular lining across the inner surface of the meshwork.[2] This "membrane" may be what Fine and his colleagues described as an accretion and compactness of the uveal meshwork in glaucoma.[16] Chaudhry also observed marked alterations in the innermost trabeculae, although his coating substance that resulted in a "pretrabecular membrane" could not be confirmed by other investigators.[2,35] The increased metabolic activity of the remaining endothelial cells may also produce excessive or unusual extracellular material, in-

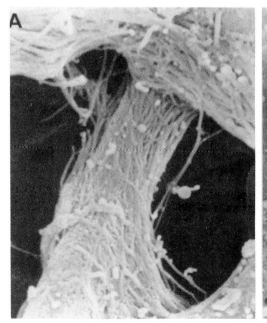
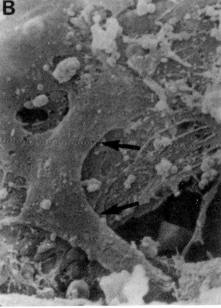

Figure 5–1. Scanning electron micrograph of trabeculae in **(A)** "early" and **(B)** "late" primary open-angle glaucoma. **(A)** shows the collagen core of a denuded trabeculae and **(B)** shows a migratory meshwork cell (*arrows*). (Original magnifications: **A** ×6000; **B** ×10,000.) (*From Grierson I. Eye. 1987;1:22, with permission.*)

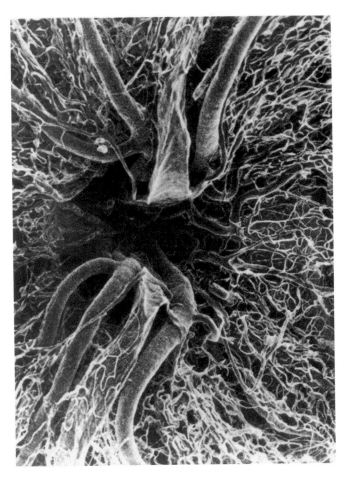

Figure 5–10. Vascular cast of optic nerve head viewed from vitreous side. Note the large number of capillaries, especially between vessels, that are poorly resolved in angiograms. Large veins are surrounded by capillaries and arteries appear to be bare. Original magnification: (Original magnification: ×90) (*Quigley HA, Hohman RM, Addicks EM. Am J Ophthalmol 93: 694, 1982. Published with permission from the American Journal of Ophthalmology, copyright by the Ophthalmic Publishing Company.*)

with angiography may simply represent a proportional loss of capillaries in advanced glaucoma and not areas of ischemia (Fig. 5–9). Therefore, filling defects may be the result of tissue loss in the optic nerve and not its cause.[56,104]

Leakage of fluorescein into the optic nerve from the surrounding choroid is seen in normal individuals and may not express a vascular abnormality from glaucoma.[99] Leakage from capillaries in the scleral lamina cribrosa would not likely present on the disc rim or the retinal edge of the disc as a splinter hemorrhages.[85] These flame-shaped hemorrhages may be an expression of abnormal forces acting on the walls of the capillaries in the optic nerve due to tissue loss, stretching, or rearrangement.[85]

So, as you can see, there remains significant debate regarding the cause of axonal transport blockage in glaucoma. More than likely both mechanical and vascular factors contribute to this damage. In some patients, one is the primary cause and the other secondary.

CONCLUSION

Glaucoma represents a disease in which abnormal levels of intraocular pressure cause a chronic, gradual destruction of ganglion cell axons by the blockage of axonal transport at the level of the scleral lamina cribrosa. This blockage could be caused by a variety of contributing factors that are mechanical, vascular, or biochemical in nature. The individual contribution of these various factors to glaucomatous damage differs from patient to patient.

Some people with very low levels of intraocular pressure develop glaucomatous optic nerve damage, whereas many individuals with elevated pressures do not. The real clinical dilemma is why an optic neuropathy from a certain level of intraocular pressure develops in some patients and not others. The answer is varying susceptibility of the optic nerve, which is most likely explained by normal variations among individuals in the anatomy and physiology of this tissue. Variation could occur in the size and support of the pores in the scleral lamina, in the blood supply to this region, including the location of the watershed zone, in the connective tissue framework of the laminar sheet, and in the composition of components of the extracellular matrix of the scleral lamina.

Understanding the etiology and pathophysiology of glaucoma is essential to an early differential diagnosis and appropriate management. Knowledge of the changes occurring in the optic nerve as a consequence of the glaucomatous process makes an appreciation of the early subtle changes in this tissue much easier to detect clinically.

REFERENCES

1. Rohen JW, Lütjen-Drecoll E. Morphology of aqueous outflow pathways in normal and glaucomatous eyes. In: Ritch R, Shields MB, Krupin T, eds. *The Glaucomas.* St. Louis: C.V. Mosby; 1989:41–74.
2. Alvarado J, Murphy C, Juster R. Trabecular meshwork cellularity in primary open-angle glaucoma and nonglaucomatous normals. *Ophthalmology.* 1984; 91:564–579.

3. Rohen JW. Why is intraocular pressure elevated in chronic simple glaucoma? Anatomic considerations. *Ophthalmology.* 1983;90:758–768.

4. Alvarado JA, Yun AJ, Murphy CG. Juxtacanalicular tissue in primary open angle glaucoma and in nonglaucomatous normals. *Arch Ophthalmol.* 1986; 104:1517–1528.

5. Rohen JW, Futa R, Lütjen-Drecoll E. The fine structure of the cribriform meshwork in normal and glaucomatous eyes as seen in tangential sections. *Invest Ophthalmol Vis Sci.* 1981;21:574–585.

6. Lütjen-Drecoll E, Futa R, Rohen J. Ultrahistochemical studies on tangential sections of the trabecular meshwork in normal and glaucomatous eyes. *Invest Ophthalmol Vis Sci.* 1981;21:563–573.

7. Lütjen-Drecoll E, Shimizu T, Rohrbach M, Rohen JW. Quantitative analysis of "plaque material" between ciliary muscle tips in normal and glaucomatous eyes. *Exp Eye Res.* 1986;42:457–465.

8. Lütjen-Drecoll E, Shimizu T, Rohrbach M, Rohen JW. Quantitative analysis of "plaque material" in the inner and outer wall of Schlemm's canal in normal and glaucomatous eyes. *Exp Eye Res.* 1986;42:443–455.

9. Tripathi RC, Tripathi BJ, Spaeth GL. Localization of sialic acid moieties in the endothelial lining of Schlemm's canal in normal and glaucomatous eyes. *Exp Eye Res.* 1987;44:293–306.

10. Floyd BB, Cleveland PH, Worthen DM. Fibronectin in human trabecular drainage channels. *Invest Ophthalmol Vis Sci.* 1985;26:797–804.

11. Quigley HA, Addicks EM. Scanning electron microscopy of trabeculectomy specimens from eyes with open-angle glaucoma. *Am J Ophthalmol.* 1980;90:854–857.

12. deKater AW, Melamed S, Epstein DL. Patterns of aqueous human outflow in glaucomatous and nonglaucomatous human eyes. *Arch Ophthalmol.* 1989;107:572–576.

13. Tawara A, Varner HH, Hollyfield JG. Distribution and characterization of sulfated proteoglycans in the human trabecular tissue. *Invest Ophthalmol Vis Sci.* 1989;30:2215–2231.

14. Lütjen-Drecoll E, Rittig M, Rauterberg J, et al. Immunomicroscopical study of type VI collagen in the trabecular meshwork of normal and glaucomatous eyes. *Exp Eye Res.* 1989;48:139–147.

15. Fink AF, Felix MD, Fletcher RC. The electron microscopy of Schlemm's canal and adjacent structure in patients with glaucoma. *Trans Am Ophthalmol Soc.* 1972;70:82–102.

16. Fine BS, Yanoff MS, Stone R. A clinicopathologic study of four cases of primary open-angle glaucoma compared to normal eyes. *Am J Ophthalmol.* 1981;91:88–105.

17. Rohen JW. Presence of matrix vesicles in the trabecular meshwork of glaucomatous eyes. *Graefe's Arch Clin Exp Ophthalmol.* 1982;218:171–176.

18. Tripathi RC. Pathologic anatomy of the outflow pathways of aqueous humor in chronic simple glaucoma. *Exp Eye Res.* 1977;25(suppl):403–407.

19. Chaudhry HA, Dueker DK, Simmons RJ, et al. Scanning electron microscopy of trabeculectomy specimens in open-angle glaucoma. *Am J Ophthalmol.* 1979;88:78–92.

20. Quigley HA, Addicks EM. Scanning electron microscopy of trabeculectomy specimens from eyes with open-angle glaucoma. *Am J Ophthalmol.* 1980;90:854–857.

21. Rohen JW, Witmer R. Electron microscopic studies on the trabecular meshwork in glaucoma simplex. V. *Graefe's Arch Clin Exp Ophthalmol.* 1972;183:251–266.

22. Grierson I, Calthorpe CM. Characteristics of meshwork cells and age changes in the outflow system of the eye: Their relevance to primary open-angle glaucoma. In: Mills KB, ed. *Glaucoma.* Proceedings of the Fourth International Symposium of the Northern Eye Institute. Manchester, UK; 1988:12–31.

23. Shirato S, Murphy CG, Bloom E, et al. Kinetics of phagocytosis in trabecular meshwork cells. *Invest Ophthalmol Vis Sci.* 1989;30:2499–2511.

24. Samuelson DA, Gum GG, Gelatt KN. Ultrastructural changes in the aqueous outflow apparatus of beagles with inherited glaucoma. *Invest Ophthalmol Vis Sci.* 1989;30:550–561.

25. Polansky JR, Wood IS, Maglio MT, Alvarado JA. Trabecular meshwork cell culture in glaucoma research: Evaluation of biological activity and structural properties of human trabecular cells in vitro. *Ophthalmology.* 1984;91:580–595.

26. Fei PF, Yue BY, Tso MOM. Effects of chondroitin sulfate on trabecular meshwork in rabbit eyes: An electron microscopic study. *Exp Eye Res.* 1984;39:583–594.

27. Yun AJ, Murphy CG, Polansky JR, et al. Proteins secreted by human trabecular cells. *Invest Ophthalmol Vis Sci.* 1989;30:2012–2022.

28. Murphy CG, Yun AJ, Newsome DA, Alvarado JA. Localization of extracellular proteins of the human trabecular meshwork by indirect immunofluorescence. *Am J Ophthalmol.* 1987;104:33–43.

29. Grierson I. What is open angle glaucoma? *Eye.* 1987;1:15–28.

30. Alvarado J, Murphy C, Polansky J, Juster R. Age-related changes in trabecular meshwork cellularity. *Invest Ophthalmol Vis Sci.* 1981;21:714–727.

31. Larina IN. On intrascleral outflow channels in glaucoma. *Vestn Oftalmol.* 1967;2:18–23.

32. Nesterov AP. Role of the blockade of Schlemm's canal in pathogenesis of primary open-angle glaucoma. *Am J Ophthalmol.* 1970;70:691–696.

33. Moses RA, Grodzki WJ, Etheridge EL, Wilson CD. Schlemm's canal: The effect of intraocular pressure. *Invest Ophthalmol Vis Sci.* 1981;70:61–68.

34. Johnson DH, Richardson TM, Epstein DL. Trabecular meshwork recovery after phagocytic challenge. *Curr Eye Res.* 1989;8:1121–1130.

35. Chaudhry HA, Dueker DK, Simmons RJ, et al. Scan-

ning electron microscopy of trabeculectomy specimens in open-angle glaucoma. *Am J Ophthalmol.* 1979;88:78–92.

36. Tripathi RC. Mechanism of the aqueous outflow across the trabecular wall of Schlemm's canal. *Exp Eye Res.* 1971;11:116–121.

37. Iwata K, Kurosawa A, Sawaguchi S. Wedge-shaped retinal nerve fiber layer defects in experimental glaucoma: Preliminary report. *Graefe's Arch Clin Exp Ophthalmol.* 1985;223:184–189.

38. Kitazawa K, Matsubara K. Optic disc changes in early glaucoma (summary). *Surv Ophthalmol.* 1989;37 (suppl):417–418.

39. Quigley HA, Sanchez RM, Dunkelberger GR, et al. Chronic glaucoma selectively damages large optic nerve fibers. *Invest Ophthalmol Vis Sci.* 1987;28:913–920.

40. Quigley HA. Reappraisal of the mechanisms of glaucomatous optic nerve damage. *Eye.* 1987;1:318–322.

41. Quigley HA. Glaucoma's optic nerve damage: Changing clinical perspectives. *Ann Ophthalmol.* 1982;611–612.

42. Radius RL, Anderson DR. Rapid axonal transport in primate optic nerve: Distribution of pressure induced interruption. *Arch Ophthalmol.* 1981;99:650–654.

43. Minckler DS. Histology of optic nerve damage in ocular hypertension and early glaucoma. *Surv Ophthalmol.* 1989;33(suppl):401–402.

44. Quigley HA, Hohman RM, Addicks EM, et al. Morphologic changes in the lamina cribrosa correlated with neural loss in open-angle glaucoma. *Am J Ophthalmol.* 1983;95:673–691.

45. Brooks DE, Samuelson DA, Gelatt KN, Smith PJ. Morphologic changes in the lamina cribrosa of beagles with primary open angle glaucoma. *Am J Vet Res.* 1989;50:936–941.

46. Quigley HA. The pathogenesis of optic nerve damage in glaucoma. Symposium on the laser in ophthalmology and glaucoma update. *Trans New Orleans Acad Ophthalmol.* 1985;111–128.

47. Hernandez MR, Andrzejewska WM, Neufeld AH. Changes in the extracellular matrix of the human optic nerve head in primary open-angle glaucoma. *Am J Ophthalmol.* 1990;109:180–188.

48. Morrison JC, Dorman-Pease ME, Dunkelberger GR, Quigley HA. Optic nerve head extracellular matrix in primary optic atrophy and experimental glaucoma. *Arch Ophthalmol.* 1990;108:1020–1024.

49. Zeimer RC, Ogura Y. The relationship between glaucomatous damage and optic nerve head mechanical compliance. *Arch Ophthalmol.* 1989;107:1232–1234.

50. Dandona L, Hendrickson A, Quigley HA. Selective effects of experimental glaucoma on axonal transport by retinal ganglion cells to the dorsal lateral geniculate nucleus. *Invest Ophthalmol Vis Sci.* 1991;32:1593–1599.

51. Quigley HA, Dunkelberger GR, Green WR. Chronic human glaucoma causing selective greater loss of large optic nerve fibers. *Ophthalmology.* 1988;95:357–363.

52. Glovinsky Y, Quigley HA, Dunkelberger GR. Retinal ganglion cell loss is size dependent in experimental glaucoma. *Invest Ophthalmol Vis Sci.* 1991;32:484–491.

53. Sossi N, Anderson DR. Blockade of axonal transport in optic nerve induced by elevation of intraocular pressure: Effect of arterial hypertension induced by angiotensin I. *Arch Ophthalmol.* 1983;101:94–97.

54. Schnabel J. Die Entwicklungsgeschichte der glaukomatosen Exkavation, Zeistchr. *Augenheilkd.* 1905;14:1.

55. Quigley HA, Addicks EM, Green WR. Optic nerve damage in glaucoma. III. Quantitative correlation of nerve fiber loss and visual field defect in glaucoma, ischemic neuropathy, papilledema, and toxic neuropathy. *Arch Ophthalmol.* 1982;100:135–146.

56. Quigley HA, Addicks EM, Green WR, Maumenee AE. Optic nerve damage in human glaucoma. II. The site of injury and susceptibility to damage. *Arch Ophthalmol.* 1981;99:635–649.

57. Airaksinen PJ, Drance SM, Douglas GR, et al. Diffuse and localized nerve fiber loss in glaucoma. *Am J Ophthalmol.* 1984;98:566–571.

58. Glowazki A, Flammer J. Is there a difference between glaucoma patients with rather localized visual field damage and patients with more diffuse visual field damage? *Doc Ophthalmol Proc Ser.* 1987;49:317–320.

59. Chauhan BC, Drance SM. The influence of intraocular pressure on visual field damage in patients with normal-tension and high-tension glaucoma. *Invest Ophthalmol Vis Sci.* 1990;31:2367–2372.

60. Caprioli J, Spaeth GL. Comparison of visual field defects in the low-tension glaucomas with those in the high-tension glaucomas. *Am J Ophthalmol.* 1984;97:730–737.

61. Drance SM. The early structural and functional disturbances of chronic open-angle glaucoma. Robert N. Shaffer Lecture. *Ophthalmology.* 1985;92:853–857.

62. Bodis-Wollner I. Electrophysiological and psychophysical testing of vision in glaucoma. *Surv Ophthalmol.* 1989;33(suppl):301–307.

63. Stamper RL. Psychophysical changes in glaucoma. *Surv Ophthalmol.* 1989;33(suppl):309–318.

64. Sommer A, Katz J, Quigley HA, et al. Clinically detectable nerve fiber atrophy precedes the onset of glaucomatous field loss. *Arch Ophthalmol.* 1991;109:77–83.

65. Miller KM, Quigley HA. The clinical appearance of the lamina cribrosa as a function of the extent of glaucomatous optic nerve damage. *Ophthalmology.* 1988;95:135–138.

66. Sakugawa M, Chihara E. Blockage at two points of axonal transport in glaucomatous eyes. *Graefe's Arch Clin Ophthalmol.* 1985;223:214–218.

67. Minckler DS, Tso MOM, Zimmerman LE. A light microscopic, autoradiographic study of axoplasmic transport in the optic nerve head during ocular hypotony, increased intraocular pressure and papilledema. *Am J Ophthalmol.* 1976;82:741–757.

68. Minckler DS, Bunt AH, Johanson GW. Orthograde and retrograde axoplasmic transport during acute oc-

ular hypertension in the monkey. *Invest Ophthalmol Vis Sci.* 1977;16:426–441.

69. Lampert PW, Vogel MH, Zimmerman LE. Pathology of the optic nerve in experimental glaucoma. *Invest Ophthalmol Vis Sci.* 1968;7:199–213.

70. Minckler DS, Spaeth GL. Optic nerve damage in glaucoma. *Surv Ophthalmol.* 1981;26:128–146.

71. Elkington AR, Inman CBE, Steart PV, Weller RO. The structure of the lamina cribrosa of the human eye: An immunocytochemical and electron microscopic study. *Eye.* 1990;4:42–57.

72. Minckler DS. Histology of optic nerve damage in ocular hypertension and early glaucoma. *Surv Ophthalmol.* 1989;33(suppl):401–402.

73. Radius RL. Distribution of pressure-induced fast axonal transport abnormalities in primate optic nerve: An audioradiographic study. *Arch Ophthalmol.* 1981;99:1257–1263.

74. Minckler DS, Tso MOM. A light microscopic audioradiographic study of axoplasmic transport in the normal rhesus optic nerve head. *Am J Ophthalmol.* 1976;82:1–15.

75. Quigley HA, Anderson DR. The dynamics and location of axonal transport blockade by acute intraocular pressure elevation in primate optic nerve. *Invest Ophthalmol Vis Sci.* 1976;15:606–616.

76. Minckler DS, Ogden TE. Distribution of axonal transport injury in the lamina in experimental glaucoma in the monkey. In: Krieglstein GK (ed). *Glaucoma Update III.* Berlin: Springer-Verlag; 1987:27–35.

77. Radius RL. Anatomy of the optic nerve head and glaucomatous optic neuropathy. *Surv Ophthalmol.* 1987;32:35–44.

78. Müller H. Anatomische Beitragezur Ophthalmologie: Veber Nervean-Veranderungen an der Eintrittsstelle des Scherven. *Arch Ophthalmol.* 1958;4:1.

79. von Jaeger E. Uber Glaucom und Seine Heilungdurch Iridectomie. *Z Ges der Aerzte zu Wien.* 1958;14:465–484.

80. Anderson DR, Hendrickson AE. Failure of increased intracranial pressure to affect rapid axonal transport at the optic nerve head. *Invest Ophthalmol Vis Sci.* 1977;16:423–426.

81. Radius RL, Bade B. Axonal transport interruption and anatomy at the lamina cribrosa. *Arch Ophthalmol.* 1982;100:1661–1664.

82. Radius RL. Pressure-induced fast axonal transport abnormalities and the anatomy at the lamina cribrosa in primate eyes. *Invest Ophthalmol Vis Sci.* 1983;24:343–346.

83. Hayreh SS. The pathogenesis of optic nerve lesions in glaucoma. Symposium: The optic disc in glaucoma. *Trans Am Acad Ophthalmol Otololaryng.* 1976;81:197–213.

84. Ochs S. Local supply of energy to the fast axoplasmic transport mechanism. *Proc Natl Acad Sci USA.* 1971;68:1279–1282.

85. Gasser P. Ocular vasospasm: A risk factor in the pathogenesis of low-tension glaucoma. *Int Ophthalmol.* 1989;13:281–290.

86. Neetens A. Autoregulation of the blood supply to the anterior optic nerve lamina cribrosa. *Trans Ophthalmol Soc UK.* 1977;97:168–176.

87. Maumene EA. Causes of optic nerve damage in glaucoma. *Ophthalmology.* 1983;90:741–752.

88. Hayreh SS. Pathogenesis of visual field defects: Role of the ciliary circulation. *Br J Ophthalmol.* 1970;54:289–311.

89. Ulrich WD, Ulrich C, Bohne BD. Deficient autoregulation and lengthening of the diffusion distance in the anterior optic nerve circulation in glaucoma: An electro-encephalo-dynamographic investigation. *Ophthalmic Res.* 1986;18:253–259.

90. Sossi N, Anderson DR. Effect of elevated intraocular pressure on blood flow; occurrence in the cat optic nerve head studied with iodantipyrine I 125. *Arch Ophthalmol.* 1983;101:98–101.

91. Hayreh SS. Interindividual variation in blood supply of the optic nerve head. *Doc Ophthalmol.* 1985;59:217–246.

92. Brooks DE, Samuelson DA, Gelatt KK. Ultrastructural change in laminar optic nerve capillaries of beagles with primary open-angle glaucoma. *Am J Vet Res.* 1989;50:929–935.

93. Novack RL, Stefánsson E, Hatchell DL. Intraocular pressure effects on optic nerve-head oxidative metabolism measured in vivo. *Graefe's Arch Clin Exp Oph thalmol.* 1990;228:128–133.

94. Radius RL, Anderson DR. Breakdown of the normal optic nerve head blood-brain barrier following acute elevation of intraocular pressure in experimental animals. *Invest Ophthalmol Vis Sci.* 1980;19:244–255.

95. Yabionski M. An analysis of the "vascular hypothesis" concerning optic disc pathology in glaucoma. *Ann Ophthalmol.* 1979;11:67–69.

96. Sebag J, Thomas JV, Epstein DL, Grant WM. Optic disc cupping in anterior ischemic optic neuropathy resembles glaucomatous cupping. *Ophthalmology.* 1986;93:357–361.

97. Robert Y, Steiner D, Hendrickson P. Papillary circulation dynamics in glaucoma. *Graefe's Arch Clin Exp Ophthalmol.* 1989;227:436–439.

98. Tuulonen A. Asymptomatic miniocclusions of the optic disc veins in glaucoma. *Arch Ophthalmol.* 1989;107:1475–1480.

99. Nanba K, Schwartz B. Nerve fiber layer and optic disc fluorescein defects in glaucoma and ocular hypertension. *Ophthalmology.* 1988;95:1227–1233.

100. Jonas JB, Naumann GOH. Parapapillary retinal vessel diameter in normal and glaucomatous eyes. II. Correlations. *Invest Ophthalmol Vis Sci.* 1989;30:1604–1611.

101. Hayreh SS. Pathogenesis of optic nerve head changes in glaucoma. *Semin Ophthalmol.* 1986;1:1–13.

102. Henkind P, Alterman M. Radial peripapillary capillaries of the retina. II. Possible role in Bjerrum scotoma. *Br J Ophthalmol.* 1968;52:26–31.

103. Henkind P. Radial peripapillary capillaries of the retina: I. Anatomy: Human and comparative. *Br J Ophthalmol.* 1967;51:115–123.

104. Quigley HA, Hohman RM, Addicks EM. Quantitative study of optic nerve head capillaries in experimental optic disk pallor. *Am J Ophthalmol.* 1982;93: 689–699.

105. Levy NS, Adams CK. Slow axonal protein transport and visual function following retinal and optic nerve ischemia. *Invest Ophthalmol Vis Sci.* 1975;14:91–97.

106. Levy NS. The effect of interruption of the short posterior ciliary arteries on slow axoplasmic transport and histology within the optic nerve of the rhesus monkey. *Invest Ophthalmol.* 1976;15:495–499.

107. Radius RL. Optic nerve fast axonal transport abnormalities in primates. Occurrence after short posterior ciliary artery occlusion. *Arch Ophthalmol.* 1980;98: 2018–2022.

108. Radius RL, Anderson DR. Morphology of axonal transport abnormalities in primate eyes. *Br J Ophthalmol.* 1981;65:767–777.

109. Shaffer RN. Nerve fiber loss and disparity of disc and field changes in glaucoma. Symposium on the laser in ophthalmology and glaucoma update. *Trans New Orleans Acad Ophthalmol.* 1985;129–133.

110. Hayreh SS, Revie HS, Edwards J. Vasogenic origin of visual field defects and optic nerve changes in glaucoma. *Br J Ophthalmol.* 1970;54:461–472.

111. Laatikainen L. Fluorescein angiographic studies of the peripapillary and perilimbal regions in simple, capsular and low tension glaucoma. *Acta Ophthalmol.* 1971;111(suppl):10–13.

112. Jonas JB, Nguyen XN, Gusek GC, Naumann GOH. Parapillary chorioretinal atrophy in normal and glaucomatous eyes. *Invest Ophthalmol Vis Sci.* 1989;30:908–918.

113. Jonas JB, Nguyen XN, Naumann GOH. Parapapillary retinal vessel diameter in normal and glaucomatous eyes. I. Morphometric data. *Invest Ophthalmol Vis Sci.* 1989;30:1599–1603.

114. Krakau T. Disc haemorrhages and the etiology of glaucoma. *Acta Ophthalmol.* 1989;67(suppl):31–33.

115. Carter CJ, Brooks DE, Doyle DL, Drance SM. Investigations into a vascular etiology for low-tension glaucoma. *Ophthalmology.* 1990;97:49–55.

116. Sebag J, Thomas JV, Epstein DL, Grant WM. Optic disc cupping in arteritic anterior ischemic optic neuropathy resembles glaucomatous cupping. *Ophthalmology.* 1986;93:357–361.

117. Harrington DO. The Bjerrum scotoma. *Trans Am Ophthalmol Soc.* 1964;62:324–348.

118. Harrington DO. The pathogenesis of the glaucoma field. *Am J Ophthalmol.* 1959;47:177–185.

119. Quigley HA, Hohman RM, Sanchez R, Addicks EM. Optic nerve head blood flow in experimental glaucoma. *Arch Ophthalmol.* 1985;103:956–962.

120. Radius RL, Schwartz EL, Anderson DR. Failure of unilateral carotid artery ligation to affect pressure-induced interruption of rapid axonal transport in primate optic nerves. *Invest Ophthalmol Vis Sci.* 1980;19:153–157.

DIAGNOSIS OF THE GLAUCOMAS

Chapter 6

EXAMINING THE PATIENT: GLAUCOMA DETECTION, DIAGNOSIS, AND EVALUATION

Linda Casser Locke

Textbooks on glaucoma traditionally and by necessity present information arranged by the clinical diagnosis of the various types of the disease. The goal of this chapter, however, is to discuss the detection, diagnosis, and evaluation of the glaucoma patient by presenting the information in the manner in which patients are most likely to present to the optometric practitioner:

- The initial routine examination
- The completion evaluation of the glaucoma patient or suspect
- The glaucoma patient presenting for acute eye care
- The glaucoma screening

For each of these types of examinations, recommendations are made as to the clinical procedures that should be performed to help ensure the appropriate evaluation for glaucoma. The tests to be performed, as well as when and why they should be done, are specified. Since most optometrists will already be familiar with the majority of these tests, the techniques will be described only as components of each examination protocol. Greater detail on performing each technique, the interpretation of the results, and the management of the glaucoma patient are included in other chapters.

INITIAL ROUTINE EXAMINATION

Rationale for Examination Protocol

To adequately detect glaucoma as well as a host of other ophthalmic conditions, the optometrist must have a thorough protocol for data collection that is consistently implemented. The protocol listed in Table 6–1 is designed for a cooperative adult patient. Protocol modification may be required if patient comprehension or cooperation levels are reduced.

Examination Protocol

History. A thorough ocular and systemic medical history may elicit findings that are significant to the diagnosis of glaucoma, may lead the optometrist to suspect glaucoma as a potential diagnosis, or may reveal one or more risk factors that affect the interpretation of subsequently elicited data.[1-3] Of course, the patient may have ocular symptoms that are completely unrelated to glaucoma, yet the diagnosis of

The author extends thanks to Felix M. Barker II, OD, MS, for his thoughtful insights and materials pertaining to restricted spectrum illumination of the nerve fiber layer and fundus biomicroscopy, and to Richard Meetz, OD, MS, for his assistance in preparation of the section on glaucoma screening.

TABLE 6–1. SUGGESTED INITIAL EXAMINATION PROTOCOL: GLAUCOMA DETECTION, DIAGNOSIS, AND EVALUATION

Patient history: ocular and systemic

Visual acuities

Pupillary reflexes

Color vision testing

Visual field screening

Blood pressure screening

Refractive analysis: distance and near

Slit-lamp examination: predilation

Applanation tonometry

Pupillary dilation

Direct ophthalmoscopy

Binocular indirect ophthalmoscopy

Slit-lamp examination: postdilation, includng fundus biomicroscopy

Fundus photography as indicated

glaucoma may be made as a result of complete data collection.

Age and Race. The prevalence of primary open-angle glaucoma is clearly age related.[4] As with systemic essential hypertension, a higher incidence is found among blacks.[5,6] Other characteristics of glaucoma found in the black population include a younger age of onset, a higher mean cup-disc ratio, greater visual field loss at the time of diagnosis, and a more severe disease that is less responsive to treatment.[7–9]

Ocular Symptoms. It is unusual for a patient presenting for routine examination to report symptoms related to glaucoma. Occasionally, however, a patient with primary or secondary open-angle glaucoma may experience pronounced periodic elevations ("spikes") in the intraocular pressure leading to symptoms of blurred vision and halos as a result of corneal edema.[10] The significance of these symptoms may be overlooked if the intraocular pressure is in the normal range at the time of examination. If the glaucoma is far advanced, the patient may complain of visual field defects, reduced visual acuity, or mobility problems.

History of Eye Surgery or Trauma. The patient may have undergone a laser or surgical procedure related to glaucoma or may have had a cataract extraction that was complicated by secondary glaucoma. Significant ocular contusion may produce a secondary glaucoma due to trabecular meshwork insult, angle recession, or other changes in the anterior chamber angle.[11,12] Frequently, signs of ocular contusion that

occurred 10 to 20 years earlier may be detected during the examination, which the patient failed to mention during the history. Specific requestioning about prior eye injuries may then elicit the pertinent information.[13,14]

Previous Diagnosis of Glaucoma. A patient may report having been previously diagnosed with primary open-angle glaucoma for which he or she is currently taking medication or is supposed to be taking medication. The patient may have been treated for glaucoma in the past, but the treatment was subsequently discontinued by another doctor or by the same doctor following reassessment of the condition. Finally, the patient may have been referred by an optometrist to another practitioner for suspected glaucoma, and, for any number of reasons, the patient may have failed to follow through with that recommendation.

Family History of Glaucoma. Patients having first-degree relatives (parents, siblings) with glaucoma have a much greater likelihood of developing glaucoma themselves.[16–18] Inquiring as to the age of the family member at the time of diagnosis as well as his or her treatment regimen may assist in identifying the type and severity of the condition. It is not unusual, however, for the patient to confuse ocular terminology and incorrectly report that a family member has glaucoma.

Significant Topical Ophthalmic Medication Use. It is uncommon for topical ophthalmic medication to contribute to the development of glaucoma. There are two groups of drugs, however, that must be considered in this regard, namely, topical steroids and topical decongestants.

In susceptible individuals, the short-term use of topical steroids for treatment of an acute ocular problem may cause an elevation of intraocular pressure.[4,19] The patient initially presenting for routine examination, however, is less likely to be using topical steroids for an acute, short-lived problem. It is possible, though, that the patient may present having used topical steroids over a relatively long period of time. For example, a dermatologist may have prescribed long-term topical steroid use for a condition such as ocular acne rosacea, requiring the application of potent steroid creams to the periocular skin. A general physician may have prescribed a topical combination steroid/antibiotic drop for a chronic red eye problem in a nursing home patient. Any health care provider may have unknowingly contributed to chronic topical steroid use through poor control of refills resulting in patient self-medication without supervision. The long-term use of systemic steroids has also been implicated in the elevation of intraocular pressure in susceptible individuals.[19]

Whatever the cause, a patient using topical steroid medication regularly over a prolonged period may be at risk for the development of a secondary open-angle glaucoma, among other complications.

The second major category of topical ophthalmic medications that may contribute to glaucoma development is decongestant drops. Several over-the-counter decongestant agents (e.g., Prefrin) contain 0.12% phenylephrine hydrochloride. Even this low concentration of phenylephrine may result in pupillary dilation in sensitive patients, especially if the corneal epithelium is disrupted allowing more effective penetration of the drug into the anterior chamber.[15,20,21] In susceptible individuals with narrow anterior chamber angles, topical decongestant drug use may result in elevation of intraocular pressure due to further narrowing of the anterior chamber angle. In the case of a patient presenting for routine examination, topical decongestant drop use may contribute to the development of intermittent acute or primary angle closure glaucoma.

It is not uncommon for a patient to fail to mention that he or she is using topical ophthalmic medications. Specifically asking the patient "Do you use any eyedrops, such as Visine or Murine?" will help to reduce underreporting by the patient.

Significant Systemic Disease. Since the integrity of the optic nerve is dependent in large measure on the integrity of its vascular supply, any systemic disease that affects the vascular system may contribute to glaucoma development. Diabetes mellitus and systemic hypertension are two of the most common and important conditions in this regard and need to be considered in treatment of the patient.[22,23] Diabetics or hypertensives with untreated or uncontrolled glaucoma may exhibit glaucomatous optic nerve damage sooner and faster in the disease process than patients who are systemically healthy. Diabetic patients with glaucoma may exhibit a different pattern of visual field loss than nondiabetic glaucoma patients.[24] Patients with rubeosis irides secondary to diabetes are at risk for developing secondary angle closure glaucoma.[4]

Vascular insufficiency to the optic nerve may be a contributing factor in the development of glaucomatous damage. Acute hypotensive episodes such as severe shock, blood loss from gastrointestinal or uterine hemorrhaging, or sustained systemic hypotension have been implicated as major factors in the production of low-tension glaucoma.[25] Migraine-related cerebral ischemia may be present in some cases of low-tension glaucoma.[26] A significant drop in blood pressure due to aggressive hypertensive therapy has also been shown to result in optic nerve head ischemia.[27] Thus, a glaucoma suspect in whom the blood pressure has been aggressively lowered may become susceptible to frank glaucomatous changes.

Significant Systemic Medication Use. Two important categories of systemic medications may alter the glaucomatous condition by lowering intraocular pressure, namely, diuretic agents and systemic beta adrenergic blocking agents.[28] The most common use of these medications is for the treatment of systemic hypertension. Systemic beta adrenergic blocking agents are also used to control angina pectoris, cardiac arrhythmias, and migraine headaches.

Since systemic diuretic agents and beta adrenergic blocking agents reduce intraocular pressure, a patient using one or both of these agents may exhibit intraocular pressure readings that are artifactually low. If these medications are reduced in dosage or discontinued, the intraocular pressure may elevate.

Table 6–2 lists the components of a thorough ocular and systemic patient history for the initial routine examination that are pertinent to the diagnosis of glaucoma.

Visual Acuity Measurement. Monocular visual acuity measurement is, of course, an integral component of each and every ophthalmic examination. Patients with early to moderate glaucoma will not typically exhibit visual acuity decrements attributable to optic nerve head and visual field changes. The retention of macular function, as measured by Snellen, acuity until very late in the glaucomatous disease process is the reason that patients with glaucoma rarely seek eye care because of poor vision. Thus, the assessment of Snellen visual acuity does not help distinguish glaucomatous from non-glaucomatous patients. Endstage

TABLE 6–2. PATIENT HISTORY COMPONENTS PERTINENT TO GLAUCOMA

Patient age
Patient race
Ocular symptoms
Previous eye surgery or trauma
Previous diagnosis of glaucoma
Family history of glaucoma
Topical ophthalmic medication use
Systemic disease history
Systemic medication usage

glaucoma with advanced optic nerve head damage and visual field loss can result in profound visual acuity loss, and, if uncontrolled, eventual blindness. Regrettably, patients with advanced glaucoma and irreversible optic nerve head damage who have not previously sought care on a routine basis may believe that new glasses will solve their visual problem.

Pupillary Reflexes. Pupillary reflexes in patients with early glaucoma are usually normal. Patients with unilateral or asymmetrical glaucoma may exhibit a subtle afferent pupillary defect on the side with more advanced disease if the test is carefully performed using a bright illumination source.[29,30] With more advanced glaucomatous disease, abnormal pupillary responses may be present consistent with the degree and symmetry of the glaucomatous optic neuropathy. Patients with endstage glaucoma may exhibit amaurotic pupillary responses.

Color Vision Testing. Routine monocular color vision testing with techniques such as the Pseudoisochromatic, Ishihara, or Dvorine plates is not sufficiently sensitive to elicit the subtle color vision defects that are suggestive of glaucoma. More detailed color vision testing, if included as part of the diagnostic battery, is easiest to perform at the completion of the glaucoma evaluation visit.

Visual Field Screening. Confrontation visual field testing, as performed during routine examination, allows for a quick "pass–fail" assessment screening of the visual field.[31,32] This technique is not sensitive enough to detect early glaucomatous field defects. Only advanced glaucoma will exhibit significant field loss through confrontation visual field testing.

In many offices, automated visual field screening is done routinely to detect neurological problems, including glaucoma. Many practitioners choose a reasonable age criterion such as 35 to begin routine automated visual field screening, since the middle age and older age groups have a higher incidence of glaucoma. Unfortunately, a number of elderly patients have difficulty responding in a reliable manner to automated visual field testing due to the attention span, posture, and manual dexterity required for this rapid sequence testing. Due to response capability, some patients may respond more favorably to manual kinetic (e.g., Goldmann bowl) perimetry techniques.

If visual field defects are suspected as a result of the visual field screening, then more detailed evaluation using threshold automated visual field testing is indicated. Detailed visual field analysis is a required component for the completion of the glaucoma evaluation visit.

Blood Pressure Screening. Studies have correlated intraocular pressure with blood pressure, particularly in an effort to predict visual field defects.[33] From the standpoint of glaucoma diagnosis, treatment, and management, blood pressure measurement in the optometrist's office serves several purposes.[34] Firstly, sphygmomanometry helps to screen for patients who have undiagnosed or undercontrolled hypertension, adding a dimension to the relative risk of developing glaucoma. Until the blood pressure is controlled, it is prudent to avoid the use of diagnostic agents such as 10% phenylephrine and glaucoma therapeutic agents such as epinephrine that may precipitate hypertensive crisis.[35]

A patient who exhibits systemic hypotension (BP ≤ 95/60) may be a poor candidate for topical beta adrenergic blocking agents or may have an inherent circulatory problem contributing to the development of low tension glaucoma.

Refractive Analysis: Distance and Near. The initial routine examination includes refractive analysis. The nature of the patient's refractive error may prove to be a risk factor for specific types of glaucoma.

If a myope with an inherently large physiological optic cup develops elevated intraocular pressures, the disc will be more susceptible to pathological changes due to the glaucomatous process.[36] Myopic patients may also have obliquely inserting optic nerves resulting in shallow, temporally sloping cups that may make visualization of the demarcation between the cup and rim difficult. Pigment dispersion syndrome, which may be associated with pigmentary glaucoma, is more commonly observed in young myopic patients. Myopia occurs more frequently in populations of patients with primary open-angle glaucoma, ocular hypertension, and low-tension glaucoma than in age-matched normal populations.[37,38]

Although hyperopia seems not to be a risk factor for primary open-angle glaucoma, it provides a definite risk factor for angle closure glaucoma. A hyperopic eye tends to have a smaller, shorter globe or flatter corneal curvature resulting in narrower anterior chamber angles. These angles will tend to become narrower as the patient ages due to thickening of the crystalline lens. Thus, the hyperope with anatomically narrow anterior chamber angles may be susceptible to spontaneous acute angle closure glaucoma later in life.[39]

Aphakic and pseudophakic patients may be susceptible to secondary open-angle glaucoma in the postoperative course. If the patient is found to have glaucoma, epinephrine-based drugs are generally avoided due to the possibility of inducing cystoid macular edema.[15]

Some unusual refractive situations may have a bearing on the evaluation of the potential glaucoma patient. If the patient has a high degree of anisometropia with one eye significantly more myopic than the other due to a difference in globe size, the optic nerve head cupping may be dissimilar between the two eyes with the more myopic eye having a significantly larger physiological cup. Since optic nerve cupping asymmetry can be an important clinical cue as to the presence of glaucoma, it is necessary to rule out an inherent contributing factor such as anisometropia.

Biomicroscopic (Slit-Lamp) Examination: Predilation. A thorough slit-lamp examination is important for patients of all ages to evaluate ocular health. It is important that the examiner have an efficient, standard slit-lamp examination routine that uses appropriate illuminations to thoroughly evaluate the anterior segment without overlooking significant findings.[40]

The most likely ocular structures involved in abnormalities associated with glaucoma are the cornea, iris, and anterior chamber. Table 6–3 indicates commonly encountered slit-lamp abnormalities that may be indicators of glaucoma.[41] The interpretation of these findings to assess for secondary glaucoma is covered elsewhere in this book. Careful evaluation of the crystalline lens using the slit-lamp is reserved until after pupillary dilation.

Certain anterior segment findings may suggest the need for additional slit-lamp examination.[40] For example, an asymptomatic patient with chronic anterior uveitis may exhibit keratic precipitates (KPs) on the corneal endothelium. It is then appropriate to specifically evaluate the anterior chamber for inflammatory cells and flare. Alternatively, if a Krukenberg's spindle is present, iris transillumination is performed to look for peripheral iris defects associated with pigment dispersion syndrome.[42–45]

Finally, every routine slit-lamp examination should include the Van Herick estimation technique ("limbal slit" technique) of anterior chamber angle depth.[40] This will help to determine whether the angle is of appropriate dimension for uneventful pupillary dilation and will be an indicator of the presence of narrow angles that may predispose the patient to chronic or acute angle closure glaucoma. Occasionally, if a patient has unilateral angle recession, lens subluxation, or aphakia without an intraocular lens implant, the involved eye may be observed to have a deeper anterior chamber using the Van Herick technique.

Applanation Tonometry. The measurement of IOP with applanation tonometry efficiently follows the complete routine slit-lamp examination. Applanation tonometry is requisite for the diagnosis and management of glaucoma. The time of day the applanation readings are measured is recorded to assess diurnal variation in IOP.

Applanation tonometry should be attempted on patients of all ages who are able to cooperate. Handheld applanation tonometers (e.g., Perkins) are available to measure the IOP of patients who are unable to be positioned in the slit-lamp.[46]

Noncontact tonometry (NCT, "air puff") may be best suited for some specific testing conditions: glaucoma screenings, IOP measurement of young children and adults who cannot cooperate for applanation tonometry, and IOP measurement in the presence of anterior segment infection or suspected globe penetration. If measurements obtained through noncontact tonometry are questionable, they must be repeated using Goldmann tonometry. As a "last resort," digital IOP assessment may be performed on the patient who is unable to cooperate for any other techniques.[47] If, however, any index of suspicion for glaucoma is observed in the patient on whom digital IOP assessment has been performed, then consultation or referral is necessary for sedation or general anesthesia so that accurate IOP measurement can be obtained.

TABLE 6–3. ROUTINE SLIT-LAMP EXAMINATION: POSSIBLE INDICATORS OF GLAUCOMA

Cornea
Opacities, especially due to penetrating injury
Krukenberg's spindle
Keratic precipitates (KPs)
Exfoliative debris on endothelium
Microcornea
Megalocornea

Iris
Atrophy
Heterochromia
Iridodialysis
Pigment release following pupillary dilation
Exfoliative debris at ruff
Posterior synechiae
Rubeosis
Superficial pigment dusting
Transillumination: at ruff or periphery

The numerical value obtained with tonometry must be evaluated in conjunction with assessment of the optic nerve head appearance as well as the results of optic nerve functional testing (e.g., visual fields) to properly evaluate whether a given IOP measurement is normal or abnormal for an individual patient. While elevated IOP is commonly associated with primary open-angle glaucoma, well over 50% of glaucomatous patients present on initial examination with IOPs in the "normal" range.[48]

Utilization of Diagnostic Pharmaceutical Agents (DPAs). Routine pupillary dilation has become the standard of care for patients of all ages.[49] Included in assessing patient suitability for dilation are estimating the characteristics of the anterior chamber angle using the Van Herick slit-lamp technique and determining, through the history, whether the patient may have a sensitivity to any of the components of dilating agents. Concurrent use of both an anticholinergic agent and an adrenergic agonist will help to ensure adequate dilation/cycloplegia for all subsequently performed techniques. Although prudent clinical judgment on the part of the practitioner must enter into the specific choice of dilating agents, the most commonly used drugs are combinations of 1% tropicamide and 2½% phenylephrine drops,[50] instilled approximately 1 minute apart.

It is not uncommon for patients who are diabetic, who have darkly pigmented irises, or who have habitually miotic pupils to dilate poorly. In this instance, since full pupillary dilation is needed to adequately perform subsequent testing, it is appropriate to instill an additional one or two drops of each diagnostic agent in an effort to produce adequate dilation. Once again, prudent clinical judgment on the part of the practitioner will determine whether or not the patient is a suitable candidate for instillation of multiple doses. For example, the anterior chamber angles must be of adequate size to permit full dilation without inducing angle closure. Even though the risk of hypertensive crisis from the use of 2½% phenylephrine drops is low, it may be prudent to avoid multiple drops of this agent in a patient in whom blood pressure was found to be high or who is known to have significant cardiovascular disease. For these patients, the use of punctal occlusion following installation will help to minimize systemic absorption of the drops.[50,51] Alternatively, a small cotton pledget placed in the inferior cul-de-sac and moistened with the drug will maximize pupillary dilation by enhancing contact time.[52] The use of 10% phenylephrine on the pledget is generally avoided, however, since the likelihood of systemic absorption using this technique is greater and 10% phenylephrine is more likely to have systemic hypertensive effects.[15]

In contrast, some patients exhibit marginally narrow anterior chamber angles using the Van Herick technique so that the routine use of dilating agents may be questioned. In these instances, it is appropriate to more thoroughly assess the anterior chamber angle to determine whether pupillary dilation is appropriate. Since topical anesthetic drops are used to measure applanation tonometry, it is relatively easy at this point in the examination to incorporate 4-mirror gonioscopy to evaluate the anterior chamber angle. (Some clinicians routinely perform 4-mirror gonioscopy following applanation tonometry for a period of time to more fully develop their 4-mirror and angle evaluative ability, a demanding skill requiring good dexterity and precise technique.[53]) The use of the newer hand-held Sussman 4-mirror goniolens may be easier to master than the handle-mounted Zeiss goniolens. Four-mirror gonioscopy requires a minimum amount of time, allows for rapid comparison between the two eyes, and is less likely to cause significant corneal disruption prior to evaluation of the fundus.

It is not uncommon for gonioscopy to reveal that the anterior chamber angle is actually larger than initially assessed using the Van Herick technique so that routine pupillary dilation may proceed uneventfully. Gonioscopy may confirm, however, that the angle is extremely narrow and susceptible to spontaneous or iatrogenic-induced closure. These patients may be considered candidates for prophylactic laser iridotomy even though it is not always possible to definitively predict from gonioscopy which patients will develop acute or primary angle closure glaucoma.[54]

The risk of inducing acute angle closure glaucoma through routine pupillary dilation in patients with marginally narrow angles is low and has probably been exaggerated. However, the practitioner may elect to modify his or her dilation regimen to further minimize the risk of angle closure, particularly if secondary or tertiary ophthalmic care is not readily available. Rechecking the angle following pupillary dilation by the Van Herrick technique will help to assess the degree of angle narrowing induced by the dilation. Frequently, the angle may actually enlarge following pupil dilation. The patient may be dilated early in the day and warned of angle closure symptoms so that additional care will be readily available if problems arise. It is even possible to ask the patient to remain in the office or return 4 to 6 hours later during the mid-dilation recovery phase to reassess the angle and remeasure the IOP.[50] The clinician may elect to dilate one eye at a time at two separate visits. Some clinicians use tropicamide drops as the only diagnostic agent in marginally narrow angle patients so that if difficulties arise and topical miotic drops are necessary, antagonistic action between pilocarpine and phenylephrine will not contribute to relative pupillary block. Others perform a prone provocative test to help predict the effect of pupillary dilation in patients with narrow angles.[55]

Patients with pigment dispersion syndrome or exfoliation syndrome may exhibit pigment release into the anterior chamber following pupillary dilation due to mechanical disruption of the iris pigment epithelium.[56,57] This sudden pigment release may result in a sharp IOP elevation several hours after pupillary dilation. Thus, for the patient with pigment dispersion syndrome or narrow anterior chamber angles, an IOP measurement several hours following pupillary dilation may provide useful diagnostic data.

Sector pupillary dilation has been described as a method for facilitating evaluation of the posterior segment while minimizing the risk of acute angle closure.[50,52,58] This technique may also be useful for pupillary dilation when precise anterior chamber angle evaluation is more difficult, such as for patients who are confined to a wheelchair or are bed bound. Instillation of an alpha adrenergic blocking agent such as 0.5% dapiprazole hydrochloride solution (Rēv-Eyes) reverses pupillary mydriasis due to phenylephrine and to a lesser degree, tropicamide, without shifting of the iris-lens diaphragm.[15] Although conjunctival hyperemia and burning on instillation are common side effects, instillation of dapiprazole or other adrenergic blocking agents may facilitate the use of mydriatic agents in patients with marginally narrow anterior chamber angles.

Patients with posterior chamber intraocular lens implants (IOLs) or anterior chamber lenses that are not iris fixed are safe candidates for pupillary dilation. However, patients who have anterior chamber IOLs that are iris fixed should not be dilated due to the risk of lens dislocation.[50]

Patients who are being treated with miotic agents present a clinical challenge relative to pupillary dilation. If there are no contraindications to discontinuing the miotic agent for a few days, such as narrow anterior chamber angles, it is helpful to do so prior to instilling mydriatic/cycloplegic agents.

Direct Ophthalmoscopy Following Pupillary Dilation.
An efficient yet systematic routine for direct ophthalmoscopy will allow for thorough evaluation of the ocular posterior pole.[59,60] Direct ophthalmoscopy is usually performed with the patient's spectacles removed. However, if the spectacle lenses are clean and in good condition, a much more satisfactory view will be obtained if the patient's glasses are left in place when significant astigmatism or moderate to high degrees of myopia are present.

The optic disc is evaluated for its shape, color, peripapillary changes, vascular abnormalities, and the presence or absence of spontaneous venous pulsation.[61–64] Monocular cues are used to specifically evaluate the integrity of the disc rim tissue.[65] Deflection of the blood vessels as they course over the surface of the optic nerve will help to delineate the edge of the optic cup. Color differentials of the optic nerve head should not be used to define cup-disc ratios. Sloping cup margins will present as less defined rim tissue compared to steep cup margins. The distribution of laminar dots may suggest nerve rim erosion.[64] The presence of splinter disc hemorrhages suggests early optic nerve head damage.[67–69] Glaucomatous optic nerve head cupping is often more profound in patients with low-tension glaucoma compared to primary open-angle glaucoma.[70] Clinical experience along with supplemental testing will help the clinician distinguish glaucomatous cupping from large but physiological cupping.[71–73]

The horizontal and vertical cup-disc ratios are noted for each eye. Convention dictates that the horizontal dimension be listed first. Significant cup-disc ratio asymmetry between the two eyes is an important possible sign of glaucomatous change.[74,75] The best evaluative technique for accurately assessing the optic nerve head incorporates the use of subsequent stereoscopic techniques.

A complete direct ophthalmoscopic examination continues with systematic scanning of the retinal vasculature, fundus, and macular area. As an indicator of systemic vascular integrity, the retinal vessels are assessed for changes such as hypertensive or diabetic retinopathy. When evaluated in conjunction with other findings such as IOP measurement, optic nerve head assessment, and visual field analysis, this information will help cue the clinician as to whether the patient may have low-tension glaucoma or systemic disease risk factors that suggest more careful monitoring of IOPs or earlier treatment intervention. Use of the red-free (green) filter in the direct ophthalmoscope will help to enhance vascular changes, especially when evaluating for diabetic retinopathy. Signs of previous ocular trauma, such as choroidal rupture or macular holes in a young adult patient, may help to explain ipsilateral monocular elevations in IOP.[76]

Since the availability of 60D, 78D, and 90D auxiliary lenses for routine indirect fundus biomicroscopy, some clinicians no longer perform direct ophthalmoscopy on each patient.[59]

Binocular Indirect Ophthalmoscopy. Examination of the peripheral retina using binocular indirect ophthalmoscopy should be performed at each initial examination and at appropriate routine intervals thereafter. Of pertinence in evaluating a patient for glaucoma is detecting the presence of chorioretinal scars, other indicators of previous traumatic incidents, and peripheral retinal disease. Specifically, a patient with prominent lattice degeneration or atrophic retinal holes may be at risk for developing retinal detachment if placed on long-term antiglaucoma miotic therapy.[15] For these individuals, prophylactic treatment of the peripheral retinal lesions may be appropriate before glaucoma therapy is instituted.

A stereoscopic view of the optic nerve head will be obtained when evaluating the posterior pole with the binocular indirect ophthalmoscope. However, the reduced magnification of this stereoscopic image compared to that obtained using adjunct slit-lamp techniques reduces its diagnostic value for optic nerve head evaluation.

Slit-Lamp Examination Following Pupillary Dilation, Including Fundus Biomicroscopy. Slit-lamp examination following adequate pupillary dilation will allow for a complete assessment of the crystalline lens as well as stereoscopic examination of the fundus. Most crystalline lens changes that are pertinent to glaucoma are usually not detectable without pupillary dilation (Table 6–4).

Blunt or penetrating ocular trauma may cause late-stage secondary open-angle glaucoma that is typically unilateral. Traumatic changes involving the crystalline lens may include subluxation and rosette cataracts.[14,77,78] Posterior subcapsular cataracts also frequently develop from trauma, often with marked asymmetry between the two eyes. Focal lens opacities may be present along with corneal scars and iris defects due to penetrating injury. A past episode of acute IOP spiking, such as occurs during acute angle closure glaucoma, can produce focal lens opacities known as glaukomflecken. Lens opacities located posteriorly along the visual axis, e.g., age-related posterior subcapsular or congenital posterior polar, may preclude the use of therapeutic miotic drops if glaucoma is diagnosed.

The characteristic capsular changes of exfoliation (pseudoexfoliation) syndrome are frequently not apparent until after pupillary dilation.[79] Patients exhibiting exfoliation syndrome have a significantly higher risk of developing secondary open-angle glaucoma. Patients with pigment dispersion syndrome may have pigment deposition on the posterior surface of the crystalline lens known as posterior capsular pigmented ring. This arcuate or annular deposit is located peripherally on the posterior capsule where the zonules insert and will be best detected when the patient fixates off primary gaze.[80]

Stereoscopic evaluation of the fundus using the slit-lamp and auxiliary lenses (fundus biomicroscopy) is critical to effectively visualize the topography of the optic nerve.[81] Use of the 60D, 78D, or 90D lens in conjunction with the slit-lamp provides an inverted and reversed image of high resolution that can be viewed under varying magnification.[60] Since use of these lenses does not involve ocular contact, quick comparison of the optic nerve head between the two eyes can be made to assess symmetry of the cup-disc ratios. The red-free (green) filter of the slit-lamp can also be used in conjunction with these lenses to enhance vascular findings.

An alternative technique for noncontact evaluation of the optic nerve head with the slit-lamp is the Hruby lens. The Hruby lens is used much less frequently since the introduction of the 60D, 78D, and 90D lenses, which are easier to use and provide a better quality image. The advantage of the Hruby lens, however, is that it provides an upright, direct image of the optic nerve head.

Another technique for viewing an upright image of the optic nerve head is with the central portion of the 3-mirror retinal contact lens. This technique is particularly valuable for prolonged study of the optic nerve. Use of the 3-mirror contact lens typically induces a transient superficial punctate keratitis. If further techniques for evaluating the posterior segment such as retinal photography are anticipated at this

TABLE 6–4. CRYSTALLINE LENS AND RETINAL FINDINGS: POSSIBLE INDICATORS OF GLAUCOMA

Crystalline lens
- Rosette cataract
- Subluxation
- Exfoliation (pseudoexfoliation) syndrome
- Posterior capsular pigmented ring
- Opacity due to penetrating injury
- Glaukomflecken

Retina
- Chorioretinal scar
- Choroidal rupture
- Traumatic macular hole
- Retinal tear
- Retinal detachment
- Vascular occlusion(s)

visit, the use of a 3-mirror contact lens may be deferred to a subsequent appointment.

Fundus Photography. Fundus photography provides objective documentation of the optic nerve head, providing information with which to judge the development of nerve head changes over time. Since the patient is dilated at this stage of the examination, fundus photography can be performed at the initial visit. Stereophotography of the optic nerve head is the preferred technique for documenting and monitoring optic nerve head changes.[82]

Restricted spectrum illumination ("red-free") photography of the peripapillary nerve fiber layer may be performed to evaluate for areas of nerve fiber layer dropout, indicative of focal or diffuse optic nerve head damage. Although not routinely performed in most offices due to technical complexities, a number of reports of success with this technique have been published.[83–89]

Examination Assessment and Plan

For the majority of patients, the results of the initial route examination will indicate the absence of glaucoma. Evaluating the collective results of the examination as a whole will determine the appropriate interval for repeated routine examination. This examination interval is shortened for patients who have risk factors that may predispose them to the development of glaucoma.

Occasionally, a patient presents for routine examination in whom the diagnosis of primary open-angle glaucoma is unmistakeable: exceptionally high IOPs, obviously abnormal optic nerve heads, and extensive visual field loss as determined with visual field screening. For these patients, the immediate institution of glaucoma therapy is appropriate.

Periodically, a patient may present for examination, specifically for a second opinion, who is being treated for primary open-angle glaucoma by another eye care provider. In order to fully assess the appropriateness of the treatment, it is useful to have the patient discontinue the medication for a short time prior to the next examination. This is especially important if miotics are used so that reasonable pupillary dilation may be achieved. Caution must be used, however, since there may be instances in which the medication should not be discontinued. For example, the patient may have been prescribed a miotic due to narrow anterior chamber angles. If the patient has significant glaucomatous optic neuropathy, even minor IOP elevation due to medication discontinuance could have adverse effects.

For the majority of patients with primary open-

angle glaucoma or who are glaucoma suspects, the diagnosis is less definitive without further testing and the need for treatment is less immediate. The patient must be fully informed of the examination results and scheduled to return for further evaluative testing at an appropriate interval based on the results obtained from initial evaluation of the visual field, IOP, and optic nerve head. Scheduling the patient at a different time of the day from the initial evaluation will help to assess diurnal pressure variation. If the index of suspicion is high that the patient does, in fact, have glaucoma, proper practice management procedures must be in place to help ensure that the patient is not lost to follow-up.[90]

Patient Education

As with all chronic asymptomatic diseases, it is sometimes difficult to convey to the patient the importance of continued evaluation to monitor their condition. The use of visual aids and patient education materials, such as a model eye, to explain aqueous flow and to illustrate the location of the optic nerve, and even using the patient's own fundus photographs and visual field results can be helpful illustrative tools. With the patient's consent, having family members present to hear the explanation/discussion can be helpful, especially if the patient is elderly.

For some patients, the word "glaucoma" is associated with imminent blindness and can have devastating psychological effects. For this reason, a brief explanation in layman's terms of the pathophysiology involved before the term "glaucoma" is introduced will help to increase understanding and, hopefully, allay inappropriate concern. It is a patient management challenge to explain to the patient at an appropriate level the findings of your examination and the need to return for necessary supplemental testing without causing undue alarm. When the need for treatment is imminent or when patient compliance is poor, more pointed discussions with the patient are needed with detailed record documentation. The use of written patient educational materials that describe glaucoma and its treatment modalities helps to reinforce in-office explanations.[91,92]

COMPLETING THE EVALUATION OF THE GLAUCOMA PATIENT OR SUSPECT

Rationale for at Least a Second Visit

As with systemic hypertension, primary open-angle glaucoma is seldom definitively diagnosed at the initial visit, although the index of suspicion may vary widely based on testing results. The follow-up evaluative appointment will allow for completion of addi-

TABLE 6–5. SUGGESTED PROTOCOL FOR COMPLETING THE EVALUATION OF THE GLAUCOMA PATIENT OR SUSPECT

Visual acuities
Threshold visual field testing
Applanation tonometry
Gonioscopy
Dilated fundus examination
Additional testing as indicated:
    Physical diagnosis
    Spatial contrast sensitivity testing
    Detailed color vision testing

tional testing that is important to the diagnosis of glaucoma but is generally not included in the initial routine examination.

As discussed in detail elsewhere in this book, one of the important outcomes of collecting clinical data on the glaucoma suspect is to determine at what point the elevated IOP has affected visual function. Intensive research efforts are underway in an effort to identify visual function tests as well as objective measures of the optic nerve head and juxtapapillary area that are sensitive and specific enough to detect early damage from glaucoma, yet are cost effective and accessible in an office setting. The use of appropriate diagnostic psychophysical tests must also take into account the nature of optic nerve axonal loss inherent in the aging process.[93]

Tests included in this section for completing the evaluation of the glaucoma patient or suspect are those most commonly performed in office at this time (Table 6–5). Table 6–6 includes a listing of visual function tests and objective assessments of structural

TABLE 6–6. VISUAL FUNCTION/ANATOMICAL ASSESSMENT TESTS UNDER STUDY FOR EARLIER DIAGNOSIS OF PRIMARY OPEN-ANGLE GLAUCOMA

Multiflash campimetry
Computerized image analysis of optic nerve head topography
Color contrast sensitivity
Flash electroretinography
Pattern electroretinography (PERG)
Photostress recovery time
Two-pulse temporal resolution
Dynamic contrast sensitivity
Peripheral contrast sensitivity
Temporal contrast sensitivity
Pattern visually evoked potential (PVEP)
Computerized image enhancement of the peripapillary nerve fiber layer
Fluorescein angiography
Quantitative neuroretinal rim assessment

optic nerve damage that are being studied in research settings to enhance the clinician's ability to detect primary open-angle glaucoma at an earlier stage. These and other tests will likely form the foundation for the in-office tests of tomorrow.[94–114]

Examination Protocol

Visual Acuity Measurement. See Visual Acuity Measurement under Initial Routine Examination above.

Perimetry. Since the introduction of automated threshold visual field testing instruments that are affordable and readily available in private offices, this technique has become the standard of care for evaluating patients for glaucoma as well as for monitoring the control of their disease while on treatment. Unfortunately, this technique is not without its shortcomings. For example, automated threshold visual field testing can prove to be tiresome for some elderly patients so that fixation losses are frequent and reliability poor. When visual field defects are present, the results will be even more variable on repeat testing so that more than one field evaluation may be necessary to confirm the presence and extent of a defect.[115,116] Interpreting the results of automated perimetry and the establishment of criteria for real changes in visual fields from glaucoma over time are issues of concern for the clinician.

For some patients, Goldmann bowl perimetry using static and kinetic techniques may be the preferred instrument for visual field analysis. Some of the newer models of automated visual field instruments also have capability for kinetic field testing. Occasionally, a patient is unable to cooperate for any detailed visual field test. In these instances, the clinician must rely primarily on data obtained from IOP measurement and optic nerve head appearance, weighing those results with risk factors in the patient's history.

Some clinicians advocate performing threshold visual field testing after pupillary dilation. This technique may allow for more consistent control of pupil size during subsequent visual field testing and will eliminate overall sensitivity reductions due to miosis, especially in the elderly patient. Whether visual field testing is done with the patient's pupils dilated or undilated, repeat testing must be conducted under the same conditions.[117]

Applanation Tonometry. Intraocular pressure measurement is repeated using applanation tonometry. Remeasuring the IOP at a different time of the day will allow for some assessment of diurnal IOP variation. The IOP may be found to be unchanged, higher or lower than the original reading. Patients with chronic open-angle glaucoma tend to exhibit exaggerated diurnal IOP variations compared to normal patients.[118,119] Patients with pigmentary glaucoma, a form of secondary open-angle glaucoma, may exhibit diurnal IOP swings as high as 10 to 20 mm Hg.

Gonioscopy. If gonioscopy was not performed during the initial examination, it must be performed at the second visit. Gonioscopy can be performed using a variety of appropriate goniolenses, but the 4-mirror goniolens allows for indentation gonioscopy to ascertain whether appositional abnormalities are present in eyes with narrow angles.[40] If narrow angles are observed through gonioscopy and glaucoma treatment is indicated, epinephrine drugs may be contraindicated due to a tendency to cause pupillary dilation. Strong miotic drops may also be contraindicated due to the potential for relative pupillary block with subsequent angle closure.

Table 6–7 lists anterior chamber angle findings that may be associated with glaucoma.[11,12,120]

Dilated Fundus Examination. Dilated fundus examination may be repeated at this visit for fundus photography, evaluation of the nerve fiber layer, or stereoscopic examination of the optic nerve head if these procedures were not included at the initial examination.

Additional Testing. Physical and psychophysical testing to complement the initial examination protocol may be added by the clinician as deemed appropriate. The tests described in this section are those that are more commonly used in the clinical setting. Much research is ongoing to determine readily available, cost-effective techniques that will reliably facilitate the early diagnosis of primary open-angle glaucoma.[121]

Physical Tests. Remeasurement of the blood pressure as part of the completion evaluation may assist in decision making for initiating glaucoma therapy. For example, patients with poorly controlled hypertension may be poor candidates for topical epinephrine therapy. Measurement of the resting pulse rate will help to detect patients with bradycardia, who may be poor candidates for treatment with topical nonselective beta adrenergic blocking agents.

Laboratory analysis, either ordered independently by the optometrist or in conjunction with the patient's primary care physician, may play an important role in the assessment and subsequent treatment of the glaucoma patient. For example, measurement of blood sugar levels will provide indication of the control of diabetes mellitus, an important risk factor in the development of glaucoma. Pulmonary function testing may be an important consideration for certain patients requiring treatment with topical beta adrenergic blocking agents. Investigators have considered laboratory tests such as blood flow measurements, coagulation tests, biochemical variables, plasma and blood viscosities, and autonomic nerve function to evaluate possible pathogenic aspects of glaucoma.[122–126]

Spatial Contrast Sensitivity Testing. Contrast sensitivity testing has evolved over the past 20 to 30 years into clinically applicable techniques that are intended to assess visual "quality" as a component of visual function. Although these tests are not yet diagnostically specific, studies have shown that certain ocular diseases produce selective spatial frequency deficits, while others result in uniform loss across a wide range of frequencies.[127] It has been reported that patients with glaucoma will exhibit deficits in the low-to-middle spatial frequency ranges. Others have noted that contrast sensitivity loss for patients with glaucoma does not exhibit spatial frequency selectivity.[128,129] Lundh suggests that central contrast sensitivity testing to static patterns possesses poor glaucoma screening potential.[95] Temporally modulated stimuli appear most sensitive in detecting glaucoma. The clinical challenge occurs when assessing the effect of glaucoma on contrast sensitivity in elderly patients. In this patient group, contrast sensitivity function may be reduced due to findings unrelated to glaucoma, such as pupillary miosis, media opacities, and macular abnormalities.[130]

Color Vision Testing. Acquired blue, blue-yellow, and blue-green color vision defects appear to be more commonly found in certain patients with ocular hypertension and glaucoma.[129,131,132] It is likely that these defects are the result of diffuse rather than localized nerve fiber layer loss.[133] A number of studies have used the Farnsworth-Munsell 100-Hue test,

TABLE 6–7. ANTERIOR CHAMBER ANGLE FINDINGS THAT MAY BE ASSOCIATED WITH GLAUCOMA

Angle recession
Dense angle pigmentation
Sampaolesi's line
Peripheral anterior synechiae
Exfoliative debris
Angle rubeosis
Angle cleavage abnormalities

which is not commonly used clinically, to assess glaucoma-related color vision defects.[133–136] One of the more sensitive clinically practical tests for detecting color vision defects is the Farnsworth D-15 panel test administered monocularly using the Macbeth lamp. A desaturated version of the D-15 test is even more sensitive to early subtle acquired defects.[131] When frank optic nerve damage is present due to asymmetrical glaucoma, red desaturation may be present in the affected eye.[137]

Provocative Testing. Provocative tests are intended to help differentiate glaucoma suspects from individuals who have or will develop some type of glaucoma. Whereas tests such as water drinking, tonography, topical steroid response testing, and phenylephrine provocative testing for pigmentary dispersion syndrome were once commonly used as diagnostic tests for primary open-angle glaucoma, their clinical usefulness today is limited.[4,19,56,138] Provocative tests for angle closure glaucoma that may be of diagnostic value in patients with narrow angles include the dark room test, the prone dark room test, and the mydriatic test.[4,39,55]

Examination Assessment and Plan

The results of this examination, viewed collectively with results from the initial routine examination, should provide the clinical information to indicate whether or not the patient requires treatment for glaucoma. If visual function tests are found to be normal with a corresponding normal appearance of the optic nerve head yet IOPs are elevated, the patient may be classified as ocular hypertensive. Depending on such issues as the degree of IOP elevation and the presence or absence of other risk factors, the patient may be monitored every 3 to 6 months. Data obtained at the initial examination as well as in the course of the completion evaluation visit will then serve as baseline information against which the results of future visits can be compared. Observed changes in testing results in the future may indicate the need for glaucoma therapy. During patient follow-up care, it is important that the optometrist monitor not only IOP readings but also the optic nerve and visual function.[3]

The initial and completion examinations may indicate that glaucoma therapy is needed. Besides the diagnostic role of these tests, the results will also provide indication as to the targeted pressure reductions desirable under treatment to prevent additional glaucomatous functional loss. The details of drug indications, contraindications, first drug of choice, multidrug therapy, and so forth are covered elsewhere in this book. However, the pneumonic "ALARM" helps

TABLE 6–8. MNEMONIC FOR PERTINENT GLAUCOMA TREATMENT CONSIDERATIONS

A = Angle:	when narrow avoid epinephrine and strong miotics
L = Lens:	avoid miotics with central cataracts
A = Aphakia:	avoid epinephrine (CME) and strong miotics (RD)
R = Retina:	avoid miotics with significant peripheral retinal disease
M = Medical/medications:	oral beta blockers, asthma, severe hypertension, cardiac abnormalities, and so forth have implications for treatment choices

to highlight important information obtained in the initial and completion evaluations that is pivotal to glaucoma drug use (Table 6–8). Appropriate first-line glaucoma treatment is generally begun at the completion evaluation with a return appointment scheduled to determine the response to medication.

Patient Education

At the conclusion of diagnostic testing, the nature of the assessment and management plan are shared with the patient, as well as family members, if appropriate. If no treatment is necessary and the patient is to be monitored, it is once again important to share sufficient information with the patient to ensure his or her return, while not instilling undue alarm. If treatment is instituted, time is taken to explain the nature of the medication, instillation technique (with in-office demonstration if necessary), as well as potential side effects. As with all therapeutic regimens, an appropriate follow-up appointment is scheduled with instructions to call or return sooner if problems are noted. Appropriate practice management procedures must be in place to help ensure that the patient is not lost to follow-up.

THE GLAUCOMA PATIENT PRESENTING FOR ACUTE EYE CARE

Although patients with primary open-angle glaucoma are usually asymptomatic, patients with secondary open-angle glaucoma or angle closure glaucoma can develop symptoms that may prompt the patient to present to the optometrist for nonroutine, acute eye care. In the course of thorough, problem-oriented clinical assessment, the specific diagnosis is then made.

Conversely, the optometrist may examine a patient for an acute eye care problem that is completely unrelated to glaucoma, such as conjunctivitis or blepharitis, and in the course of evaluation, clinical signs suggestive of undiagnosed primary open-angle glaucoma are detected. Inclusion of IOP measurement and direct ophthalmoscopic examination of the posterior pole in the acute eye care protocol allows the optometrist to provide a valuable service to the patient.

The optometrist's office staff must be properly trained so that patients requiring acute eye care are scheduled appropriately, based on the nature and duration of their symptoms.

Rationale for Examination Protocol

A systematic routine for evaluation of a patient presenting for acute eye care helps to ensure that no findings are overlooked and that appropriate differential diagnosis is made. The protocol indicated in this section is suggested for a patient new to the office. It can be modified based on the professional judgment of the optometrist to add or eliminate tests, particularly if the patient has been previously examined.[139] Table 6–9 lists the components of a suggested Acute Eye Care Protocol.

For each of the protocol components listed below, some of the anticipated results related to glaucoma are included, but these are by no means all inclusive.

Examination Protocol

History. History taking is directed toward symptomatology associated with the acute problem. Patients presenting with secondary open-angle glaucoma or acute angle closure glaucoma often have one or more of the following signs and symptoms, typically in only one eye: ocular pain, blurred vision, conjunctival injection, headaches, and nausea or vomiting. Pertinent ocular and systemic history should be elicited, such as recent trauma or pre-existing eye conditions. Stress has been suggested as a precipitant of acute angle closure glaucoma.[140]

Visual Acuity Measurement. Visual acuity may be normal or it may be reduced in the affected eye. Pinhole measurement is taken if the entering visual acuity is less than expected.

Pupillary Reflexes. The involved pupil may be observed to be fixed and dilated in acute angle closure glaucoma. Iridoplegia may be observed following ocular trauma. An eye with uveitic glaucoma may exhibit miosis.

Versions. No direct diagnostic value for glaucoma is expected with this test. However, it is an important consideration for the patient who has sustained acute eye or head trauma. Pain experienced on extraocular muscle movement may be associated with optic neuritis.

Auxiliary Tests As Indicated. Confrontation visual field screening quickly assesses for gross visual field loss. Red desaturation in one eye is suggestive of optic nerve dysfunction. A red lens held over one eye during versional testing helps to identify a paretic extraocular muscle.

External Examination with Penlight or Transilluminator. This preliminary ocular health evaluation will provide for an overview assessment of globe injection, discharge, lid edema, and so forth.

Preauricular Lymph Node Palpation. Although not related to glaucoma diagnoses, palpation of the preauricular lymph node is important in differentially diagnosing anterior segment infectious conditions.

Slit-Lamp Biomicroscopy. Corneal edema is usually present in acute angle closure glaucoma. Keratic precipitates and an active anterior chamber reaction may suggest uveitic glaucoma when severe or glaucomatocyclitic crisis when mild if the IOP is found to be elevated.[141] Hyphema may precipitate hemolytic glaucoma. Rubeosis irides may herald neovascular glaucoma, a result of conditions such as diabetes mellitus, central retinal vein occlusion, and carotid artery disease. Van Herick angle assessment will suggest the presence of acute angle closure glaucoma.

TABLE 6–9. SUGGESTED ACUTE EYE CARE EXAMINATION PROTOCOL

History
Visual acuity measurement
Pupillary reflexes
Versions
Auxiliary tests as indicated, such as:
Confrontation field screening
Red desaturation test
Red lens test
External examination with penlight or transilluminator
Preauricular lymph node palpation
Slit-lamp biomicroscopy
Tonometry as indicated
Gonioscopy if indicated
Direct ophthalmoscopy
Dilated fundus examination if indicated

VISION SCREENING PATIENT INFORMATION FORM
WALKER EYE CLINIC/IU SCHOOL OF OPTOMETRY

DATE: _____ SCREENING LOCATION: _____

NAME: LAST_____ FIRST_____ MID. INT. _____

ADDRESS: _____ CITY: _____

STATE: _____ ZIP: _____ BIRTH DATE: _____ SEX: _____

HOME TELEPHONE: _____ WORK TELEPHONE: _____

OCCUPATION/HOBBIES: _____

Do you now have glasses or contact lenses?   YES   NO   If yes, which? _____

How old are they? _____ When do you use them? _____

Approximately how long has it been since your last eye examination? _____

Where was it done? _____

Are you having any problems with your eyes? YES   NO   If yes, briefly describe:

_____

Do you have frequent headaches?   YES   NO

Have you ever had any eye injuries, infections, surgery, etc.?   YES   NO

Have you ever been told that you have glaucoma or any other serious eye problem?   YES   NO

Have there been any serious eye problems in your immediate family?   YES   NO

Are you now under a doctor's medical care?   YES   NO   Doctor's name: _____

When was your last visit? _____ Are you due to go back soon? _____

Are you taking **ANY** medication?   YES   NO

Do you have any allergies, including allergies to medicine?   YES   NO

If yes, list briefly_____

How did you hear about the vision screening program? _____

I give permission for my self/child to participate in a vision screening conducted by the Walker Eye Clinic.
I understand that this is not a complete eye examination and that no prescription will be given.

PATIENT/GUARDIAN SIGNATURE: _____

WITNESS: _____

Figure 6–2. A sample patient information form that may be used for glaucoma screenings. Note the consent statement at the bottom. This is the front of a two-sided form with Figure 6–1.

it is helpful to schedule patients every few minutes to provide for smooth and regular "flow."

Patient Demographics and History. In the screening setting, this information is usually best collected by having the patient complete the first part of a screening examination form on which the questions have been written in layman's terms (Fig. 6–2). If available, the on-site screening coordinator may distribute forms to the participants as they present for testing, ensuring that the information is completed. The history is an abbreviated one to elicit key informational points:

- Patient name, age, sex, race, and address
- Chief complaint, if any
- Length of time since last eye examination

- Significant general health problems, such as diabetes or high blood pressure
- Family history of glaucoma
- Current medication usage

More detailed or comprehensive patient history information may be elicited if time permits or if desired by the optometrist. This questionnaire may also serve as a consent form so that the patient acknowledges his or her understanding of the limitations of scope of the glaucoma screening (Fig. 6–2).

Visual Acuity Measurement. Monocular distance and near visual acuities are tested using standard Snellen visual acuity charts. If available, lay personnel may be trained to conduct this component of the screening.

Referral for full examination is usually recommended if the visual acuity is measured to be 20/40 or less in either eye.

Tonometry. The noncontact tonometer (NCT, American Optical) is the instrument of choice for most glaucoma screenings.[160] It has good reliability, requires no ocular contact, and, with moderate training, can be operated by lay people. For maximum accuracy, a minimum of three readings per eye is suggested.[158] Averaging three readings with a spread of 3 mm Hg or less, or using the median of three readings has been suggested.[161] An accepted NCT referral criterion for public screenings is 24 mm Hg and above. Regardless of the absolute reading, referral is also indicated if a difference of more than 5 mm Hg between the two eyes is obtained.

Additional noncontact tonometers have become available in recent years, such as the Pulsair by Keeler.[46] This instrument has several advantages over the standard NCT, including portability, easier usage with children, and greater accuracy of readings on distorted corneas. However, due to instrument variability, an averaging of four readings per eye is necessary to ensure accurate IOP measurement.

Optic Nerve Head Assessment. Assessment of the optic nerve head during a glaucoma screening is typically performed with a direct ophthalmoscope. Although direct ophthalmoscopy through an undilated pupil may be challenging, it can usually be accurately performed by an experienced practitioner.[59] Investigators in one study used black and white photographs taken with a non-mydriatic fundus camera to screen for glaucomatous optic nerve head changes.[162]

Referral criteria for optic nerve head assessment are typically based on a cup-disc ratio of 0.5 or greater in the vertical dimension, or an overall cup-disc ratio difference greater than 0.2 between the two eyes.[157] Despite the observed cup-disc ratio size, the presence of other monocular cues that suggest glaucomatous changes, such as a splinter hemorrhage or rim notching, also warrants referral for full stereoscopic evaluation. Lastly, if visualization of the optic nerve head is impossible during the glaucoma screening due to factors such as pupil size or media opacity, referral for further examination is recommended.

Visual Field Screening. Automated visual field screening may be incorporated into the glaucoma screening protocol when appropriate personnel and equipment are available.[3,157] For example, a glaucoma screening conducted in the optometrist's office might include an automated visual field screening. For the most part, however, the inclusion of visual field testing has not lent itself well to efficient glaucoma screenings in mass populations. Other types of psychophysical tests that are rapid, inexpensive, "patient friendly," and easy to interpret may be developed in the future and can be incorporated into glaucoma screenings as a more sensitive assessment of visual function.[48]

Referral is indicated if visual field screening results suggest glaucomatous changes.

Patient Education/Referral and Follow-Up

At the conclusion of the glaucoma screening, the testing results are reviewed with the patient. It is very important that the patient participating in a glaucoma screening once again understand the limitations of the screening and that it does not substitute for thorough, in-office eye care. A written statement to that effect should be included on any screening-related materials distributed to the patient. Most screening results can be categorized as follows:

- "Pass"—Screening results are within normal limits; continue regular routine care
- "Fail/Referral Indicated"—Advised to seek further care
- "Under active care"—Continue doctor's recommendations

A patient may "fail" the glaucoma screening due to visual acuity results, tonometry measurement, optic nerve head assessment, visual field findings, an inappropriately long period of time since the last routine examination, or by reporting a chief complaint that should be investigated. Certainly, other detected abnormalities that are not directly related to glaucoma may also warrant referral.

Ideally, a written copy of the results is given to the patient at the conclusion of the screening (Fig. 6–3). If he or she "passed" the screening and is established with an eye care provider, this written information can be provided to the practitioner by the patient.

To maximize effectiveness, glaucoma screenings should include some means for follow-up of recommendations or referrals made as a result of the screening process. Budgetary considerations and personnel availability may determine how thoroughly this aspect can be implemented. If a recommendation of "Fail/Referral" is made, the patient may be given a completed glaucoma screening referral form to take to an eye care provider (Fig. 6–4). The evaluating doctor's office then completes the referral report form and returns it to the screening individual/organization. After an appropriate length of time, if no report

159. Werner DL, Field S. A mammoth vision screening—Public relations and public service. *J Am Optom Assoc.* 1982;53:731–737.
160. Olander KW, Higuchi B, Zimmerman TJ. Update on screening for glaucoma. *Ann Ophthalmol.* 1987;19:366–367.
161. Brown B, DaRin D. Comparison of Keeler and Reichert non-contact tonometers. *Clin Exp Optom.* 1989;72:98–101.
162. Tuulonen A, Airaksinen PJ, Montagna A, Nieminen H. Screening for glaucoma with a non-mydriatic fundus camera. *Acta Ophthalmol (Copenh).* 1990;68:445–449.

Chapter 7

TONOMETRY

Peter A. Lalle

The introduction of the Maklokof and Schiotz tonometers at the turn of the century allowed the measurement of intraocular pressure (IOP) to become a simple, in-office procedure. Further improvement in design and accuracy occurred in the late 1950s with the introduction of Goldmann tonometry. The dawn of the "electronic age" in the late 1960s introduced the McKay-Marg tonometer, quickly followed by the noncontact tonometer (AONCT) in the early 1970s. The 1980s introduced microchip capability, allowing reduction in size and improvement in ease of operation of the electronic tonometers. Yet despite these advances in design and technology, tonometers are still usually based on one of two techniques: indentation or applanation.

PRINCIPLES OF TONOMETRY

Indentation

Indentation tonometry is similar in concept to pushing your thumb into a basketball to check the pressure, the more air in the ball the greater the amount of effort required to indent its surface. Indentation tonometry involves measuring the resisting force of the IOP to pushing on the cornea with a known weight or force until it bows backwards. The amount of indentation will vary inversely to the IOP. The results of indentation tonometry are influenced by the rigidity of the cornea and sclera to indentation (the stiffness of the rubber skin of the basketball). This rigidity varies from eye to eye and introduces a potential measurement error. With indentation tonometry, there is a simultaneous, significant outflow of aqueous reducing the IOP and causing repeated tonometry readings to decrease.

Applanation

The Imbert-Fick formula states that:

$$\text{Pressure (IOP)} = \text{force/area}$$

Intraocular pressure is determined by measuring either force or area while holding the other variables constant. For instance, Goldmann tonometry takes a given area of the cornea and measures the force required to flatten it to a plano surface. Therefore, IOP is directly related to the force needed to flatten (not indent) the cornea.

The area of the cornea that is flattened (applanated) is always the same for every patient. However, the amount of force that is necessary to push against the patient's cornea to flatten it to a known

TABLE 7–3. ADVANTAGES AND DISADVANTAGES OF NCT

Advantages	Disadvantages
Accurate when compared to a Goldmann tonometer, varies slightly when IOP is >30 mm	Some patients are apprehensive of the "puff," and refuse measurement
Requires no anesthetic	Expensive
Displaces virtually no aqueous, allowing repeatable readings	Bulky, heavy, requires separate table
Can be delegated to technician with little training	Cannot be calibrated or fixed by user
No damage to corneal epithelium	Cannot be used on restricted patients (Reichert version)
Takes little time with a cooperative patient	Uncooperative patients can be time consuming
Can measure cornea through soft lens, allowing edematous corneas to be measured	Repeat readings required since single reading may be measuring height of ocular pulse
Portable model (Keeler) can be used for restricted patients	Edematous corneas cannot be measured (see above)

electromechanically braked and the instrument then computes the IOP based on the amount of air pressure at the time of applanation. In previous designs, the piston did not stop and a forceful puff was delivered to every eye. Since the piston now stops at the instant of applanation, most eyes receive a puff of air with less force than on prior models.

Because the instrument takes an instantaneous reading, it will measure the IOP at various points along the ocular pulse. With Goldmann, the "average" reading is taken by visually midpositioning the mires. With the XPERT version of the NCT, three readings are taken per eye, and the machine will automatically print all three as well as the average. In large scale screenings, it is not necessary to take all three readings if at least one measurement is less than 20 mm Hg.

Like the Goldmann tonometer, poor results are obtained with an edematous cornea. However, IOP can be determined through a soft contact lens.[11,12] In the case of an irregular or edematous cornea, a thin, soft contact lens can be placed on the eye (in effect giving a smooth surface) and IOP then measured by either the Goldmann or noncontact tonometer. The only contraindication is if the cornea cannot tolerate a contact lens (Table 7–3).

The method for checking calibration in the office is only an electronic verification, which still needs to be validated with another instrument. Check the patient with the NCT first and immediately verify the reading with a Goldmann tonometer. Studies have shown that when comparing two Goldmann tonometers, they will agree within 1 to 3 mm Hg of each other.[7] Therefore, the averaged NCT reading should be within 2 to 3 mm Hg of the Goldmann reading. It is recommended that this check be performed quarterly, more often if the instrument has recently been transported, e.g., to a screening.

Only the chin and forehead rest need to be wiped with alcohol after every use; there is nothing to sterilize. Occasionally, the video lens should be cleaned, since it can become soiled by lashes and tears.

Pneumotonometer. This instrument also arrived in the 1970s and has the ability to measure IOP with the patient in any position.[3] Its main use has been in hospitals and clinics where patients frequently present in wheelchairs and stretchers. It is also valuable for measuring the IOP of infants. A tired, hungry baby is first given anesthetic drops and then its bottle. Most infants will soon fall asleep. The sleeping baby can be held over a parent's shoulder, the lids held open, and a reading taken. It is also used in the immediate postoperative period on patients whose corneas are irregular or edematous since it is more accurate than the Goldmann tonometer in these situations.

The instrument consists of a source of pressurized gas, a handpiece, and a console (Fig. 7–8). A piston with a hollow core is driven out of a handpiece by gas pressure. The gas can be supplied by either a pressurized can or a small compressor that uses room

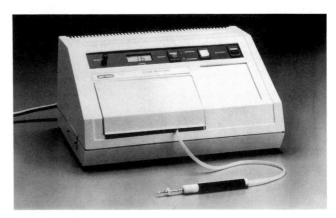

Figure 7–8. Digilab pneumotonometer. Console with a digital readout. Probe is in the foreground. (*Courtesy of BIO-RAD, Cambridge, MA.*)

air. Gas flows down the inside of the piston into a small, flexible tube before entering a tiny pancake-shaped chamber. The ocular-surface side of this chamber is a flexible membrane, 5 mm in diameter with the other side being a round disc with holes in which the gas escapes. As the membrane is pushed against the convex cornea, it bows back into the chamber until it covers up the escape holes. This creates a back pressure in the hollow core of the piston that is electromechanically measured in the console. The pressure inside the piston increases until it pushes the front of the membrane and the cornea back, reopening the escape holes and restoring the flow of gas (Fig. 7–9). The IOP is determined at this point, reflecting the amount of pressure needed to maintain a flow of gas when against the cornea. It can be displayed as a printed waveform or a digital read-out at the console. The waveform gives a continuous, on-going reading, while the digital display gives an on-going average.

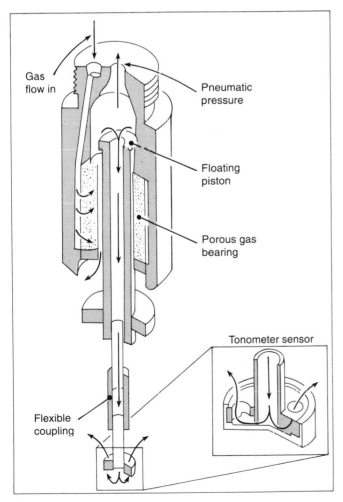

Figure 7–9. Digilab pneumotonometer. Cross-section of pneumotonometer probe tip.

The technique requires the eye be anesthetized with proparacaine. Avoid viscous combination drops as they can clog the membrane's escape holes. The piston in the handpiece will jump forward when pressurized and, therefore, it should be facing away from the patient when the gas is turned on. The lids are controlled if necessary and the probe tip is pressed lightly against the apex of the cornea. The probe tip must be held against the cornea for a minimum of 5 seconds, but no more than 10 seconds. The reading is initially higher in the first 1 to 2 seconds. On average, the pneumotonometer will slightly overestimate the IOP as compared to Goldmann tonometry. Although considered an applanation tonometer, this instrument will displace a significant amount of aqueous with each reading. Repeated readings, therefore, will be lower than the initial one and care should be taken in patients with shallow or flat anterior chambers[13] (Table 7–4).

For calibration, the instrument is provided with a pressurized membrane connected to a pressure gauge. The probe tip is positioned against the pressurized membrane and the instrument's reading is compared to the pressure gauge. However, there is a wide variability between machines and it is strongly recommended that frequent comparisons be made with another tonometer to verify calibration.

The tip should be liberally swabbed with alcohol to disinfect. It is not practical to remove the tip for cleaning after each use.

TABLE 7–4. ADVANTAGES AND DISADVANTAGES OF PNEUMOTONOMETER

Advantages

More accurate than Goldmann with irregular corneas (not as accurate as McKay-Marg)

Very quick with a cooperative patient

Can be used in any position, especially with restricted patients. Used extensively in infants and patients in wheelchairs and stretchers

Compact, light-weight, portable

Can be delegated, easy to use

Minimal, if any, epithelial damage

Permanent copy of readings available

Disadvantages

Not as accurate as Goldmann or NCT

Anesthesia required

Moderately expensive instrument

Expensive supplies (gas and membranes)

Displaces a significant amount of aqueous, inaccurate for repeat readings

Calibration is tedious; if out of calibration, must go back to factory

Patient must be able to hold eye still for at least 5 seconds

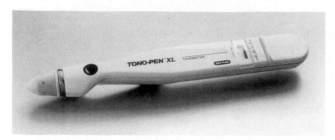

Figure 7–10. Oculab Tono-Pen. Disposable probe covering in place. (*Courtesy of BIO-RAD, Cambridge, MA.*)

MacKay-Marg Tonometer and Tono-Pen. The MacKay-Marg tonometer was first introduced for the purpose of taking IOP readings through the sclera without the need for anesthesia. These readings were not accurate and only those taken through an anesthetized cornea proved valid.[14] The original instrument's readings were in the form of a printed waveform that was difficult to obtain and interpret. A lot of skill was required to master this instrument and many users became quickly discouraged.

The principles of the MacKay-Marg tonometer have been incorporated into a new instrument, the Tono-Pen. The advent of microchip technology has allowed many internal refinements and miniaturization.[15] The entire instrument is contained within a large, tubular handpiece that has a small footplate at the end (Fig. 7–10). Within the footplate is a small, protruding plunger (a sensitive electrical position transducer). As the instrument is pushed against the cornea, both the corneal rigidity and the IOP resists indentation and the plunger is forced back into the footplate. When the cornea is flattened by the foot-

plate, corneal rigidity is largely negated and an equilibrium exists between the plunger's force and IOP. The IOP is determined when the tip of the plunger is in the same plane as the footplate.

Four valid readings per eye are taken, with internal circuits determining if a reading was valid or not. The readings are displayed as a digital readout eliminating the waveform printout. The digital display also shows a percent indication as to how much the lowest and highest readings vary.

Each instrument is internally calibrated by the factory, but should be periodically checked against another tonometer. The Tono-Pen tends to overestimate low IOPs and underestimate high IOPs. Like the original instrument, the probe tip is covered with a single-use, disposable cover to insure a sterile tip for each use.

Its accuracy when compared to the Goldmann tonometer is only fair, making it not recommended for routine office use.[16] However, its greatest asset is that it is the most accurate of all tonometers when used on a scarred or edematous cornea, especially with postoperative patients. It can also be performed on patients in any position. Combined with its portability, it is very useful for hospital or nursing home rounds (Table 7–5).

Schiotz. From the early 1900s through the late 1960s, Schiotz tonometry was the accepted standard. However, the need for anesthesia kept it out of most optometrists' offices. By the time diagnostic drugs became available, the Goldmann tonometer had replaced it as the standard. Because of this, most optometrists are not familiar with the instrument. Its simple, highly portable, and inexpensive design makes it the ideal back-up tonometer for the modern office (Table 7–6).

TABLE 7–5. ADVANTAGES AND DISADVANTAGES OF THE TONO-PEN

Advantages	Disadvantages
Most accurate tonometer with a scarred or edematous cornea	Accuracy not reliable enough for routine office use
Fairly quick with a cooperative patient	Since the instrument interprets the waveform, there is no way to verify the accuracy of a reading
Minimal disruption to corneal epithelium (usually)	Calibration of the handpiece is factory set, must be checked frequently by comparison to other instrument
Can be used in restricted patients	No user serviceable parts, expensive to repair
Portable, compact, light-weight, ideal for hospital and nursing home rounds	Requires anesthesia to obtain reliable results
	Expensive instrument, requires supplies (tonotips)
	Displaces significant amount of aqueous, may affect repeatability
	Influenced by external pressure of fingers or lids

TABLE 7–6. ADVANTAGES AND DISADVANTAGES OF SCHIOTZ TONOMETRY

Advantages	Disadvantages
Reliable, mechanically simple, no electronic component	Patients very apprehensive with procedure
Very inexpensive to buy and maintain	Anesthesia required
Calibration simple to check	Patient positioning is cumbersome and time consuming
Can be used on restricted patients	Good patient cooperation is required
	Corneal abrasion a distinct possibility with uncooperative patients
	Readily influenced by external pressure or poor technique
	Must be disassembled after each use to clean and disinfect
	Must be performed by doctor, rarely delegated
	Displaces significant amount of aqueous, affecting repeatability

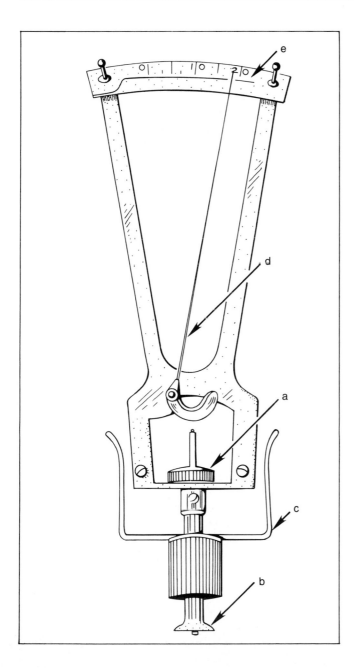

Of all tonometers, the Schiotz, since it is an indentation tonometer, is most influenced by ocular rigidity requiring that measurements on a high myope or high hyperope patient be confirmed with an applanation instrument.

A weighted plunger inside of a footplate surrounded by an outer sleeve is brought in contact with and indents the cornea (Fig. 7–11). The amount of indentation is related to the weight of the plunger and inversely related to IOP and ocular rigidity. The amount of indentation is measured by a lever resting on top of the plunger, with a pointer connected to the lever. For each 0.05 mm that the plunger indents the cornea, the pointer moves up one marking on the scale. With an IOP of 16 mm, the scale reading is 5.5, which represents only 0.275 mm of indentation. Eyes with elevated IOPs will have smaller scale readings. The measuring scale is logarhythmic with the lower scale values representing a disproportionate range of IOP values. Therefore, eyes with increased IOP need more weight on the plunger to further indent the cornea and get a higher, more accurate scale reading.

The tonometer is assembled with the 5.5-gram weight attached to the plunger. If additional weights are needed, they are added on top of the 5.5-gram weight. The eye is anesthetized with proparacaine. Viscous combination drops can affect accuracy by gumming up the cylinder in which the plunger travels. The patient is reclined so that the eyes are able to look straight up. The doctor stands either behind the patient or to one side. Have the patient hold up his or

Figure 7–11. Schiotz tonometer: (a) weighted plunger; (b) footplate; (c) outer sleeve; (d) pointer; (e) scale.

her hand and look at the thumb for fixation. Make sure the measuring scale is visible before placing the tonometer on the eye. Gently place the footplate on the cornea and continue to bring the tonometer a few millimeters further down so that the outer sleeve of the tonometer is floating freely. Note the scale reading and gently remove the tonometer. The needle may be seen to pulsate in some patients (ocular pulse), and the midpoint between the highest and lowest reading should be used. A table is supplied to convert the scale reading to pressure in mm Hg.

Any scale reading below 3 needs to be repeated with a heavier weight. Place the 7.5-gram weight on top of the initial 5.5-gram weight. (The weight marked "7.5" is actually a 2-gram weight that equals 7.5 grams when added on top of the 5.5. The "10" gram weight is likewise added on top of "5.5" and "7.5" to equal 10 grams.) Increasing weight is added until a scale reading of at least 3 is obtained.

Before each use, calibration should be checked by placing the tonometer on the metal block provided. Its front curvature exactly matches the curvature of the footplate and prevents the plunger from protruding. The scale reading should be zero and no error is tolerated.

The tonometer should be completely disassembled after use and swabbed with alcohol. A pipe cleaner dipped in alcohol is used to ream out the cylinder. Dried tears or anesthetic will cause the plunger to bind up and give erroneous readings. The tonometer should be stored disassembled, to indicate to the next user that it was carefully cleaned before storage.

FINAL CONSIDERATIONS

The choice of instruments is an individual preference, as all will perform reasonably well if used within their limitations. From a theoretical standpoint, that which displaces the least amount of aqueous and is least affected by ocular rigidity should be the most accurate, i.e., the Goldmann or NCT. Also, it is important for every office to have at least one back-up instrument so that if one tonometer is broken, another is available. The back-up tonometer can also be used to double check suspicious findings. Ideally, the primary instrument should be accurate and easily used (Goldmann or NCT). The back-up instrument does not have to be as accurate and should be relatively inexpensive since it will be rarely used.

Accurate and legible tonometry readings must be placed in the patient's chart. The numerical measure-

ments are recorded in millimeters of mercury. The use of "wnl" or "normal" is never acceptable and leaves the practitioner vulnerable to malpractice claims. If different types of tonometers are used in the office, the type of tonometer should be recorded next to the reading. The time at which tonometry is performed is also recorded. This will provide useful information concerning a patient's diurnal fluctuations.

The age at which tonometry should be performed on a patient is open to debate. Waiting until a patient is 40 to perform tonometry is no longer acceptable. Since tonometry has minimal complications, the best advice is to measure the IOP of every patient, regardless of age. The exception would be infants and small children who do not display any signs of congenital glaucoma. Because of the medical and legal importance of taking accurate readings on glaucoma patients, it is recommended that only the doctor perform tonometry on these patients.

If a patient refuses tonometry, the chart should well document that the risk of not doing tonometry was explained and that the patient understands and accepts the risk. Some doctors even make the patient sign a waiver. Likewise, whenever it is not possible to obtain a reliable reading (e.g., edematous cornea, blepharospasm), the circumstances should be documented in the patient's record. Therefore, it is incumbent on each practitioner to perform tonometry on every patient capable of being tested regardless of age or physical limitations. Tonometry, even with its limitations, remains a key test in the diagnosis and treatment of glaucoma.

REFERENCES

1. Drance SM. The significance of the diurnal tension variations in normal and glaucomatous eyes. *Arch Ophthalmol.* 1960;64:494–501.
2. Stamper RL. Intraocular pressure: Measurement, regulation, and flow relationships. In: Duane TD, Jaeger EA, eds. *Biomedical Foundations of Ophthalmology.* Vol. 2. Philadelphia: Harper & Row; 1987:1–30.
3. Buchanan RA, Williams TD. Intraocular pressure, ocular pulse pressure, and body position. *Am J Optomet Phys Opt.* 1985;62:59–62.
4. Passo MS, Goldberg L. Exercise training reduces intraocular pressure among subjects suspected of having glaucoma. *Arch Ophthalmol.* 1991;109:1096–1098.
5. Forbes M, Pico G, Grolman B. A noncontact applanation tonometer. *Arch Ophthalmol.* 1974;91:134–140.
6. Ohrstrom A, Kattstrom O, Palland W, et al. Oral and topical beta-receptor blockers in glaucoma treatment. A

multi-center study. *Acta Ophthalmol (Copenh)*. 1984;62: 681–695.

7. Phelps CD, Phelps GK. Measurement of intraocular pressure, a study of reproducibility. *Graefe's Arch Clin Exp Ophthalmol*. 1976;198:39–43.

8. Pepose J, Linette G, Lee S, et al. Disinfection of Goldmann tonometers against human immunodeficiency virus type I. *Arch Ophthalmol*. 1989;107:983–985.

9. Lingel N, Coffey B. Effects of disinfecting solutions recommended by the Centers for Disease Control on Goldmann tonometer biprisms. *J Am Optom Assoc*. 1992;63:43–48.

10. Meyers K, Lalle P, Litwak A, et al. XPERT NCT: A clinical evaluation. *J Am Optom Assoc*. 1990;61:863–869.

11. Rubenstein JR, Deutsch TA. Pneumotonometry through bandage contact lenses. *Arch Ophthalmol*. 1985; 103:1660–1661.

12. Khan JA, LaGreca BA. Tono-Pen estimation of intraocular pressure through bandage contact lenses. *Am J Ophthalmol*. 1989;108:422–425.

13. Quigley HA, Langham ME. Comparative intraocular pressure measurements with the pneumotonograph and Goldmann tonometer. *Am J Ophthalmol*. 1975;80: 266–273.

14. Moses RA, Marg E, Oeschli R. Evaluation of the basic validity and clinical usefulness of the MacKay-Marg tonometer. *Trans Am Acad Ophthalmol Otolaryngol*. 1962; 66:88–95.

15. Boothe WA, Lee DA, Panek WC, et al. The Tono-Pen: A manometric and clinical study. *Arch Ophthalmol*. 1988;106:1214–1217.

16. Kao SF, Lichter PR, Bergstrom TJ, et al. Clinical comparison of the Oculab Tono-Pen to the Goldmann applanation tonometer. *Ophthalmology*. 1987;94(12):1541–1544.

Chapter 8

GONIOSCOPY

Anthony B. Litwak

The diagnosis of primary "open"-angle glaucoma is one of exclusion, differentiating it from primary and secondary angle closure glaucomas as well as secondary open-angle glaucoma. Gonioscopy is used to view the anterior chamber angle, diagnose narrow angles, and define anterior chamber angle abnormalities. The management and treatment regimen will differ depending on the type of glaucoma diagnosed. Gonioscopy should therefore be performed on all glaucoma and glaucoma suspect patients.

PRINCIPLES

Since light emanating from the anterior chamber angle exceeds the critical angle at the corneal interface and is internally reflected back into the eye, visualization of the anterior chamber angle requires the use of a goniolens or gonioprism to overcome these optical properties.

There are basically two types of gonioscopy systems: direct and indirect. Direct gonioscopy uses a high convex lens to directly examine the anterior chamber angle. Indirect gonioscopy incorporates the use of mirrors or prisms in conjunction with the bio-microscope to view the anterior chamber angle anatomy. There are many types of gonioscopic lenses and prisms available; however, only the most common will be discussed (Table 8–1).

INSTRUMENTS AND TECHNIQUE

Direct Gonioscopy—The Koeppe Prototype Goniolens

The prototype for direct gonioscopy is the Koeppe lens, a 50-diopter convex lens available in 17 to 22.5-mm diameters. Direct gonioscopy gives broad, panoramic views of the angle. The image contains less distortions and artifacts than with indirect gonioscopy.

Technique. When performing direct gonioscopy, the patient is lying down, face up. Both corneas are anesthetized and the lens is inserted onto the cornea with the aid of goniogel or a balanced salt solution. A hand-held magnifier with an external light source is used to examine the anterior chamber angle through the Koeppe lens. The examiner rotates around the patient to view the entire 360° of the angle without interruptions. With two lenses, the angles can be tilted slightly away from the mirror or the patient asked to look towards the mirror in use to look deeper into the angle or over a convex iris contour (Fig. 8–3). If excessive lens tilt or patient gaze is required to view the anterior chamber angle structures, the angle should be considered narrow and at risk for possible closure. Conversely, if the lens is tilted toward the mirror or if the patient's gaze drifts away from the mirror used, then the angle will artificially appear more narrow. This may result in an incorrect

diagnosis of a narrow angle. As the lens is being rotated, the practitioner must be making mental notes to be used for documentation. After the entire angle has been viewed, the patient is asked to look up and the suction seal is broken by gently pressing through the lower lid just below the edge of the lens, allowing air to enter and break the seal (*see* Fig. 8–2.C.). After both eyes have been examined, the patient's eyes should be lavaged with a eye wash or sterile isotonic saline solution.

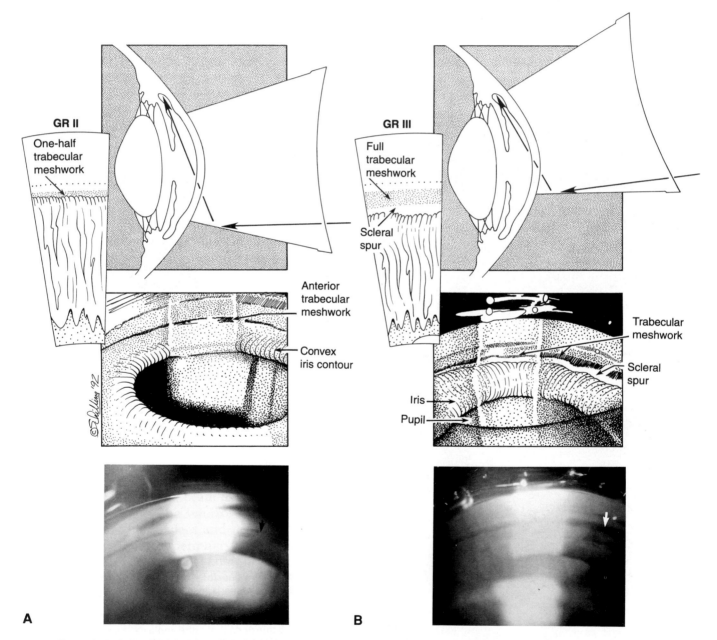

Figure 8–3. Lens tilting to view deeper into the angle. **A.** Angle view in the primary gaze position. Note convex iris contour with only anterior trabecular meshwork visible. **B.** Angle view tilting the goniolens away from the mirror or having the patient look slightly into the mirror. Note deeper view into the angle with full trabecular meshwork and scleral spur visible.

Indirect Gonioscopy— The 4-Mirror Goniolens

The Zeiss 4-mirror goniolens contains four identical 64° angled mirrors and a central fundus lens all mounted in a removable Unger holder. The Posner goniolens is a lighter version of the Zeiss lens and has a permanently mounted, steeper angled handle. The Sussman 4-mirror gonioprism is a hand-held version of the Zeiss lens (Fig. 8–4). The posterior surfaces of these lenses coincide with the anterior curvature of the cornea and do not require a coupling gel and therefore will not interfere with subsequent fundus examination or photography.

The four quadrants of the angle are evaluated by moving and rotating the slit beam onto the four mirrors without rotation of the lens, allowing for rapid examination of the anterior chamber angle (Fig. 8–5). The small lens footplate allows the examiner to press lightly on the cornea, directing aqueous peripherally into the angle and pushing the peripheral iris backwards (Figs. 8–6 and 8–7). Pressure (indentation) gonioscopy can help differentiate angle apposition (narrow angles) from angle adhesions (peripheral anterior synechia) (Fig. 8–6). The Goldmann-type goniolens has a larger footplate and greater posterior curvature and is not suited for pressure gonioscopy.

The disadvantages to the 4-mirror systems are that the lens can easily slip off the cornea, the patient can easily blink the lens off the eye, and the technique is more difficult to master. If inadvertent pressure is placed on the eye with the lens, the angle may

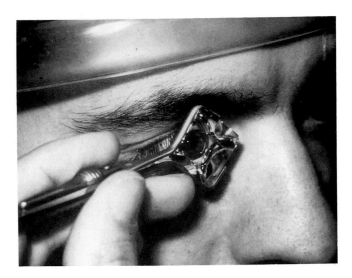

Figure 8–5. Four-mirror gonioscopy using the Zeiss goniolens. The slit beam is moved into the four mirrors to view the four angle quadrants.

be artificially deepened and mistaken for a more opened angle. The 4-mirror lens is easiest to learn initially on cooperative patients with deep anterior chambers. The procedure can be performed routinely after tonometry. With experience, the technique can be used on all patients. It can also be performed over a soft contact lens.

Technique. Anesthetize both corneas, explain the test to the patient, position the patient in the slit-lamp, and give them a fixation target to keep their eyes in the primary position. The gonioprism is inserted directly onto the cornea (*see* Fig. 8–5). No goniogel or fluid is required. The slit-lamp beam is moved vertically and laterally into each of the four mirrors. Tilting the lens away from the mirror being viewed will again give a deeper view into the angle. The patient's gaze position should not be changed because this results in the disruption of the tear film seal. Gently pressing perpendicularly onto the cornea (pressure gonioscopy) will cause the peripheral iris to fall back and deepen the angle (*see* Figs. 8–6 and 8–7). Excessive pressure on the lens will cause folds in the cornea and distort the image. After all four quadrants of the angle are examined, the lens is removed from the eye. If the lens should slip off of the cornea or if the tear film/goniolens interface is broken, reposition the lens outside the slit lamp. Once the lens is in the proper position, focus through the oculars. To the novice examiner, use of the 4-mirror lens can be quite frustrating; however, with experience and fortitude the technique is extremely rewarding.

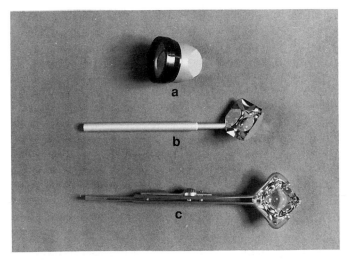

Figure 8–4. Four-mirror goniolens. (a) Sussman hand-held 4-mirror lens. (b) Posner 4-mirror with a permanently mounted handle. (c) Zeiss 4-mirror with a Unger holding fork. (*Used with permission from Fingeret M, Casser L, Woodcome HT: Atlas of Primary Eyecare Procedures. Norwalk, CT: Appleton & Lange; 1990.*)

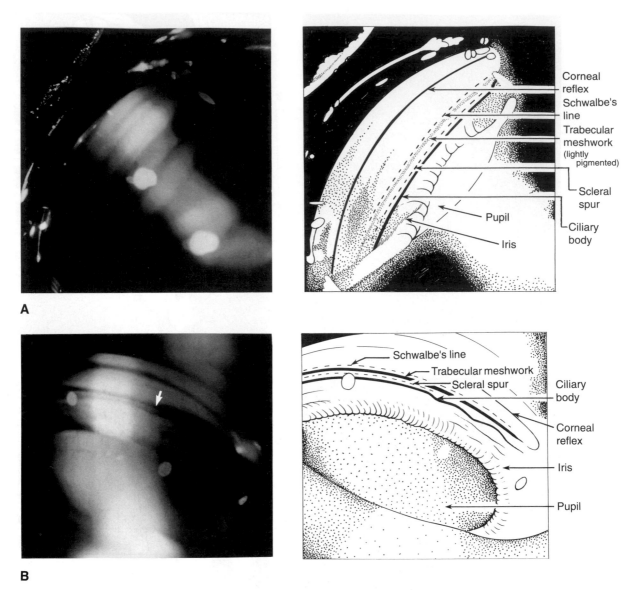

Figure 8–8. Normal angle anatomy. Note ciliary body, scleral spur, trabecular meshwork, and Schwalbe's line. The patient in **(A.)** has very little pigmentation in the trabecular meshwork. The patient in **(B.)** has a heavily pigmented trabecular meshwork. There may be considerable variation in the clinical appearance of the normal angle. (*See also* Color Plate 8–8.)

Schlemm's canal. The posterior two thirds of the trabecular meshwork is the filtering portion and will often have a more pigmented appearance than the anterior one third, which does not filter aqueous. The appearance of pigmentation in the trabecular meshwork can vary from no coloration to a heavy black band (*see* Fig. 8–8).

The anterior border of the angle is Schwalbe's line. Schwalbe's line represents the end of Descemet's membrane and the beginning of the trabecular meshwork. It often has a slightly elevated ridge, which aids in its identification; however, in some patients it is very difficult to distinguish. Schwalbe's line usually has an opaque white color, but may also

have a light brown appearance secondary to pigment deposition (Sampaolesi line). It is important not to confuse a pigmented Schwalbe's line for the trabecular meshwork in a narrow angle patient. It is also an important structure to identify in narrow angle patients, because the other angle structures may not be seen.

ANGLE GRADING SYSTEMS

The most common grading systems for evaluation of the anterior chamber angle are the Scheie, Schaefer, and Spaeth classifications. The Scheie system[1] grades

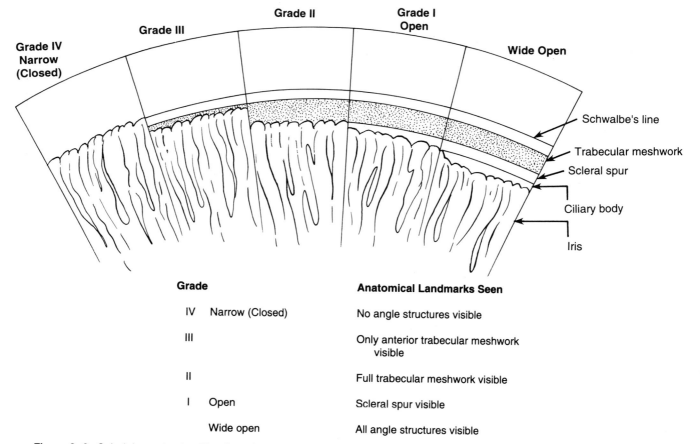

Grade		Anatomical Landmarks Seen
IV	Narrow (Closed)	No angle structures visible
III		Only anterior trabecular meshwork visible
II		Full trabecular meshwork visible
I	Open	Scleral spur visible
	Wide open	All angle structures visible

Figure 8–9. Scheie's angle classification; the grading system is based on the anatomical landmarks seen. *(Modified from Shields MB. Textbook of Glaucoma. 2nd ed. Baltimore: Williams & Wilkins; 1987, 172.)*

the angle based on the angle structures visualized (Fig. 8–9). When the ciliary body is visible, the angle is graded wide open. If no angle structures are visualized, the angle is grade IV (narrow). This simplistic system does not predict angle closure with dilation and its grading scale is opposite to the usual terminology. The Schaefer classification[2] estimates the corneal-iris angle and predicts angle closure with dilation (Fig. 8–10). An estimated angle greater than 20° is graded wide open with minimal chance of angle closure (grade 4). An angular width of 10 to 20° is graded moderately narrow with a possibility of induced angle closure (grade 3). Less than 10° angular width is judged extremely narrow and with a high probability of angle closure with dilation (grade 2). Grade 1 represents a partially or totally closed angle.

The Spaeth classification[3,4] is an extension of the Schaefer system where the iris contour and the insertion of the iris into the angle are designated along with an estimation of the cornea-iris angle. The iris contour is described as steep (convex), regular (straight), or queer (concave) and the apparent location of the iris insertion into the angle is identified from Schwalbe's line to ciliary body (Fig. 8–11). In the final analysis, the clinician should be aware of the multiple parameters and variables involved in interpreting the anterior chamber angle. I prefer to use a grading system that incorporates the amount of lens tilting or redirection of patient gaze required to visualize the angle structures (Table 8–2).

ANGLE DOCUMENTATION

The angle grading and classification system should be recorded along with any variations or abnormalities of the angle. The amount of pigmentation in the angle must also be recorded and can vary from individual to individual. Most often the pigmentation is confined to the posterior two thirds of the trabecular meshwork, because of the location of the filtering portion of the angle. However, pigment may also be deposited on Schwalbe's line or throughout the angle. The amount of pigmentation is graded from 0 to

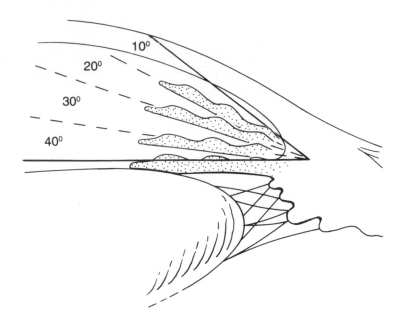

Grade	Angular Width	Risk of Angle Closure
4	Closed angle	Closure present
3	Extremely narrow angle (<10°)	Closure probable
2	Moderately narrow (10 to 20°)	Closure possible
1	Wide open angle (20° to 45°)	Closure unlikely

Figure 8–10. Schaefer angle classification. The grading system is based on the angular width between the posterior corneal surface and the anterior surface of the iris. The system also predicts the risk of angle closure. *(Modified from Shields MB.* Textbook of Glaucoma. *2nd ed. Baltimore: Williams & Wilkins; 1987, 173.)*

4, with 0 representing no pigmentation and 4 designating extensive pigment deposition (*see* Fig. 8–8). When excessive pigmentation is noted in the angle, it is important to transilluminate the iris, looking for peripheral iris transillumination defects and pigment deposited on the posterior surface of the corneal endothelium (Krukenberg's spindles). Patients with

large depositions of pigment in the angle may develop pigmentary glaucoma (see Chapter 10).

An abnormality of the angle that frequently occurs as a result of chronic inflammation or appositional angle closure is peripheral anterior synechia (PAS), broad adhesions of the peripheral iris tissue to the trabecular meshwork (Fig. 8–12). Peripheral ante-

TABLE 8–2. ANGLE GRADING SYSTEM (LITWAK)

Angle Grade	Clinical Appearance	Risk of Angle Closure With Dilation
Grade IV	All angle structures seen (ciliary body) without lens tilt/patient gaze	Minimal
Grade III	All angle structures seen (ciliary body) with minimal lens tilt/patient gaze	Low
Grade II	Only trabecular meshwork seen with minimal lens tilt/patient gaze	Moderate
Grade I	Only trabecular meshwork seen with moderate lens tilt/gaze	High
Grade 0	Angle closed; perform pressure gonioscopy to determine if PAS[a] is present	Angle closed

[a] PAS: Peripheral anterior synechia.

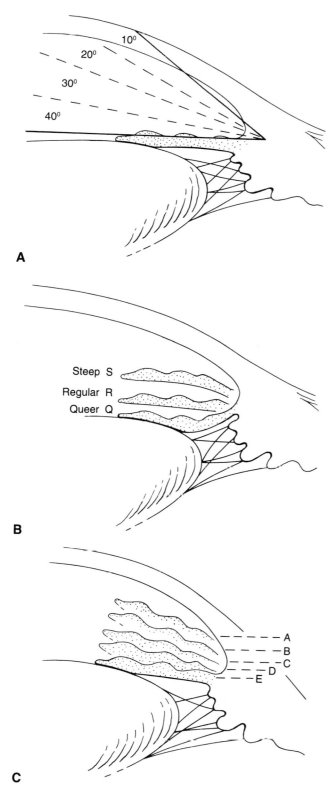

Figure 8–11. Spaeth's angle classification. The Spaeth system is a modification of the Schaefer classification. In addition to estimation of the angular width **(A.)**, the classification adds the configuration of the iris contour **(B.)** and the insertion of the iris root into the angle **(C.)**. *(Modified from Shields MB. Textbook of Glaucoma. 2nd ed. Baltimore: Williams & Wilkins; 1987, 174.)*

rior synechia should not be confused with iris process. There are many causes of PAS (Table 8–3). In the superior angle PAS is associated with chronic primary angle closure glaucoma, because the superior angle is usually the narrowest and the first to develop PAS from appositional closure. It is important to perform pressure gonioscopy to differentiate appositional angle closure without PAS from actual synechia. Likewise, it is important to perform gonioscopy yearly on all patients with narrow angles or angle closure glaucoma, especially those taking miotics. Patients with appositional angle closure (primary angle closure glaucoma) without PAS will benefit from a peripheral iridotomy. Extensive PAS represents permanent angle blockage that may require anti-glaucoma therapy or filtering surgery if the intraocular pressure cannot be controlled.

Angle neovascularization frequently develops after a hypoxic event or disease to the retina, such as a central retinal vein occlusion or proliferative diabetic retinopathy. A vasoproliferative substance is produced by the hypoxic retina and diffuses into the anterior chamber resulting in the development of rubeosis irides. These fragile tiny vessels usually form at the iris pupillary border (Fig. 8–13.A.) and grow across the iris surface into the trabecular meshwork (Fig. 8–13.B.). Fibrous tissue grows with the vessels and can contract, pulling the peripheral iris surface into the trabecular meshwork (PAS), which blocks the outflow of aqueous, resulting in an increase in intraocular pressure (neovascular glaucoma) (Fig. 8–13.C.). It is extremely important to perform gonioscopy on all patients at risk for the development of neovascular glaucoma since a small percentage may develop angle neovascularization before vessels are seen on the iris surface. Intraocular pressure does not increase until one half to three quarters of the angle is occluded. The treatment for angle neovascularization is pan-retinal photocoagulation (PRP) to the hypoxic retina.

Blunt trauma to the eye may cause a tear between the longitudinal and circular muscles of the ciliary body, known as angle recession. Gonioscopy will reveal an irregular band of the ciliary body, which is abnormally wide in the area of angle recession (Fig. 8–14). Angle recession may involve a small portion of the angle or the entire 360°. It is important to compare the width of the ciliary body between eyes to establish the diagnosis in subtle cases.

Not all patients with angle recession develop glaucoma. In fact, angle recession is only an indicator that the eye suffered blunt trauma. If a patient with angle recession develops glaucoma, it may be because the trabecular meshwork is often concurrently

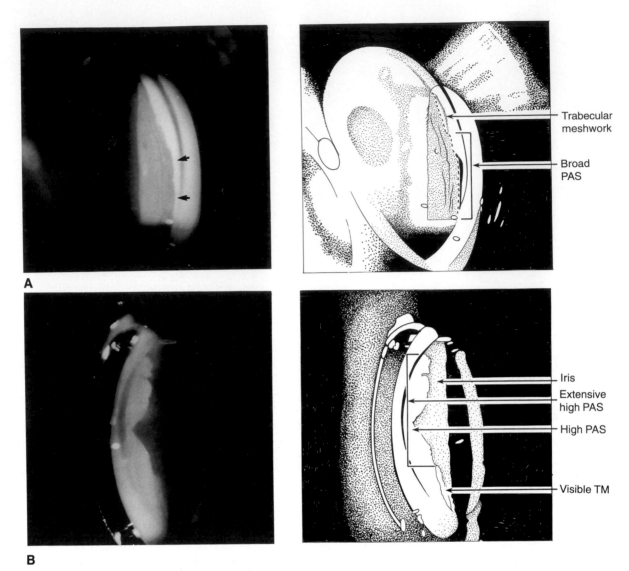

Figure 8–12.A. Peripheral anterior synechia (PAS) in a patient with chronic uveitis; PAS are broad adhesions of the peripheral iris into the trabecular meshwork. **B.** High PAS in a patient with a previously flat anterior chamber after glaucoma filtering surgery. The PAS extend well above Schwalbe's line.

TABLE 8–3. ETIOLOGY OF PERIPHERAL ANTERIOR SYNECHIA (PAS)

Chronic iritis or uveitis

Chronic apposition angle closure

Angle neovascularization

Blunt trauma

Hyphema

Irido-corneal endothelia (ICE) syndromes[1]

Congenital anomalies

Complicated intraocular surgery

Flat anterior chamber after filtering surgery

Penetrating trauma

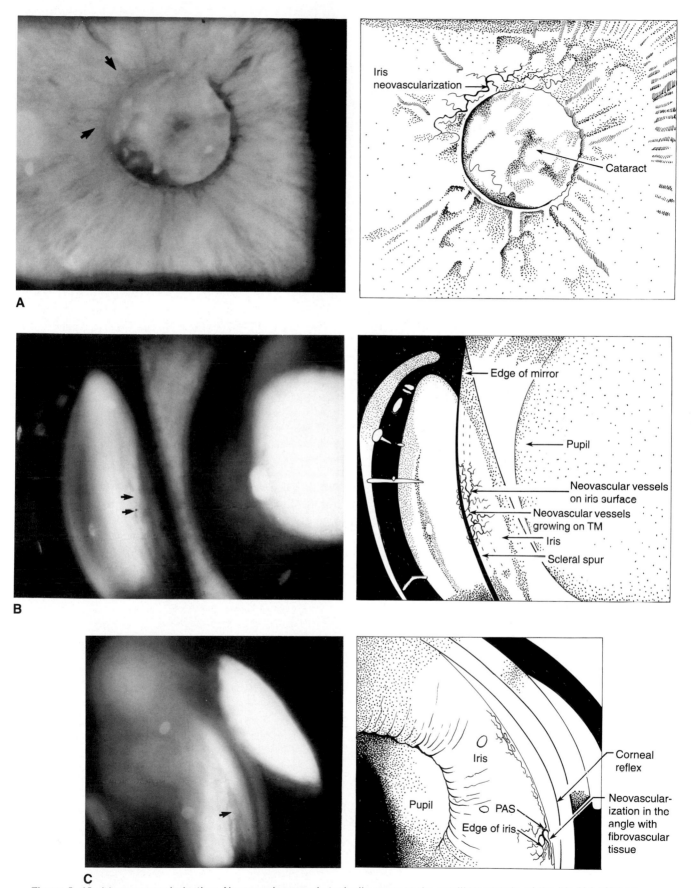

Figure 8–13. Iris neovascularization. Neovascular vessels typically occur at the pupillary margin of the iris **(A.)** after an ischemic event to the retina. These vessels may grow into the angle **(B.)** along with fibrovascular tissue forming PAS **(C.)** and neovascular glaucoma. (*See also* Color Plate 8–13.)

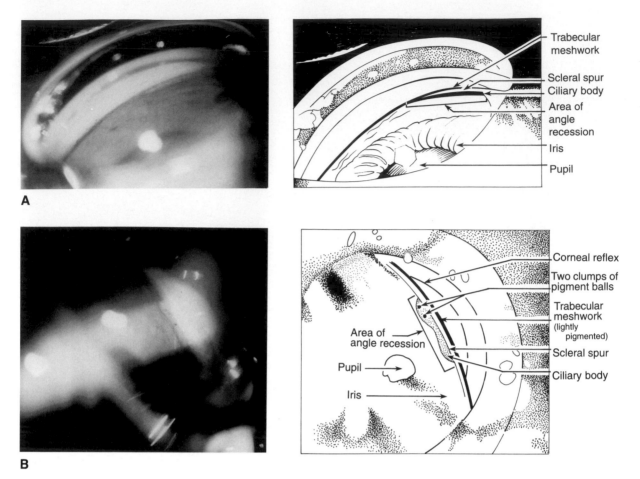

Trabecular meshwork

Scleral spur
Ciliary body

Area of angle recession

Iris

Pupil

A

Corneal reflex

Two clumps of pigment balls

Trabecular meshwork (lightly pigmented)

Scleral spur

Ciliary body

Area of angle recession

Pupil

Iris

B

Figure 8–14. Angle recession after blunt trauma. **A.** Note visibility of scleral spur and ciliary body in area of angle recess. **B.** Angle recession or clumps of pigment in the angle are indicators of possible damage to the trabecular meshwork and development of traumatic glaucoma. (*See also* Color Plate 8–14.)

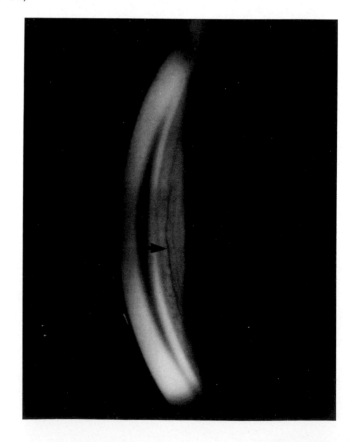

Figure 8–15. Blood in Schlemm's canal, a sign of elevated episcleral venous pressure. Schlemm's canal lies directly behind the trabecular meshwork and is not normally visible unless blood is present. (*See also* Color Plate 8–15.)

damaged, which results in a decrease of aqueous outflow. (See angle recession glaucoma in Chapter 10.) The increase in intraocular pressure may develop soon after the traumatic event or several years later. Another sign of trauma is pigment balls seen in the angle (Fig. 8–14.B.). These balls represent clumps of pigment released after a blow to the eye or breakdown products of red blood cells from an iris bleed (hyphema). These eyes are also at risk for the development of traumatic glaucoma.

An increase in episcleral venous pressure may cause blood reflux into Schlemm's canal (Fig. 8–15). Elevated episcleral venous pressure may be a sign of thyroid eye disease, superior vena cava syndrome, retrobulbar tumor, Sturge-Weber syndrome, arteriovenous fistulas, or orbital varices.[5] Other associated ocular findings include dilated, tortuous episcleral and conjunctival vessels, proptosis, chemosis, orbital bruit, and elevated intraocular pressure. However, blood in Schlemm's canal is often found in normal patients without elevated episcleral venous pressure.[6]

CONCLUSION

Gonioscopy should be performed on all glaucoma patients, glaucoma suspects, and narrow-angle patients. The anterior chamber angle size and configuration should be documented in the patient's chart (Fig. 8–16). In addition, the amount of pigmentation in the trabecular meshwork should be recorded. It is important not only to identify the abnormal findings in gonioscopy but also to document the negative findings (i.e., no PAS, no angle neovascularization, no angle recess). Finally, be sure to identify which type of glaucoma you have diagnosed. The diagnosis of primary open-angle glaucoma is one of exclusion. Gonioscopy is the key test to make the differential diagnosis.

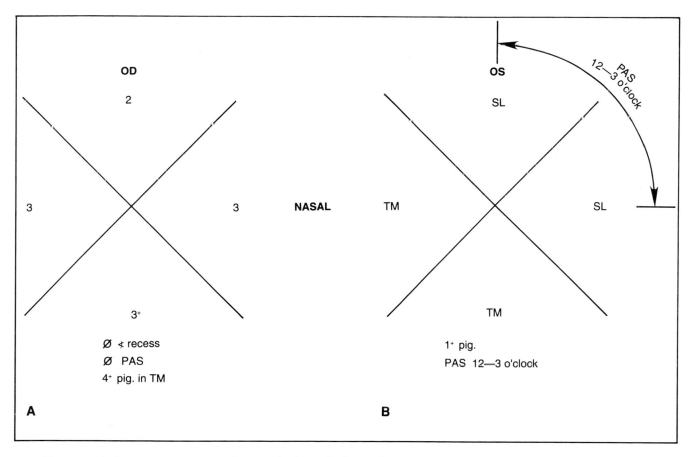

Figure 8–16. Documentation of gonioscopy findings. **A.** Crossed lines can be used for entering numerical grading classifications corresponding to the superior, temporal, inferior, and nasal quadrants. **B.** The most posterior angle structure seen can be recorded in a similar manner. Abnormal angle findings (such as pigmentation in the trabecular meshwork, PAS, angle neovascularization, angle recess) should be recorded. When not present, negative documentation is important.

REFERENCES

1. Scheie HG. Width and pigmentation of the angle of the anterior chamber. A system of grading by gonioscopy. *Am J Ophthalmol.* 1957;58:510.
2. Schaefer RN. Symposium: Primary Glaucomas. III. Gonioscopy, ophthalmoscopy and perimetry. *Trans Am Acad Ophthalmol Otol.* 1960;62:112.
3. Spaeth GL. The normal development of the human anterior chamber angle: A new system of descriptive grading. *Trans Ophthalmol Soc UK.* 1971;XCI:709.
4. Spaeth GL. Distinguishing between the normally narrow, the suspiciously shallow, and the particularly pathological, anterior chamber angle. *Perspect Ophthalmol.* 1977;1:205.
5. Shields MB. *Textbook of Glaucoma.* 2nd ed. Baltimore: Williams & Wilkins; 1987.
6. Ritch, R, Shields MB. *The Secondary Glaucomas.* St. Louis: C.V. Mosby; 1982.

Chapter 9

EVALUATION OF THE OPTIC NERVE IN GLAUCOMA

Anthony B. Litwak

Glaucoma is a chronic progressive optic neuropathy characterized by atrophy of ganglion cell axons from obstruction of axoplasmic flow at the level of the scleral lamina cribrosa. Structural changes to the optic nerve head and the surrounding retinal nerve fiber layer (NFL) have been shown to precede visual field defects in glaucoma.[1] Therefore, one of the most important aspects in the evaluation of a glaucoma or glaucoma suspect patient is the examination of the optic disc and the retinal NFL.

TECHNIQUES TO EXAMINE THE OPTIC NERVE

There are many instruments and techniques that can be used to examine the optic nerve (Table 9–1). Stereoscopic methods are superior to monocular methods because the optic nerve topography is more easily appreciated. The degree of optic nerve excavation or cupping has been shown to be underestimated with monocular instrumentation such as the direct ophthalmoscope.[2,3] This is the result of using color rather than topographical changes in evaluating the size of the excavated area on the surface of the disc.

Most of the stereoscopic methods for assessing the optic nerve involve the use of the slit-lamp and an auxillary lens. This combination permits adequate magnification along with binocularity.[4] Direct auxillary lenses include the Hruby lens and a variety of Goldmann contact lenses. Both create an upright virtual image of the fundus.

The Hruby lens (-55 D) is mounted on a slit-lamp and placed approximately 1 to 2 mm in front of the patient's eye[4,5] (Figs. 9–1 and 9–2). Once the patient is adequately dilated, the instrument is aligned so that the beam of light from the slit-lamp passes through the Hruby lens and is centered in the pupil. Focusing with the joystick permits a limited view of the fundus. Additional areas of the fundus can be examined by directing the patient's gaze with the fixation light. The Hruby lens is a rapid and easy method to stereoscopically view the optic nerve without placing a lens directly on the eye. It requires precise fixation by the patient and is not easily adapted for photography.[6]

Fundus contact lenses occur in a variety of styles. The most commonly used is the Goldmann 3-mirror

The editors would like to thank Felix Barker, OD, for his help in the preparation of this chapter.

TABLE 9–1. FUNDUS EXAMINING LENSES

Fundus Lens	Image	Goniogel Required[b]	Advantages	Disadvantages
90 Diopter lens	Inverted, reversed	No	Stereo[a]; works with small pupils	Lack of magnification; inverted image
78 Diopter lens	Inverted, reversed	No	Stereo; ideal mag[b] and field of view	Inverted image
60 Diopter lens	Inverted, reversed	No	Stereo; high mag	Reduced field of view; inverted image
Yellow filter 90, 78, 60 diopter lenses	Inverted, reversed	No	More comfortable for patients	Obscures disc pallor; difficult to examine NFL
Fundus contact lens	Direct, upright	Yes	Stereo; truest image of optic disc	Gel impairs corneal clarity for photography; requires eye contact
Center Zeiss 4-mirror	Direct, upright	No	Stereo; high resolution	Difficult to master; requires patient cooperation and eye contact
Hruby lens	Direct, upright	No	Stereo	Limited field of view; requires good fixation
Direct ophthalmoscope	Direct, upright	No	Works with small pupils; no slit-lamp required	No stereo; underestimates cup-to-disc ratio

[a] Stereo: stereopsis; mag: magnification.
[b] Less viscous solutions such as Soaclens or Celluvisc can be substituted for goniogel to reduce corneal impairment following the procedure.

lens (Fig. 9–3). It is placed on the eye with gonioscopic gel or solutions such as Celluvisc or Soaclens following topical anesthesia. The patient is instructed to look upward and the lower edge of the lens is tucked into the inferior cul-de-sac using gentle downward pressure.[7,8] The top of the lens is then tilted forward to contact the surface of the eye. The patient is asked to look straight ahead and the clinician moves the joystick of the slit-lamp forward until the focus is achieved. The 3-mirror lens gives an upright image, good resolution, and a larger field of view than the Hruby lens.[6] It requires contact with the eye and the use of a bonding solution that may be toxic to some patients' eyes.

A stereoscopic view of the optic nerve can also be achieved with indirect biomicroscopy through a high

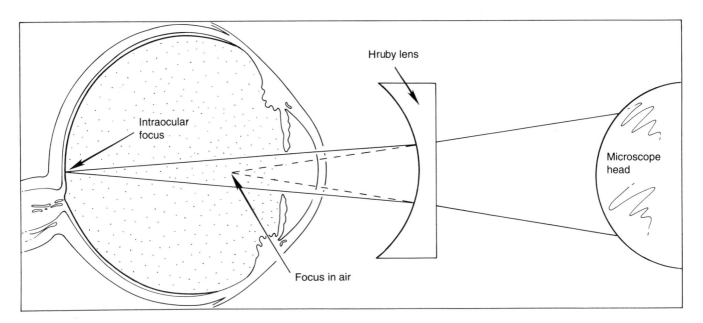

Figure 9–1. Schematic diagram of the Hruby lens used in direct biomicroscopy of the posterior fundus.

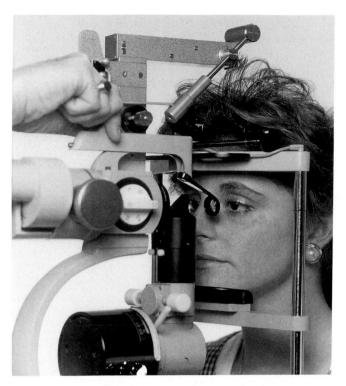

Figure 9–2. Use of the Zeiss mounted Hruby lens. The lens is pulled down from the overhead storage position. The lens is then released to travel forward against the headrest guard.

plus (60 D, 78 D, 90 D) lens.[9] This technique creates an inverted and reversed image similar to indirect ophthalmoscopy. Indirect biomicroscopy is a convenient, relatively easy technique that gives a much wider field of view (>40°) compared to the direct methods previously discussed.[6] It does require some initial mastering of the technique and interpretation.

The technique is similar to that described for the Hruby lens except the condensing lens is usually

hand held about 1 cm in front of the patient's eye (Fig. 9–4). Steady mount holders are available to attach to the slit-lamp that make the fundus image more stable. The optic nerve is viewed by focusing the light through the condensing lens and dilated pupil with the joystick (Figs. 9–5 and 9–6). Alignment of the lens can be assisted by observing the image of the filament focused in the plane of the pupil.[8,10]

The condensing lenses are available in clear or yellow glass. Clear is preferable when examining for glaucoma since it does not distort the color of the disc tissue. The +60 D lens gives the greatest magnification and may be best for optic nerve assessment. The +78 D lens provides excellent magnification and an optimum field of view. The +90 D lens gives a larger field of view and can be helpful in patients with small pupils. Photographing the optic nerve is possible with indirect fundus biomicroscopy, although significant skill and patient cooperation is required.

OPTIC NERVE EVALUATION

The outer rim tissue of the optic nerve head is composed primarily of bundles of ganglion cell axons (nerve fiber layer) that travel in an organized arrangement from ganglion cell bodies in the retina to the optic disc. At the optic disc, the axons make a 90° turn and exit through the fenestrated lamina cribrosa. Ganglion cell axons comprise 90% of the neuroretinal rim area.[11] Capillaries, astrocytes, and glial cells make up the remaining 10%. The capillary beds and axons give the outer rim tissue of the optic nerve head its orange-red appearance while the astrocytes and glial cells give connective tissue support to the axons. The optic cup is the pale, slightly oval depression in the center of the optic disc, which is devoid of axons and

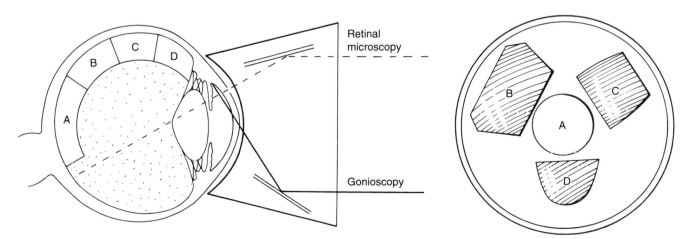

Figure 9–3. Schematic diagram of the Goldmann 3-mirror lens used to examine the posterior pole.

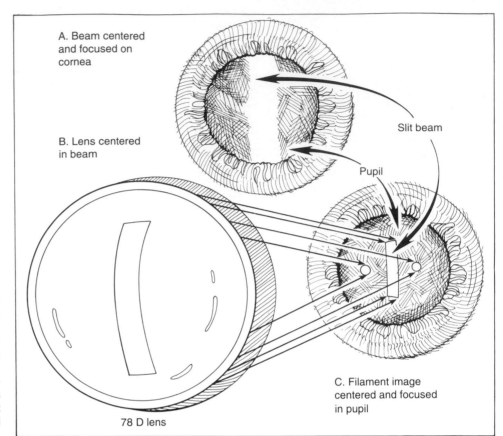

Figure 9–4. Alignment procedure for indirect biomicroscopy. A. Slit-lamp is aligned and centered with the corneal apex. B. Lens is positioned centrally in the beam and at about 1 cm from the cornea. C. If a steady mount is used, the clinician should view the image of the filament in the pupil behind the lens and adjust the lens position so that the filament is finely focused and centered in the pupil.

A. Beam centered and focused on cornea

B. Lens centered in beam

Slit beam

Pupil

78 D lens

C. Filament image centered and focused in pupil

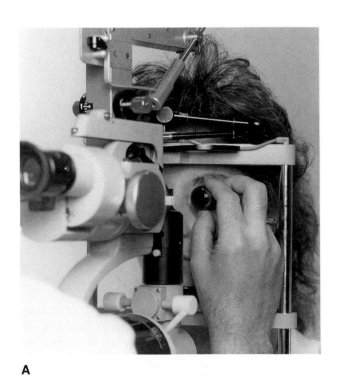

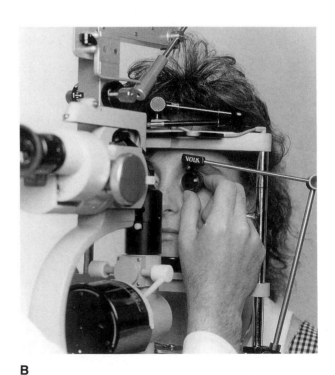

A

B

Figure 9–5. Technique of fundus indirect biomicroscopy. **A.** The slit beam is aligned with the central cornea. While controlling the lids with the middle and ring fingers, the lens is placed centrally in the slit-beam at 1 cm from the eye. **B.** Use of steady mount holder.

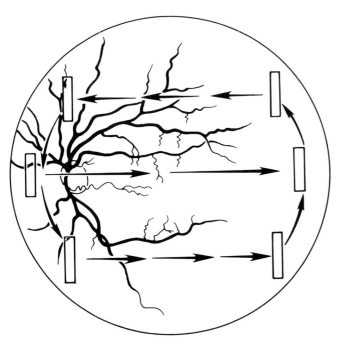

Figure 9–6. Suggested pattern of scanning the posterior pole in indirect fundus biomicroscopy.

capillaries. Dots in the center of the cup represent fenestrations in the exposed lamina cribrosa. These fenestrations are seen in one third of patients with myopia and may increase in appearance with progressive glaucomatous damage.[12] Small arterioles enter the eye from the nasal half of the optic cup, bifurcate, and follow the topography of the neuroretinal rim tissue.

There is considerable variation in the size, shape, and clinical appearance of the optic disc in normal patients. Stereoscopic observation of the optic nerve reveals that the average cup-to-disc ratio is 0.4.[2] However, large physiological optic cups of 0.7 or greater occur in approximately 2% of the normal popula-

tion.[2,3,13,14] It would be ideal if all patients were born with the same cup-to-disc ratio. Glaucomatous damage could be identified at the initial examination. Unfortunately, there is considerable variation in the size of the scleral foramen, which results in different sizes to the optic disc and in turn to the cup in normal individuals.[15,16] Physiological cup size is genetically determined and dependent on the size of the disc. (Fig. 9–7).

It may be helpful to examine other family members when differentiating a patient with large physiological cupping from glaucomatous atrophy. However, asymmetry between the two eyes in the size of the optic disc or cup is uncommon and when present should raise the suspicion of glaucoma.[2,17,18]

There have been several reports of loss of ganglion cell axons and an increase in the cup-to-disc ratio with age in the normal population.[19,20] This loss of axons may explain why retinal sensitivity decreases with age.[21] However, other studies have not found this correlation.[22] Airaksinen and colleagues did not find a significant decrease in the neuroretinal rim area with age.[23] Repka and Quigley point out that endstage glaucoma patients may show progressive visual loss despite controlled intraocular pressure because of normal age-related loss of axons.[22]

SIGNS OF OPTIC NERVE DAMAGE IN GLAUCOMA

Progressive Excavation of the Optic Cup

The most typical pattern of early optic nerve damage in glaucoma is progressive, concentric excavation of the optic nerve head (optic cupping)[24] (Fig. 9–8). In actuality, there is a thinning of the neuroretinal rim tissue of the optic disc from atrophy of the ganglion cell axons. Evaluation of the optic nerve requires ex-

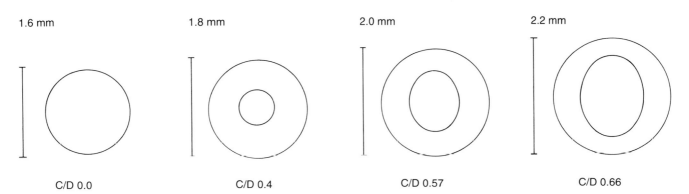

1.6 mm	1.8 mm	2.0 mm	2.2 mm
C/D 0.0	C/D 0.4	C/D 0.57	C/D 0.66

Figure 9–7. Physiological disc and cup sizes. The physiological cup size will become larger as the physiological disc size is increased (assuming the same number of ganglion axons in each nerve). Physiological cup and disc size is genetically determined.

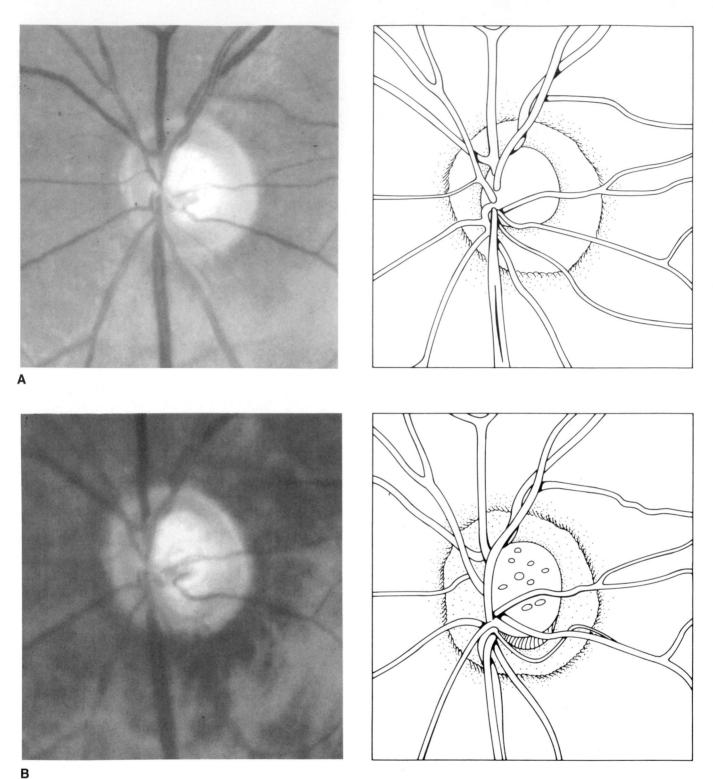

A

B

Figure 9–8. Serial disc photographs of a glaucoma suspect taken 4 years apart. Note progressive enlargement of the cup with localized deflection towards the inferior pole with shifting of the disc vessel at 4:30 **(B.)**. (*See also* Color Plate 9–8.)

amining the contour changes of the optic cup and disc vessels and not the area of pallor in the center of the optic disc. The outer edge of the central area of cup pallor may lag behind the leading edge of cup saucerization. Saucerization is the progression of diffuse, shallow cupping extending towards the disc margins without concurrent change to cup pallor.

This is an early sign of glaucomatous damage and is frequently overlooked without stereoscopic examination.

Glaucomatous damage usually occurs without the development of *significant* pallor to the remaining neuroretinal rim tissue. Pallor of the neuroretinal rim, regardless of the pattern of visual field loss, re-

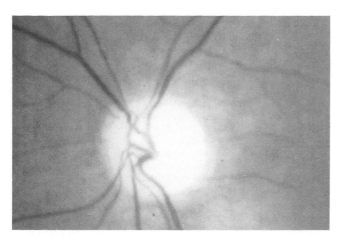

Figure 9–9. Optic cupping and diffuse pallor of the remaining neuroretinal rim tissue in an elderly patient with giant cell arteritis with anterior ischemic optic neuropathy. In glaucoma, the remaining neuroretinal rim tissue is a healthy orange-red color. (*See also* Color Plate 9–9.)

quires the investigation of a compressive lesion or a sudden ischemic event to the optic nerve such as anterior ischemic optic neuropathy (Fig. 9–9).

It has been shown in a number of clinical studies that a progressive increase in cupping of the optic disc can precede a visual field defect in glaucoma.[1,24,25] Progressive cupping, even in the absence of visual field loss, should be considered strong evidence for glaucomatous damage.

Cup-to-Disc Asymmetry

The two eyes of a normal individual will have the same disc and cup size in 99.5% of the population.[17] Therefore, a cup-to-disc asymmetry of 0.2 or greater not caused by unequal disc sizes (Fig. 9–10) or anisometropia should be considered highly suspicious for glaucoma, especially if the eye with the larger cup has a higher intraocular pressure reading. Primary open-angle glaucoma may be more advanced in one eye resulting in this appearance, or a secondary glaucoma may be present (*see* Chapter 17).

Focal Notching of the Optic Disc

As glaucomatous damage progresses, there may be selective loss of ganglion cell axons to the superior and inferior quadrants of the optic nerve with relative sparing of the nasal and temporal portions, until late in the disease process. Extension of cupping vertically, with localized deflection towards either the inferior or superior poles of the optic disc is a common pattern in glaucomatous damage (*see* Fig. 9–8.B.). Thinning of the neuroretinal rim in this region may result in the appearance of a notch (Fig. 9–11.A.). The inferior temporal pole of the optic nerve head is the most frequent location for localized disc damage.[26]

Disc Vessel Changes

Changes to the neuroretinal rim topography from ganglion cell axon loss may cause secondary changes

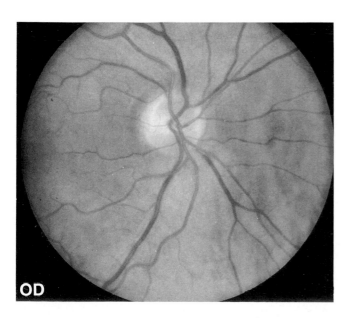

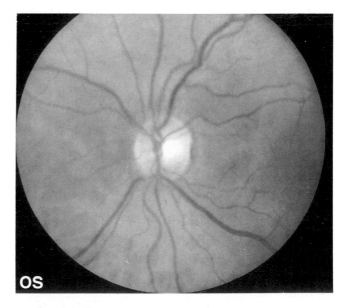

Figure 9–10. Cup-to-disc asymmetry secondary to unequal disc sizes. Photographs taken at same magnification with similar refractive errors, K readings, and axial lengths. Note larger cup and disc size in left eye compared to right eye. Cup-to-disc asymmetry of 0.2 or greater not due to unequal disc size should raise the suspicion of glaucoma. (*See also* Color Plate 9–10.)

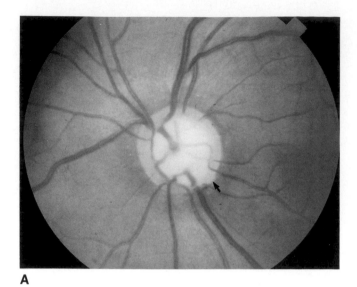

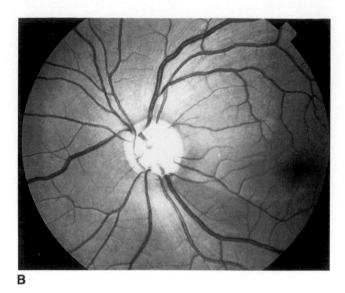

A   **B**

Figure 9–11. A. Notching of the inferior temporal pole of the optic disc in a glaucoma patient. Notches are usually associated with a wedge NFL defect and a corresponding visual field defect. (*See also* Color Plate 9–11.) **B.** Wedge NFL defect of the same patient. Wedge defects become broader away from the disc and narrower towards the optic nerve head.

to the optic disc vessels. Shifting of disc vessels documented with serial optic nerve photographs is suggestive of progressive loss of neuroretinal rim tissue (*see* Fig. 9–8.B.). Loss of neural retinal rim tissue may leave a horizontally oriented disc vessel suspended, unsupported from the margin of the cup.[27] This is

known as baring of a circumlinear blood vessel (Fig. 9–12). An overhanging disc vessel may develop in a similar fashion from deepening of the cup beneath a vertically oriented disc vessel. However, baring of the circumlinear vessel or overhanging of a disc vessel occurs in a minority of glaucoma patients and may be

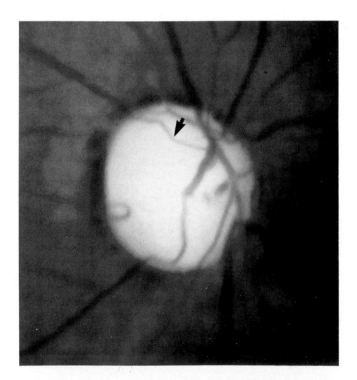

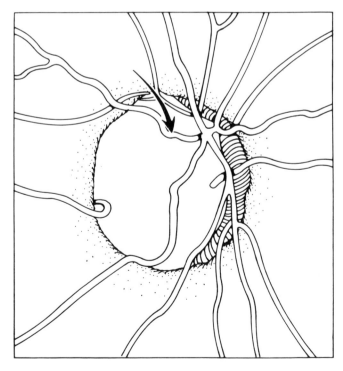

Figure 9–12. Baring of the circumlinear disc vessel. A horizontally positioned disc vessel may be left suspended without support as glaucomatous loss of neuroretinal rim tissue progresses.

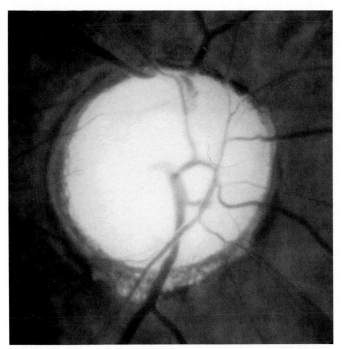

A

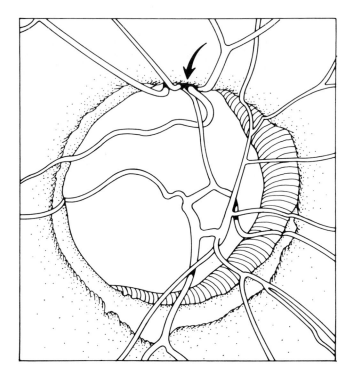

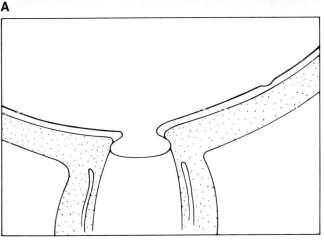

B

Figure 9–13. A. Undermining of the neuroretinal rim. Disc vessels may segmentally disappear beneath the neuroretinal rim and follow the contour of the laterally excavated cup. Note bayoneting of the retinal vein at 12 o'clock as it crosses over the sharpened neuroretinal rim. **B.** Cross-sectional view of the same patient showing beam potting of the optic disc.

seen in normal patients.[28] In endstage glaucoma, optic disc vessels may disappear segmentally beneath the scleral lip and then reappear around the sharpened edge of the cup margin creating a bayoneting of the vessel (Fig. 9–13). This is the result of the lateral extension of disc excavation beneath the scleral lip and posterior displacement of the lamina cribrosa (bean potting). Undermining of the disc margin is pathognomonic for advanced glaucoma.

Peripapillary Pigmentary Changes

Peripapillary crescents or atrophy have been reported as a sign of glaucomatous damage.[29–31] This is not to be confused with the scleral halo seen in histoplasmosis or high myopia. A mottling or ratty appearance to the retinal pigment epithelium (RPE) is seen around

the disc, usually corresponding to a thinned neural retinal rim on the temporal aspect of the optic nerve (Fig. 9–14). This sign is usually associated with advanced optic nerve damage. There is some debate as to whether this crescent is the result of ischemia to the optic nerve or secondary to a shift in the neuroretinal rim tissue due to the atrophy of ganglion cell axons. Peripapillary atrophy associated with glaucoma is found more commonly in patients with normal-tension rather than high-tension glaucoma.[32–35] Pigmentary changes around the optic disc are not specific for glaucoma.

Optic Disc Hemorrhage

Hemorrhages on the surface of the optic disc are not pathognomonic for glaucoma and can occur after a

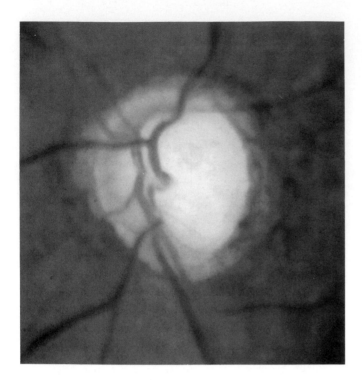 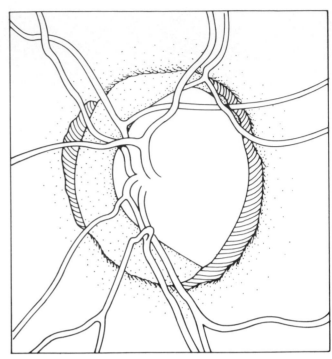

Figure 9–14. Peripapillary crescent associated with glaucoma. Note moth-eaten appearance of peripapillary crescent adjacent to thinning of the temporal rim in a normal-tension glaucoma patient. The specificity of this sign in glaucoma is unknown. (*See also* Color Plate 9–14.)

posterior vitreous detachment with avulsion of a superficial disc vessel, a resolving branch vein occlusion, anterior ischemic optic neuropathy, and in hypertensive or diabetic retinopathy. Patient history, clinical symptoms, and fundus examination help establish the diagnosis.

Optic disc hemorrhages associated with glaucoma were described by Drance in 1970[36] (Fig. 9–15). These hemorrhages can be located on or adjacent to the optic disc and are easily overlooked (Fig. 9–16). The hemorrhage is flamed-shaped when it is located off the disc in the nerve fiber layer and blot-like when located on the disc. Not surprisingly, the inferior pole of the optic nerve head, which is the most susceptible to glaucomatous damage, is the most frequent location of a Drance hemorrhage.[37,38] Less commonly, Drance hemorrhages may occur superior, temporal, or nasal to the disc. The location of a hemorrhage is often associated with a corresponding notch in the neuroretinal rim and a visual field defect. The pathophysiology of Drance hemorrhages may be ischemic[39] or mechanical due to a shifting of the disc capillaries from the loss of neuroretinal rim tissue.[40]

The reported prevalence of optic disc hemorrhages in primary open-angle glaucoma varies from 2 to 23%.[41,42] Disc hemorrhages will resolve on the av-

erage in 10 weeks with a range of 2 to 35 weeks.[41] Recurrences of Drance hemorrhages are common and usually appear in the same quadrant within 6 months of the original disc hemorrhage.[41] Patients with normal or low-tension glaucoma are more likely to develop a disc hemorrhage than patients with high-tension glaucoma.[38,41,43,44] Kitazawa and colleagues found a five times greater prevalence of disc hemorrhages in low-tension compared to high-tension glaucoma patients.[41]

Disc hemorrhages can be an early indicator of glaucomatous damage and may precede nerve fiber defects,[45] structural changes to the optic disc,[38] and visual field defects[46,47] (see Fig. 9–15.A.). Glaucoma suspects who develop a disc hemorrhage should be given strong consideration for medical therapy.[48] Optic disc hemorrhages can also be an indicator of progressive or advanced glaucomatous damage[37] (see Fig. 9–15.B.). The patient's current medical therapy should be re-evaluated and upgraded when an optic disc hemorrhage is discovered. In addition, patient's medicine compliance should be questioned when a disc hemorrhage appears in an apparently controlled patient. The presence of a disc hemorrhage in an advanced glaucoma patient holds an unfavorable prognosis.

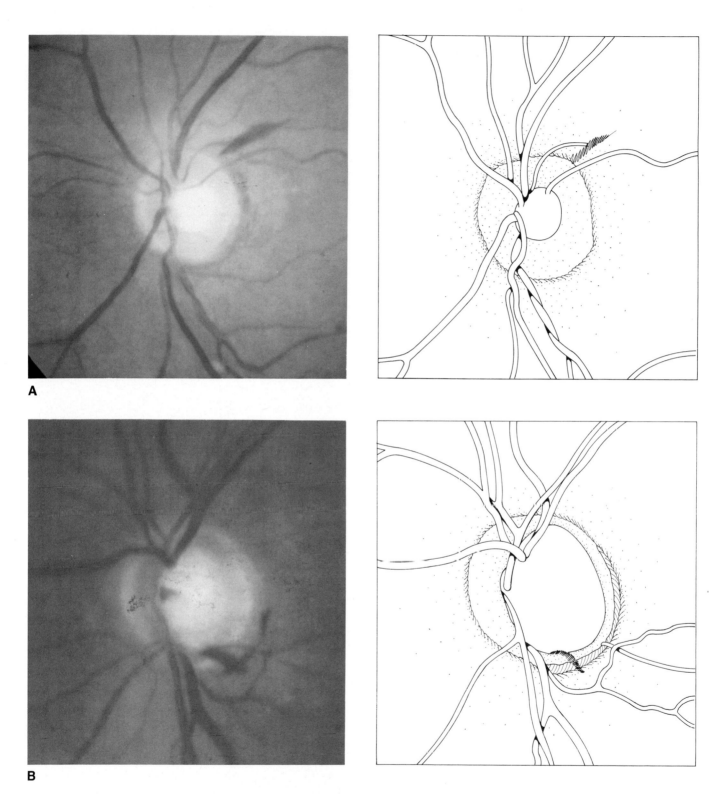

Figure 9–15. Disc hemorrhage (Drance hemorrhage) in glaucoma. Splinter hemorrhages on or adjacent to the optic nerve head usually in the inferior or superior temporal pole may be a sign of early glaucomatous damage **(A.)** or an indication of progressive glaucomatous damage **(B.)**. Disc hemorrhages are not pathognomonic for glaucoma. (*See also* Color Plate 9–15.)

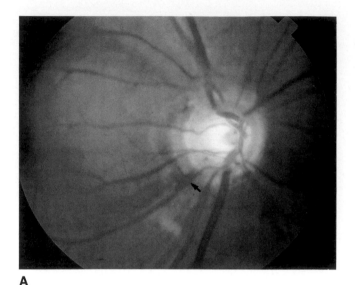
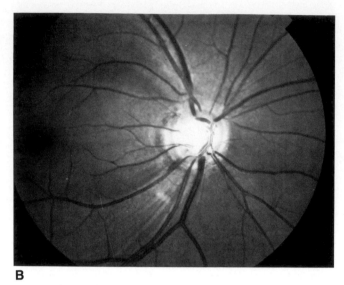

A   **B**

Figure 9–16. Drance hemorrhage with associated NFL defect. Note subtle disc hemorrhage at the 7 o'clock position **(A.)** with an accompanying slit NFL defect **(B.)**. Also note slit defects at 6:30 and 10:30 o'clock positions. (*See also* Color Plate 9–16.)

OPTIC NERVE DOCUMENTATION

There are several methods employed for documentation of the optic nerve, including the recording of a cup-to-disc ratio, drawings of the optic nerve, serial optic disc photographs, and computer image analysis of the optic nerve head.

Recording a cup-to-disc ratio gives some information in understanding optic nerve physiology and pathology. The cup-to-disc ratio is an indirect assessment of the neuroretinal rim area. Unfortunately, early glaucomatous damage cannot be adequately predicted by the initial estimation of the cup-to-disc ratio because of the wide range of normal physiological cup and disc sizes. A change in the cup-to-disc ratio is evidence of glaucomatous damage; however, interobservation variability makes serial disc comparison arduous.[49–51] An experienced observation using the same technique dramatically improves consistency.[2,52] In addition to recording the cup-to-disc ratio, it is beneficial to describe the slope of the cup, the presence of disc notching or hemorrhage, disc vessel abnormalities, and peripapillary pigmentary changes.

Drawing the optic disc provides an efficient means of documenting and following changes to the optic nerve head. Drawings of the optic nerve require the doctor to carefully study the disc topography. In addition to drawing the area of neural retinal rim tissue and optic cup, the clinician should include the slope of the cup with contour lines, the position and contour of disc vessels, and any peripapillary pigmentary changes or hemorrhages. However, even the most meticulous drawings do not give the same amount of information that can be obtained from a set of stereoscopic disc photographs.

The most accurate method to determine progressive cupping of the optic nerve is with serial stereoscopic fundus photographs of the optic disc.[52,53] Glaucoma suspects and patients are followed over a long period of time. It is extremely helpful to have an initial set of stereoscopic photographs for subsequent comparisons. Stereoscopic documentation can be performed with a stereoscopic fundus camera or with a regular fundus camera by using the standard decentration technique. The latter takes two sequential 35-mm slides of the optic nerve with a fixed amount of decentration, one slightly offset to the left causing a white crescent along the right side of the image and one slightly offset to the right causing a white crescent to the left of the image. Any change in patient fixation or deviation from the fixed amount of decentration will produce an erroneous three-dimensional image when comparing subsequent photographs. The two photographs are placed side by side (left crescent slide on the left and right crescent slide on the right) on a light box and viewed with a stereoscopic viewer. Subtle changes to the optic nerve, such as a shifting of disc vessels, can be uncovered by a careful comparison of serial stereoscopic fundus photographs (*see* Fig. 9–8). Fundus cameras that take two photographs simultaneously at a fixed angle have recently been introduced to remove decentration errors.

Computerized topographic image analysis has been used to measure the disc rim area in order to differentiate early glaucomatous cupping from a normal physiological cup.[54,55] Unfortunately, the outer edge of the optic cup is an arbitrary point and the slope of the cup varies considerably among individuals. The area of neuroretinal rim tissue has also been shown to vary within the normal population.[56] These drawbacks along with an expensive price tag has limited the use of computer imaging analysis in clinical practice.

Computer image analysis research has been applied to the quantitative study of the thickness of retinal nerve fiber layer in glaucoma.[57] Preliminary studies indicated that the height of juxtapapillary NFL may be a useful measurement to detect glaucomatous damage at an early stage and to recognize progressive nerve damage over time.[58,59] Computer image analysis has also been used to construct contour maps of the optic disc vessels. These contour drawings can be compared over time to detect subtle changes in disc topography.[60]

EVALUATION OF THE NERVE FIBER LAYER (NFL) IN GLAUCOMA

Evaluation of the retinal NFL is a useful technique to identify optic nerve damage in glaucoma patients.[61] Abnormalities in the NFL can occur in any optic neuropathy; however, in glaucoma there is selective damage to the NFL in the superior and inferior arcuate bundles with relative preservation of the papillomacular bundle until late in the disease process.[62]

Defects in the retinal NFL may be one of the earliest signs of glaucomatous damage.[63–65] NFL loss has been shown to precede visual field loss and structural changes to the optic disc.[1,65,66] The NFL examination may also be used to confirm visual field defects and to differentiate a large physiological cup from glaucomatous optic nerve damage.[67] The technique is easy to learn and does not require expensive equipment. With practice and experience, the NFL evaluation can give important adjunctive information in the diagnosis and management of glaucoma.

Normal Nerve Fiber Layer Appearance

The NFL lies superficial in the retina just beneath the internal limiting membrane. The normal NFL will cast a white haze over the underlying retinal vessels and choroidal structures. Reflections of light off the nerve fiber bundles give a bright striated appearance to the NFL. The brightness of these reflections is directly related to the thickness of the NFL.[68] The normal NFL is brightest (and thickest) in the superior and inferior arcades close to the optic disc (Fig. 9–17). The NFL becomes less prominent towards the papillomacular and nasal bundles and as you move further away from the optic disc (Fig. 9–17.A.). In fact, one should only pay attention to the NFL within one or two disc diameters from the optic nerve head. Outside this range there is gradual thinning of the NFL, which should not be mistaken for NFL atrophy. Therefore, the normal NFL appearance should be bright in the superior arcades with gradual dimming in the papillomacular area and a gradual increase in brightness towards the inferior arcades (Fig. 9–17). The brightness pattern should be fairly symmetrical between the superior and inferior arcades and also between the two eyes.

Evaluation Technique of the Nerve Fiber Layer

After examination of the optic nerve head with a clear 78-diopter lens, click in the red-free filter in the biomicroscope and turn the light illumination to maximum. Look slightly above and below the optic disc for bright striations from the reflections off the NFL (see Fig. 9–17.C, D.). Note the bright-dimmer-bright pattern.

Red-free illumination is used because the green light is absorbed by the pigment in the RPE and choroid, and the shorter wavelengths of light are reflected by the NFL. Bright reflections contrasted against a dark background provide optimum viewing of the NFL. Any clear fundus viewing lens can be substituted for the 78-diopter lens; however, the yellow fundus lenses are poorly suited for the NFL examination. The direct ophthalmoscope with the red-free filter can also be used, because stereopsis is not necessary for the examination of the NFL.

Evaluation of the NFL may not be possible in all patients. A blonde fundus does not provide a dark background to highlight NFL reflections. Media opacities such as cataracts will scatter the shorter wavelengths of light making the NFL examination difficult. Poor focusing techniques will frustrate the novice NFL observer. However, with practice and experience, the NFL evaluation can provide additional information to the practitioner in the majority of cases.

Photography of the Nerve Fiber Layer

In most situations, the clinical assessment of the NFL is adequate and photography of the NFL is not necessary. Photographs do provide the added advantage

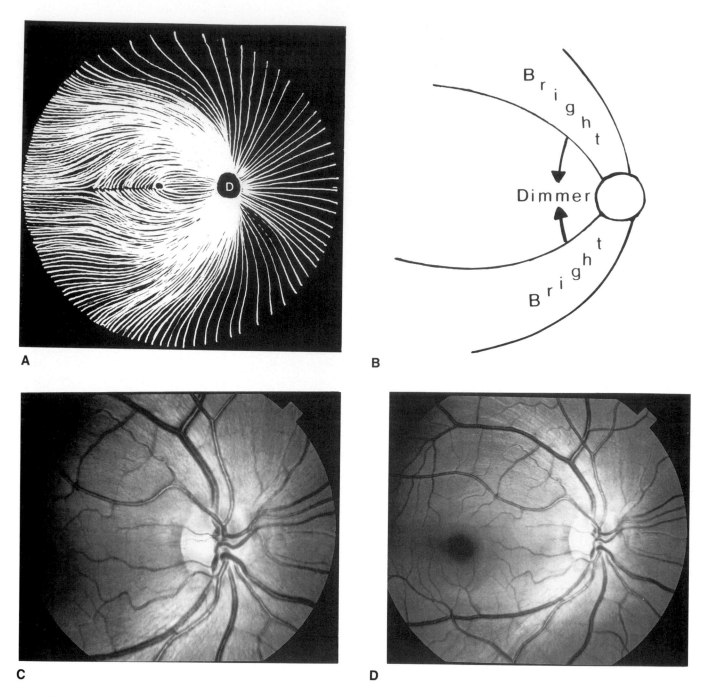

Figure 9–17. A. Anatomical position of retinal nerve fibers in the right eye. Note how temporal fibers arc around the macula and converge towards the superior and inferior poles of the optic nerve head. **B.** Brightness pattern of the retinal NFL. There should be a bright NFL pattern in the superior and inferior arcades and a gradual dimming as the papillomacular zone is approached. Any discontinuity in the brightness pattern represents an abnormality in the NFL. **C.** Clinical appearance of the normal NFL. The NFL is brightest in the superior and inferior arcuate zones and becomes dimmer towards the papillomacular zone. Notice how the NFL casts a white haze over the smaller retinal vessels. **D.** Wide angle photograph of the normal NFL. Note normal thinning of the NFL striations away from the optic nerve head. (*From Litwak AB. Evaluation of the retinal nerve fiber layer in glaucoma.* J Am Optom Assoc. *1990;61:390–397. Copyright American Optometric Association.*)

of being able to meticulously inspect the NFL without patient blinking or having to maintain steady fixation. Photographs also allow for comparison of the NFL between the inferior and superior arcades of the same eye and between corresponding quadrants in the fellow eye. Serial NFL photographs can be compared over time to determine progressive NFL loss.

Technical Pan black and white slide film is preferred for NFL photography.[61] The Technical Pan film is a slow speed, high contrast film. The red-free filter built into most fundus cameras can be used or a 560-nm cut filter available from Ditric Optics (312 Main Street, Hudson, MA 01749) can be placed into an empty filter slot in the camera. The flash setting for the Topcon TRC 50 V fundus camera with a 35° angle setting is 150 watt/second. Several shots should be bracketed to obtain the optimal flash setting, which may vary depending on the media clarity, the amount of fundus pigmentation, and the prominence of the NFL. Media clarity and proper focus of the NFL is critical. The film is developed in a HC 110 developer dilution B for 8 minutes at 68°F. Contact printing is used to convert a negative slide into a positive photograph or transparency. Color photography is preferred for optic nerve documentation but does not provide adequate contrast for NFL evaluation.

Damage of the Nerve Fiber Layer in Glaucoma

There are three patterns of NFL defects seen in glaucoma damage.[61] (Table 9–2). *Slit defects* represent focal damage of the optic nerve at the lamina cribrosa with retrograde degeneration of the ganglion cell axon back to its cell body in the retina. These dark slits are larger than an arteriole width in size and travel all the way back to the optic disc (Fig. 9–18). Slits smaller than an arteriole width in size or that do not go all the way back to the optic disc may be an early sign of damage but may also represent a variation seen in normal individuals. Follow-up for progressive atrophy of these types of defects is recommended.

Wedge defects represent an expanding loss of ganglion axons in the same area of the optic nerve. Wedge defects become narrower towards the disc and broader away from the disc. These defects are usually associated with a notch in the optic nerve head (*see* Fig. 9–11) and a corresponding visual field defect (Fig. 9–19). Wedge defects are the easiest type of NFL loss to identify; unfortunately, they are the least common pattern seen.

The most common abnormality of the NFL in glaucoma is *diffuse atrophy* to the NFL in the superior and inferior arcades. The arcuate zones look thinned or raked with more widely spaced NFL striations (Fig. 9–20). There is a discontinuity of the normally bright and gradually dimmer appearance from the arcades to the papillomacular bundle. The smaller tertiary blood vessels in the superior and inferior arcades, which are normally obscured by the overlying NFL, become more visible with NFL loss (Fig. 9–21).

Often the diffuse thinning of the NFL is difficult to determine. It is helpful to compare the superior and inferior poles of the same eye (*see* Fig. 9–21) and

TABLE 9–2. NFL DEFECTS IN GLAUCOMA

	Slit	Wedge	Diffuse
Clinical appearance	Slit defect larger than an arteriole in size at the optic disc	NFL defect one clock hour or greater in size at the optic disc	Raked or thinned NFL in arcuate bundles; striations are more spaced apart
Characteristics	Slits must travel all the way back to the disc	NFL defect narrow at disc, broader towards periphery	Tertiary retinal vessels are more easily seen in area of diffuse loss
IOP	More common in normal-tension glaucoma	More common in normal-tension glaucoma	More common in high-tension glaucoma
Optic disc	Focal deflection of cup excavation towards the poles; may show no disc abnormality	Disc notching at corresponding pole	Thinning of the corresponding neuroretinal rim tissue
Visual field	May show no visual field abnormality	Focal scotoma in corresponding visual field	Diffuse depression or constriction of corresponding field
Comments	Slit defects seen in 10% of normals; beware of pseudoslits	Least common NFL defect; easiest NFL defect to identify	Most common NFL defect in glaucoma; compare superior and inferior arcades and between the two eyes in subtle cases

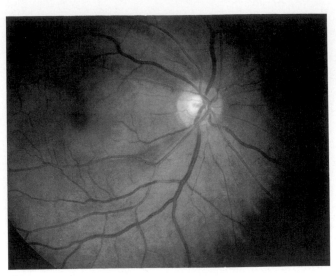

A

Figure 9–18. A. Glaucoma suspect with elevated IOP, non-glaucomatous cupping, and normal visual fields. NFL slit defects can be appreciated in the inferior and superior arcades with normal white light. (*See also* Color Plate 9–18.) **B.** Same patient using Technical Pan film and a 560 nm cut-off filter. Note the multiple NFL slit defects at the 7, 10, and 11 o'clock positions. These slits are larger than an arteriole width in size and travel all the way back to the optic nerve head. (*From Litwak AB. Evaluation of the retinal nerve fiber layer in glaucoma. J Am Optom Assoc. 1990;61:390–397. Copyright American Optometric Association.*)

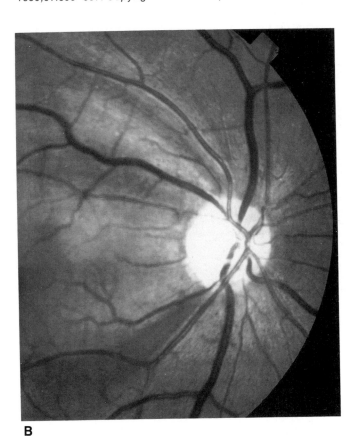

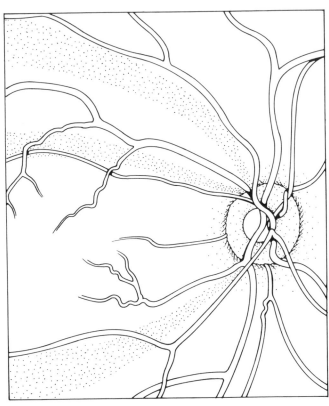

B

also to compare between eyes. Discrepancies in the brightness of the NFL in these zones can be a sign of diffuse damage.

Interpretation of the Nerve Fiber Layer

The interpretation of the NFL requires experience in judging the amount of diffuse NFL atrophy. It is important when learning the technique to evaluate the NFL in all normal patients. Look for a striated pattern in the superior and inferior arcades within one or two disc diameters of the optic nerve head. One should observe the continuous bright-dimmer-bright pattern of the NFL (*see* Fig. 9–17). Note how only the larger blood vessels are seen and small tertiary vessels are buried beneath the NFL.

After becoming familiar with the normal NFL pattern, begin to evaluate the NFL in known glaucoma patients with visual field loss (*see* Fig. 9–19).

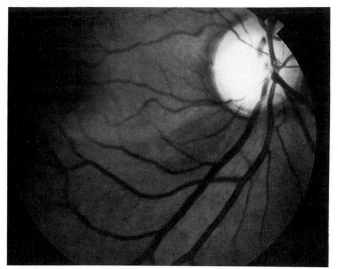

A

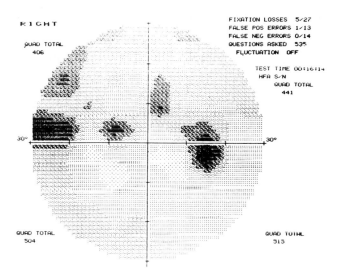

B

Figure 9–19. A. Inferior wedge NFL defect in the right eye of a glaucoma patient. Wedge defects are the easiest type of NFL loss to identify; however, they are also the least common. **B.** Automated visual field of the same patient. Note the early superior nasal step and paracentral scotoma which corresponds to the inferior wedge NFL defect. (*From Litwak AB. Evaluation of the retinal nerve fiber layer in glaucoma. J Am Optom Assoc. 1990;61:390–397. Copyright American Optometric Association.*)

The NFL should be atrophied in the area corresponding to the visual field loss and optic nerve damage. In advanced glaucoma damage, the papillomacular bundle may become brighter than the superior and inferior arcades (Fig. 9–22). This is known as NFL reversal and is the result of relative atrophy of the NFL in the arcuate zones. In endstage glaucoma, little or no

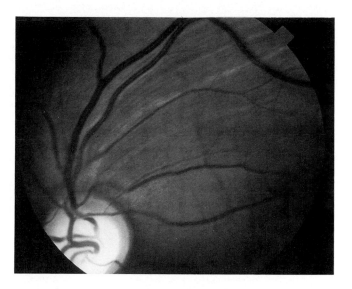

Figure 9–20. Diffuse loss pattern of the NFL in the left eye of a glaucoma patient. Note the thinned or raked appearance of the NFL, which allows the tertiary retinal vessels to be more visible. Also note the more widely spaced NFL striations and the discontinuity in the brightness pattern from 12 to 2 o'clock. (*From Litwak AB. Evaluation of the retinal nerve fiber layer in glaucoma. J Am Optom Assoc. 1990;61:390–397. Copyright American Optometric Association.*)

NFL striations are seen, the blood vessels are dark and prominent, the outer walls of blood vessel whiten, and the granular appearance of the deep retina is visible[61] (Fig. 9–23).

After one becomes comfortable in differentiating between normal and abnormal NFL patterns, the NFL examination can be used to evaluate the status of the optic nerve in glaucoma suspect patients (*see* Figs. 9–18 and 9–21). Quigley has shown that between 20 and 50% of the optic nerve may be damaged before a visual field defect appears on automated perimetry or conventional perimetry.[62,66] Sommer confirmed that NFL loss may precede visual field defects by 6 years.[65] Once a reproducible visual field defect appears on automated perimetry, sequential automated visual fields will be more sensitive in identifying progressive sequential changes to the optic nerve or retinal NFL. However, early changes to the retinal NFL may identify those glaucoma suspects (without visual field loss) who are suffering damage to their optic nerve.[65] Hopefully, earlier diagnosis and treatment of these patients may prevent them from developing subsequent visual field loss. The practitioner needs to incorporate the information from all testing results in making diagnosis and treatment decisions. The NFL examination gives one additional piece of information in the glaucoma evaluation.

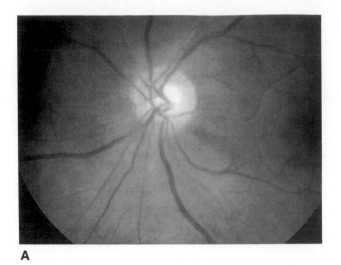

A

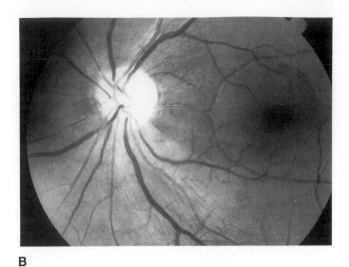

B

Figure 9–21. A. Glaucoma suspect with elevated intraocular pressure, nonglaucomatous cupping and a normal visual field. (*See also* Color Plate 9–21.) **B.** NFL photograph of same patient. Note the diffuse NFL loss in the superior arcades by comparison with the inferior arcades. Tertiary blood vessels are easily seen in the area of diffuse NFL loss. Also note the slit NFL defect at 4 o'clock position.

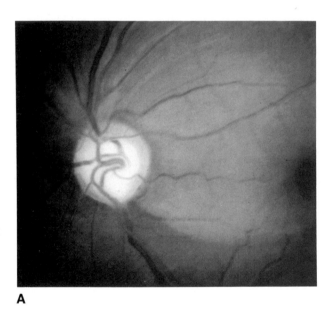

A

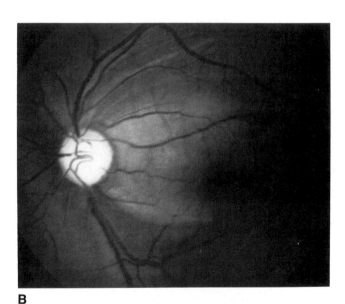

B

Figure 9–22. A. Advanced glaucoma patient with large cupping and an inferior notch of the optic disc. NFL loss inferiorly is visible. (*See also* Color Plate 9–22.) **B.** NFL reversal pattern. In advanced glaucoma, the papillomacular bundle may appear brighter than the superior and inferior arcades (reversal NFL pattern). Note the diffuse NFL loss in the superior arcuate zone and complete NFL loss in the inferior arcuate zone. **C.** Automated visual field of the same patient. Note the dense superior altitudinal defect that corresponds to the complete dropout of NFL in the inferior arcades. There is a relative paracentral scotoma in the inferior arcuate zones, which corresponds to the diffuse NFL loss in the superior arcades. Patient's visual acuity was 20/20. (*From Litwak AB. Evaluation of the retinal nerve fiber layer in glaucoma.* J Am Optom Assoc. *1990;61:390–397. Copyright American Optometric Association.*)

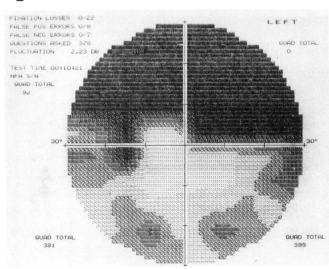

C

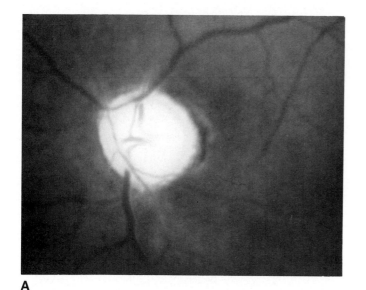

A

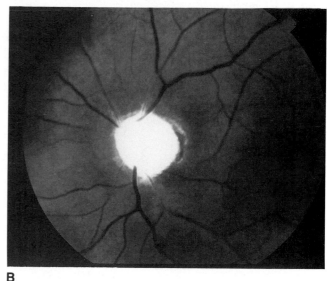

B

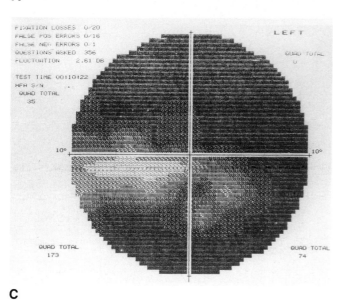

C

Figure 9–23. A. Endstage glaucomatous damage. Note complete cupping of the optic nerve. (*See also* Color Plate 9–23.) **B.** Complete loss of striations of NFL of the same patient. Note the prominent retinal blood vessels and the granular appearance of the retinal pigment epithelium in the peripapillary area. Also notice the pseudosheathing effect of the retinal vessels near the optic disc due to the greater visibility of their outer walls. **C.** Automated visual field of the patient using the central 10° program. Note the extensive field loss except for a small central island of vision. Patient's visual acuity was 20/20. (*From Litwak AB. Evaluation of the retinal nerve fiber layer in glaucoma. J Am Optom Assoc. 1990;61:390–397. Copyright American Optometric Association.*)

REFERENCES

1. Caprioli J. Correlation of visual function with optic nerve fiber layer structure in glaucoma. *Surv Ophthalmol.* 1989;33(suppl):319–330.
2. Carpel EF, Engstrom PF. The normal cup-disk ratio. *Am J Ophthalmol.* 1981;91:588–597.
3. Schwartz B. Cupping and pallor of the optic disk. *Arch Ophthalmol.* 1973;89:272–277.
4. Goldman H. Biomicroscopy of the eye. *Am J Ophthalmol.* 1968;66:789–804.
5. Barker FM. Vitreoretinal biomicroscopy: A comparison of techniques. *J Am Optom Assoc.* 1987;58:985–992.
6. Gutner R, Cavallerano A, Wong D. Fundus biomicroscopy: A comparison of four methods. *J Am Optom Assoc.* 1988;59:388–390.
7. Thurschwell L. How to perform gonioscopy and peripheral retinal examination with a Goldmann three-mirror contact lens. *So J Optom.* 1983;1:18–24.
8. Fingeret M, Casser L, Woodcome HT. *Atlas of Primary Eyecare Procedures.* Norwalk, CT: Appleton & Lange; 1990.
9. Rosen E. Biomicroscopic examination of the fundus with a +55D lens. *Am J Ophthalmol.* 1959;48:782–787.
10. Cavallerano A, Gutner R, Garston M. Indirect biomicroscopy techniques. *J Am Optom Assoc.* 1986;57:755–758.
11. Minckler DS. The organization of nerve fiber bundles in the primate optic nerve head. *Arch Ophthalmol.* 1980; 98:1630–1636.
12. Read RM, Spaeth GL. The practical clinical appraisal of the optic disc in glaucoma. The natural history of cup

progression and some specific disc-field correlations. *Trans Am Acad Ophthalmol Otol.* 1974;78:255–274.

13. Quigley HA, Brown AE, Morrison JD, Drance SM. The size and shape of the optic disc in normal human eyes. *Arch Ophthalmol.* 1990;108:51–57.

14. Jonas JB, Gusek GC, Naumann GO. Optic disc, cup and neuroretinal rim size configuration and correlation in normal eyes. *Invest Ophthalmol Vis Sci.* 1988;29:1151.

15. Jonas JB, Guseck GC, Guggenmoos-Holzmann I, Naumann GO. Size of the optic nerve scleral canal and comparison to intravital determination of optic disk dimensions. *Graefe's Arch Clin Exp Ophthalmol.* 1988;226: 213–215.

16. Bengtsson B. The variation and covariation of cup and disc diameters. *Acta Ophthalmol.* 1976;54:804–818.

17. Armaly MF. Genetic determination of cup/disc ratio of the optic nerve. *Arch Ophthalmol.* 1967;78:35–45.

18. Schwartz JT, Reuling FH, Garrison RJ. Acquired cupping of the optic nerve head in normotensive eyes. *Br J Ophthalmol.* 1975;59:216–221.

19. Dolman CL, McCormick AQ, Drance SM. Aging of the optic nerve. *Arch Ophthalmol.* 1980;98:2053–2058.

20. Johnson SM, Miao M, Sadun AA. Age-related decline of human optic nerve axon population. *Age Ageing.* 1987;10:5–9.

21. Katz J, Sommer A. Asymmetry and variation in the normal hill of vision. *Arch Ophthalmol.* 1986;104:65–68.

22. Repka MX, Quigley HA. The effect of age on normal human optic nerve fiber number and diameter. *Ophthalmology.* 1989;96:26–32.

23. Airaksinen PJ, Drance SM, Schulzer M. Neuroretinal rim area in early glaucoma. *Am J Ophthalmol.* 1985; 99:1–4.

24. Pederson JE, Anderson DR. The mode of progressive disc cupping in ocular hypertension and glaucoma. *Arch Ophthalmol.* 1980;98:490–495.

25. Odberg T, Riise D. Early diagnosis of glaucoma: The value of successive stereophotography of the optic disc. *Acta Ophthalmol.* 1985;63:257–263.

26. Quigley HA, Dunkelberger GR, Green WR. Chronic human glaucoma causing selectively greater loss of large optic nerve fibers. *Ophthalmology.* 1988;95:357–363.

27. Herschler J, Osher RH. Baring of the circumlinear vessel. An early sign of optic nerve damage. *Arch Ophthalmol.* 1980;98:865.

28. Sutton GE, Motolko MA, Phelps CD. Baring of a circumlinear vessel in glaucoma. *Arch Ophthalmol.* 1983; 101:739.

29. Honrubia F, Calonge B. Evaluation of the nerve fiber layer and peripapillary atrophy in ocular hypertension. *Int Ophthalmol.* 1989;13:57–62.

30. Primrose J. Early signs of the glaucomatous disc. *Br J Ophthalmol.* 1971;55:820–825.

31. Jonas JB, Nguyen XN, Gusek GC, Naumann GO. Parapapillary chorioretinal atrophy in normal and glaucoma eyes. I. Morphometric data. *Invest Ophthalmol Vis Sci.* 1989;30:908–918.

32. Caprioli J, Spaeth GL. Comparison of visual field defects in low-tension glaucoma. *Am J Ophthalmol.* 1984; 97:730–737.

33. Buss DR, Anderson DR. Peripapillary crescents and halos in normal-tension glaucoma and ocular hypertension. *Ophthalmology.* 1989;96:16–19.

34. Wilensky JT, Kolker AE. Peripapillary changes in glaucoma. *Am J Ophthalmol.* 1976;81:341–345.

35. Primrose J. The incidence of the peripapillary halo glaucomatosus. *Trans Ophthalmol Soc UK.* 1969;89:585–587.

36. Drance SM, Begg IS. Sector hemorrhage: A probable acute ischaemic disc change in chronic simple glaucoma. *Can J Ophthalmol.* 1970;5:137–141.

37. Shihab ZM, Lee PF, Hay P. The significance of disc hemorrhage in open-angle glaucoma. *Ophthalmology.* 1982;89:211–213.

38. Airaksinen PJ, Mustonen E, Alanko HI. Optic disc hemorrhages: Analysis of stereophotographs and clinical data of 112 patients. *Arch Ophthalmol.* 1981;99:1795–1801.

39. Begg IS, Drance SM, Sweeney VP. Ischaemic optic neuropathy in chronic simple glaucoma. *Br J Ophthalmol.* 1971;55:73–90.

40. Quigley HA, Addicks EM, Green WR, et al. Optic nerve damage in human glaucoma. II. The site of injury and susceptibility to damage. *Arch Ophthalmol.* 1981;99:635–649.

41. Kitazawa Y, Shirato S, Yamamoto T. Optic disc hemorrhage in low-tension glaucoma. *Ophthalmology.* 1986;93: 853–857.

42. Diehl DL, Quigley HA, Miller NR, Sommer A, Burney EN. Prevalence and significance of optic disc hemorrhage in a longitudinal study of glaucoma. *Arch Ophthalmol.* 1990;108:545–550.

43. Chumbley LC, Brubaker RF. Low tension glaucoma. *Am J Ophthalmol.* 1976;81:761–767.

44. Drance SM. Some factors in the production of low tension glaucoma. *Br J Ophthalmol.* 1972;56:229–242.

45. Airaksinen PJ, Mustonen E, Alanko HI. Disc hemorrhages precede retinal nerve fiber layer defects in ocular hypertension. *Acta Ophthalmol.* 1981;59:627–641.

46. Drance SM, Fairclough M, Butler DM, Kottler MS. The importance of disc hemorrhage in the prognosis of chronic open angle glaucoma. *Arch Ophthalmol.* 1977; 95:226–228.

47. Susanna R, Drance SM, Douglas GR. Disc hemorrhages in patients with elevated intraocular pressure: Occurrence with and without field changes. *Arch Ophthalmol.* 1979;97:284–285.

48. Drance SM. Disc hemorrhages in the glaucomas. *Surv Ophthalmol.* 1989;33:331–337.

49. Lichter PR. Variability of expert observers in evaluating the optic disc. *Trans Am Ophthalmol Soc.* 1976;84:532–572.

50. Kahn HA, Leibowitz H, Ganley JP, et al. Standardizing diagnostic procedures. *Am J Ophthalmol.* 1975;79:768–775.

51. Schwartz JT. Methodologic differences and measurement of cup-disc ratio. *Arch Ophthalmol.* 1976;94:1101–1105.

52. Tielsch JM, Katz J, Quigley HA, Miller NR, Sommer A. Intraobserver and interobserver agreement in measurement of optic disc characteristics. *Ophthalmology.* 1988;95:350–356.

53. Somner A, Pollack I, Maumenee AE. Optic disc parameters and onset of glaucomatous field loss. I. Methods and progressive changes in disc morphology. *Arch Ophthalmol.* 1979;97:1444–1448.

54. Caprioli J, Miller JM. Correlation of structure and function in glaucoma. *Ophthalmology.* 1988;95:723–727.

55. Caprioli J, Miller JM. Videographic measurements of optic nerve topography in glaucoma. *Invest Ophthalmol Vis Sci.* 1988;29:1294–1298.

56. Caprioli J, Miller JM. Optic disc rim area is related to disc size in normal subjects. *Arch Ophthalmol.* 1987;105:1683–1685.

57. Caprioli J, Ortiz-Colberg R, Miller JM, Tressler C. Measurements of peripapillary nerve fiber layer contour in glaucoma. *Am J Ophthalmol.* 1989;108:404–413.

58. Caprioli J. The contour of the juxtapapillary nerve fiber layer in glaucoma. *Ophthalmology.* 1990;97:358–366.

59. Caprioli J, Miller JM. Measurement of relative nerve fiber layer surface height in glaucoma. *Ophthalmology.* 1989;96:633–641.

60. Varma R, Spaeth GL, Hanau C, et al. Positional changes in the vasculature of the optic disc in glaucoma. *Am J Ophthalmol.* 1987;104:457–464.

61. Litwak AB. Evaluation of the retinal nerve fiber layer in glaucoma. *J Am Optom Assoc.* 1990;61:390–397.

62. Quigley HA, Addicks EM, Green WR. Optic Nerve Damage in Human Glaucoma. III. Quantitative Correlation of nerve fiber loss and visual field defects in glaucoma, ischemic optic neuropathy, papilledema, and toxic neuropathy. *Arch Ophthalmol.* 1982;100:135–146.

63. Sommer A, Miller NR, Pollack I, et al. The nerve fiber layer in the diagnosis of glaucoma. *Arch Ophthalmol.* 1977;95:2149–2156.

64. Sommer A, Quigley HA, Robin AL, et al. Evaluation of nerve fiber layer assessment. *Arch Ophthalmol.* 1984;102:1766–1771.

65. Sommer A, Katz J, Quigley HA, et al. Clinically detectable nerve fiber atrophy precedes the onset of glaucomatous field loss. *Arch Ophthalmol.* 1991;109:77–83.

66. Quigley HA, Dunkelberger GR, Green WR. Retinal ganglion cell atrophy correlated with automated perimetry in human eyes with glaucoma. *Am J Ophthalmol.* 1989;107:453–464.

67. Jonas JB, Zach FM, Gusek GC, Naumann GO. Pseudoglaucomatous physiologic large cups. *Am J Ophthalmol.* 1989;107:137–144.

68. Quigley HA, Addicks EM. Quantitative studies of retinal nerve fiber layer defects. *Arch Ophthalmol.* 1982;100:807–814.

Chapter 10

VISUAL FIELDS

Peter A. Lalle

OVERVIEW OF VISUAL FIELDS

A visual field examination maps out the extent that a fixating eye can see. There are different methods used to measure the visual field with the sensitivity varying depending on the instrument used. The most recent advance, automated perimetry, has become the standard method used in the diagnosis and management of glaucoma. In this chapter, visual fields will be reviewed with an emphasis placed on automated perimetry. This chapter will also discuss the incorporation of the assessment of visual fields into the diagnosis and management of glaucoma, with special emphasis on automated perimetry.

Historically, the presence of a visual field defect was necessary for a patient to be classified as having true glaucoma, while those with suspicious optic nerve cupping and/or elevated intraocular pressure (IOP) were considered as "ocular hypertensives" or "glaucoma suspects" until they developed visual field loss.[1] Thus, perimetry has long played a key role in establishing the diagnosis of glaucoma. Furthermore, since a significant number of glaucoma patients will show progressive field loss despite apparently good "control" of the IOP, continued monitoring for visual field changes has been crucial in the management of glaucoma.[2]

Despite the critical role perimetry plays in the diagnosis and management of glaucoma, visual field testing is not without its clinical limitations. It is a subjective psychophysical test that is greatly influenced not only by disease but also by the response patterns of the patient. The inability of some patients to give reliable responses limits the use of perimetry in these patients.[3] Also, confounding variables may be introduced in the interpretation by the concomitant presence of other disease or anomalies. For example, it may be impossible to monitor the visual fields of patients with other anterior chiasmal diseases, such as drusen of the optic disc, vaso-occlusive disease, or ischemic optic neuropathy, since the associated field defects may be indistinguishable from those of glaucoma.

Further limitation is imposed by the very complex and indirect method used in perimetry to assess visual function. A stimulus of variable size or brightness, stationary or moving, is presented against a background of variable luminance. The light from the stimulus, properly focused, must pass through the cornea, aqueous, lens, vitreous, and outer retinal layers before finally stimulating the rods and cones. If excited, the photoreceptors send a signal via several neurons, which must traverse across the retina, a vascular minefield, through the lamina cribosa, to the chiasm, and eventually to the occipital cortex, where perception of a stimulus is elicited. When a light just bright or large enough to be seen half the time is presented, the threshold of perception is reached. The task of seeing a target against a luminated background is called the differential light threshold.

The *variability* in responses when determining the threshold in normal individuals is what makes it extremely difficult to differentiate early disease from inherent fluctuation (noise). *Fluctuation* occurs during (intratest or short-term) and between (intertest or long-term) visual field tests. An increase in fluctuation may be the earliest sign of a visual field defect. Fluctuation also increases in normal individuals with age, increasing eccentricity from fixation and in the superior visual field. Unless these factors are taken into consideration, accurate interpretation of the results of perimetry is limited.

Perhaps the greatest limitation of perimetry in glaucoma is the recent recognition that a substantial portion of the optic nerve is irreversibly damaged before visual field loss is identified clinically. Quigley has shown that up to 20% of the optic nerve is lost in glaucoma before automated perimetry can detect a defect.[4] Goldmann perimetry fared worse, with up to 40% of nerve gone before a defect occurred (Fig. 10–1).[5] This limitation continues to spur research into other psychophysical tests with greater sensitivity,

although none of these techniques have gained widespread acceptance.

With these limitations of perimetry in mind, it is useful to recall that visual field loss is not even necessary for the diagnosis and treatment of glaucoma. Progressive cupping,[6] the presence of disc hemorrhages[7] or nerve fiber layer defects[8] can all occur before visual field loss. Unfortunately, these changes are even more difficult to detect and impossible to quantify, leaving us with the admittedly imperfect visual field examination as the key test in the diagnosis and management of glaucoma.

HILL OF VISION

Traquir's classical and elegant description of the hill of vision (HOV) as an island of vision arising from a sea of blindness endures in the age of automated visual field testing. Every point in space (the visual field) is represented by a corresponding point on the retina (Fig. 10–2).

Think of the various heights on the island as representing different levels of brightness, with sea level as a large bright light and the top of the hill as the smallest, dimmest light you can see. Think of each circumference as a mapping of the visual field, showing where the target was seen. A large, bright light will be seen everywhere in the field of vision whereas a smaller, dimmer light will only be seen by the small, central part of vision. If you could look down from above on the island and see the circumferences at the

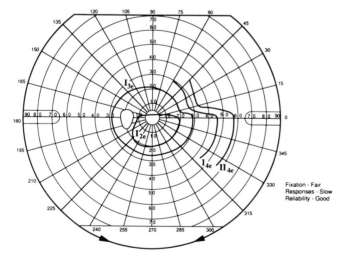

Figure 10–1. This patient with a cup-to-disc ratio of 0.8 has an inferior notch with a corresponding superior field defect. The broad superior nasal step just encroaches on the central 30°. Despite the large cup with no visible inferior rim, there is minimal field loss, illustrating the need for extensive axonal loss before a Goldmann perimeter (GVF) defect appears.

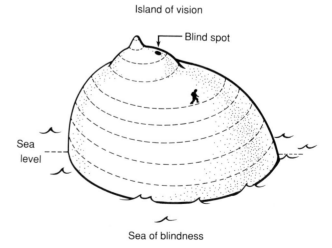

Figure 10–2. On the hill of vision, the circumferences represent the isopters that are plotted in a visual field examination. The higher the circumference is measured (smaller stimuli, greater sensitivity), the smaller it becomes (smaller area of field responding to stimuli).

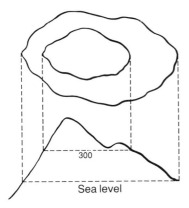

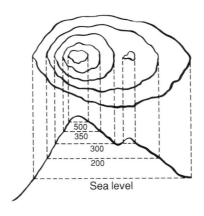

Figure 10–3. Isopters are similar to the contour lines that make up a topographical map. The greater the number of lines (isopters) plotted, the better the definition of the hill of vision.

various heights, you would suddenly recognize that it looks like both a contour map and a visual field print out. They look the same because they are the same. A contour or topographical map is a two-dimensional representation of three-dimensional land masses. Likewise, the isopter lines (circumferences) of the perimetry tell us about the topography of the HOV (Fig. 10–3). Visual field defects represent changes in the shape and contour of the HOV. Therefore, it is important to know the appearance of the normal HOV.

The normal HOV, in addition to showing the fluctuation previously described, also undergoes changes with age. As an individual ages, the HOV is depressed by 0.5 decibels (dB) per decade, as if the HOV were sinking into the sea of blindness. In addition, the variability or fluctuation also increases with age. Since glaucoma is basically a geriatric disease, these changes in the HOV become important clinically.

TECHNIQUES FOR MEASURING THE HILL OF VISION

Principles of Kinetic Testing

Basic Concept. For most of the past century, kinetic perimetry has been the standard for clinically assessing the HOV. In its simplest form, a stimulus of a certain size and brightness is selected, which determines how high on the HOV it can be seen. The stimulus is moved from outside the hill of vision (non-seeing) towards the center of the island (seeing). When the edge of the hill is located, the patient sees the stimulus.

Tangent Screen Perimetry

In a tangent screen visual field examination, small, white, round discs are moved against a black back-

ground, testing the central 30° of the visual field. With a tangent screen, a small part of the retina projects onto a very large circular area of the screen. This magnification allows small visual field defects to be found, provided the time is taken to carefully explore the central visual field. The tangent screen was the test of choice up until the late 1960s and is still used in neuro-ocular disease evaluation when looking for small, shallow scotomas. The tangent screen has several inherent limitations. The peripheral visual field, important in glaucoma to explore for a nasal step, cannot be tested by tangent screen. Also, constant, uniform background illumination, vital for obtaining reproducible fields, is difficult to achieve. Patients' responses are influenced by the motion of the perimetrist's arm and hand as well as the placement of marking pins on the screen.

Goldmann Bowl Perimetry

The design of the Goldmann perimeter eliminated many of the shortcomings of the tangent screen by standardizing the instrument testing conditions. A spot of light is projected onto a hemisphere with a 33-cm radius, allowing uniform illumination from a single light source. The full visual field can be tested against a uniform background. Both kinetic and modified static testing technique can be used with the Goldmann perimeter. In kinetic testing, a spot of light is moved from non-seeing to seeing. With modified static testing, the spot is switched off, moved to another location, and then turned back on. Modified static testing is usually employed while exploring the central area of the visual field, using one stimulus of a fixed size and brightness for all tested points.

Although it eventually became the standard for visual field testing, the introduction of the Goldmann perimeter in the early 1960s met with initial resistance.[9] Some thought their patients would miss the presence of the perimetrist. Other clinicians failed to see the advantage of testing the peripheral nasal field

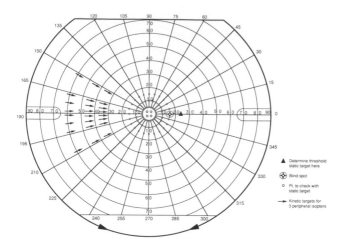

Figure 10–4. The modified Armaly-Drance technique provides a rapid suprathreshold screening of the full visual field, employing both static and kinetic targets.

in glaucoma, while still others thought the test was too long and taxing for most patients.

In the late 1960s, Armaly devised a glaucoma screening test to standardize the assessment of the visual field with the Goldmann perimeter.[9] Only the essential areas of the field were tested with a few selected targets, employing both static and kinetic techniques, and taking only about 7 minutes per eye.

Armaly initially tested only the central visual field, using static targets inside 20° and kinetic targets for the nasal field between 20 and 30°. Rock and Drance increased the sensitivity of the technique by testing the peripheral nasal field as well.[10] Armaly called the technique "selective perimetry" but it has become known as the Armaly-Drance test (Fig. 10–4; Table 10–1). The Armaly-Drance screening test has proven to have good sensitivity and specificity in identifying patients with glaucomatous visual field defects, quickly becoming the standard perimetric test for glaucoma suspects. Using this technique, the nature of glaucomatous defects was defined: which are the most common, which are significant, and what constitutes a significant change on follow-up

TABLE 10–1. BASIC ARMALY-DRANCE TECHNIQUE

1. Size I target used, placed at 25° temporally, increase brightness until just seen
2. Statistically check 76 designated points inside 20° with target determined in Step 1
3. Kinetically plot blind spot with I3e target
4. Kinetically plot several partial isopters in nasal field from 25 to 60° with larger, brighter targets

TABLE 10–2. SIGNIFICANT DEFECTS: GOLDMANN VISUAL FIELD

1. Nasal step of at least 10° if isolated
2. Nasal step of 5° if accompanied by adjacent scotoma
3. Paracentral scotoma of at least 5° in size and at least 0.5 log unit (5 decibels) in depth

(Tables 10–2 and 10–3). Its speed and accuracy allowed large numbers of patients to be examined.

The typical appearance of the earliest visual field defects in glaucoma is well documented.[11] In 90% of glaucoma cases, small, shallow paracentral scotomas and/or central nasal steps are the earliest defects seen. This is sometimes preceded by an increase in fluctuation in these areas while they still have normal threshold values. These scotomas usually appear in an area extending from the blind spot and arc out to the nasal field, following the course of the arcuate nerve fiber bundles in the retina. As the paracentral scotomas enlarge, they can form a complete arcuate defect that points to the blind spot, crosses the vertical midline, and ends up forming a "step" in the nasal periphery. Rock and Drance found that about 10% of the glaucoma suspects will have a peripheral (outside 30°) nasal step as the first discernible defect.[10] Also noted was the propensity of glaucoma to affect either the superior or inferior half of the nasal visual field first, creating an incongruity in this hemisphere.[12,13] Large arcuate defects, destroying the nasal half of the visual field can be present with only minimal involvement temporally. In advanced glaucoma, the entire visual field will be involved.

Principles of Static Perimetry

Basic Concept. Another approach to measuring the shape and contour of the HOV uses static testing. Instead of picking a given height as determined by the stimulus size and brightness and moving it towards the center of the HOV until it is seen, the target can remain stationary and change in size or brightness until it is visualized (Fig. 10–5). Static perimetry presents many stimuli of varying brightness or size, one at a time, at a given point until the patient just sees the light. This is different from kinetic pe-

TABLE 10–3. SIGNIFICANT CHANGES IN FIELD DEFECTS: GOLDMANN VISUAL FIELD

1. Enlargement of nasal step by at least 10°
2. Increase in depth of scotoma by at least 0.5 log unit
3. New significant defects

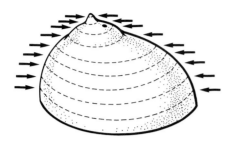

Kinetic perimetry

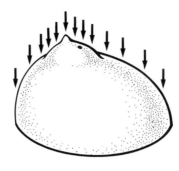

Static perimetry

Figure 10–5. With kinetic plotting, a stimulus of given size and brightness (height of the hill of vision) is selected and moved toward the edge of the hill of vision until it is first detected. By contrast, static perimetry picks the location first and varies the stimulus brightness and size until it is detected.

rimetry, which rarely tests the same location with more than one stimulus. Thus, kinetic perimetry explores a large area of the field but does not give very detailed information, while static perimetry examines a smaller area in more detail.

Static Perimeters

The Tubinger perimeter is a manually operated instrument that explores one meridian of the visual field 1° at a time. This gives detailed information that allows a static profile or "cross-section" of the HOV to be constructed. It is a time-consuming and laborious procedure that can only test one meridian before the patient becomes fatigued. It was used primarily for research. The advent of computers allowed the automation of the static visual field testing procedure, improving the psychometric properties of the test by allowing randomization of the presentation of stimuli.

Automated static perimeters have evolved into two types, depending on the method used to present the stimuli: light emitting diodes (LEDs) or projection. Perimeters using LEDs have preplaced lights on the surface of the bowl of the perimeter. The diodes are placed at the points commonly tested, with the better LED perimeters having more points. Projection perimeters mimic the Goldmann perimeter in that the target can be projected onto any point in the bowl. The better LED perimeters are effective in detecting the presence of a visual field defect when using a screening strategy. When quantification and monitoring of a visual field defect are warranted, threshold testing is needed. Most early LED perimeters could not vary their intensity enough to do adequate threshold perimetry. Modern LED perimeters, such as the Dicon 4000, do threshold testing. Projection static perimeters, while more costly, excel at threshold perimetry, which is the technique of choice for the management of glaucoma.

Ironically, many of the same arguments used during the transition from the tangent screen to the Goldmann perimeter are being used again in the transition from manual to automated instruments. These arguments point to the advantage of a technician who controls the testing procedure. However, the advantages of manual perimetry are only present if a competent technician is performing the test. One study found only 69% of manual fields performed in private offices were done correctly.[14] The best perimetrists were usually based at institutions or major hospitals. One of the main advantages of automated visual field testing, therefore, is its ability to bring reliability, reproducibility, and accuracy to visual field testing in any private office.

There are many good automated perimeters available and the practitioner is encouraged to research which instrument best suits the individual's needs. Whereas many of the concepts that will be discussed are common to all perimeters, because each perimeter speaks a different "language," it is beyond the scope of a single chapter to discuss each instrument. Therefore, while acknowledging the merits of all perimeters and, specifically projection instruments, it is necessary to select one perimeter for discussion. The standard in the United States at present is the Humphrey Field Analyzer (HFA), if for no other reason than it has the most units in operation. This chapter will present the basic principles of the HFA and use examples of patients tested with this instrument.

PRINCIPLES OF AUTOMATED VISUAL FIELD TESTING

Unlike Goldmann perimetry that uses different size stimuli, the HFA uses the size III (0.42°) unless otherwise instructed. The stimulus is varied in intensity from 0.8 to 10,000 apostilbs, a range of about 5 log units. The differential retinal threshold is inversely related to the intensity of the stimulus and is recorded in decibels (dB). Decibels are a logarithmic expression of the sensitivity of the retina and range from 0 to 50. The threshold at a given point in the visual field is determined by a staircase method of increasing and decreasing the luminance of the stimulus. If the stimulus is seen at a given point, the light is made 4 dB dimmer. This is repeated until the stimulus is not seen and then made 2 dB brighter until seen again. This is known as double crossing of the threshold. A newer testing strategy (FASTPAC) has an option that uses 3-dB steps and crosses the threshold only once. This reduces the test time of threshold fields up to 40%. Thus, multiple presentations of the stimulus with varying luminance is required to determine threshold at each point.

For all threshold and most screening tests, the HFA will first "initialize" the field to compensate for visual fields that are uniformly depressed secondary to age-related changes such as cataracts and miosis. Four points around fixation are thresholded and the second most sensitive point is selected to predict the overall height of the HOV. This is now known as the central reference level and will indicate if the visual field is normal or depressed. With all screening tests and threshold tests interpreted without STATPAC, the central reference level for the patient has the effect of raising or lowering the expected HOV, affecting the presentation of the results. STATPAC, which will be discussed in greater detail later in the chapter, is a statistical program that uses a data base to analyze each visual field.

The algorithm used by the instrument to generate the HOV for non-STATPAC tests has a fixed cone shape that decreases 3 dB in sensitivity for every 10° away from fixation. The slope of this fixed-shape HOV is the same in all four quadrants and does not change with age, only raising or lowering its height according to the central reference level.

TEST STRATEGIES

Screening Fields

The first decision with automated perimetry is to determine whether a screening test or a threshold test is necessary. A screening test is quick and simple for the patient, but will only indicate if the field is normal or abnormal. It does not quantify and characterize the defect. The threshold test is longer and harder for the patient, but yields greater information, exactly quantifying the level of defects. Screening tests are referred to as "suprathreshold" tests, since each stimulus is presented as a brightness greater than what is expected to be necessary to see at each point tested.

In order for a screening test with an automated perimeter to have a high sensitivity and specificity, several principles must be followed. To minimize the number of false-positives, each missed point must be tested a second time. To reduce false-negatives, the brightness of the suprathreshold stimulus must be varied to always closely parallel the HOV, using brighter targets peripherally and dimmer targets centrally.

The HFA can employ a variety of strategies to perform a screening test.

Single Intensity. Every test point is shown the same stimulus with no change in brightness, eliminating the initialization phase. For this strategy, the HFA will automatically select a stimulus of 24 dB unless another is selected. Remembering the model of the HOV, it becomes apparent that this strategy is flawed. Testing the most and the least sensitive areas with the same stimulus will cause central defects to be missed because the stimulus is too bright to detect shallow scotomas, and incorrectly label the peripheral regions as defective because the stimulus is too dim for the reduced sensitivity in the periphery. It will also erroneously label defects in patients with small pupils or cataracts that have a general depression. Worse yet, for patients identified at risk for glaucoma, it is not sensitive enough and therefore not recommended for screening glaucoma suspects. This strategy was commonly employed in early LED perimeters and may still be useful for routine testing of new patients for base-line visual fields.

Threshold Related. After the initialization phase, each point is tested with a stimulus 6 dB brighter than predicted by the HOV. Central points will be tested with dimmer lights, while more peripheral points will be tested with brighter stimuli. This is known as eccentricity-compensation. The HFA with FASTPAC can allow the instrument to select the central reference level based on stored, predicted values for different age groups thus skipping initialization and saving about 1 minute of test time. While saving time, this age-reference level option will probably result in too many false-positives on elderly patients with small pupils or significant cataracts and therefore may not be worth the time saving in this age group. The printout will be a map of points seen and missed. Points seen will be assigned an "O." If a point is missed, it will be retested and if still missed will be marked with a black box on the printout. If a point is missed, it is a scotoma of at least 6 dB in depth; 6 dB just exceeds the Goldmann visual field standard of 5 dB for a scotoma to be considered significant. Similar to a 20/40 visual acuity screening with 20/40 as the cutoff, missed points might be 20/50 (i.e., a 7-dB defect), or could be absolute scotomas.

Three Zone. This strategy is a modification of the threshold-related strategy, retesting all missed points with the light as bright as possible (10,000 Asb). If a point is missed with the brightest stimulus, it is marked with a black box and considered an absolute defect. If missed only by the 6-dB suprathreshold stimulus but seen by the brightest light, it is marked with an "X" and considered a relative defect. While not exactly quantifying the defect, it gives a little extra information and assurance that the point is not totally blind.

Quantify Defects. This strategy yields to the temptation of trying to get additional information about the exact depth of the missed points by thresholding all missed points at the expense of time. Adding time to a screening test defeats its purpose.

Threshold Fields

Unlike screening tests that simply compare the patient's responses to an expected "normal" HOV, threshold tests determine the exact shape and contour of the patient's HOV. While time consuming, they provide detailed information that allows a patient's visual field to be quantified and monitored closely for change. Since this is a cornerstone in the management of glaucoma, threshold testing is the only appropriate method for following glaucoma patients.

Full Threshold. After initialization, each point is tested by thresholding, starting 4 dB above the expected value for the HOV. The process is accelerated by the computer in the instrument adjusting its starting point based on data from neighboring points; that is, if one point is severely depressed, the HFA will no longer expect the neighboring point to be close to the predicted HOV. The testing procedure is randomized but, in general, central points are tested first and the periphery last.

Full From Prior. This strategy is available if previous threshold visual fields have been stored using a disc drive. Instead of initializing the field and developing an expected HOV, the HFA will use stored values from the previous visual field test. The results of the current test are then used for the next test. The printout is the same as that for the threshold strategy. This strategy should not be used with the original version of STATPAC since the data base for this statistical analysis was not generated using this technique. Subsequent versions of STATPAC have validated its use. Since the HFA "learns" from adjacent points during a test, full threshold from prior data decreases testing time minimally.

Fast Threshold. Again using stored results, the HFA presents stimuli 2 dB brighter at each point than the value found at the previous test. If the stimulus is seen, it will be considered as stable and no thresholding will be done. If missed, the point will be thresholded. The printout will show stable points as an "O." For unstable points, the amount of change in decibels from the last visual field test is noted. In one sense, this strategy is a modified version of the quantify defects" screening strategy. Unlike quantify defects that add time to a screening test, fast threshold speeds up a threshold test. More importantly, it uses the patient's own HOV for comparison, rather than one generated by the instrument from an algorithm.

Visual fields using the "fast" strategy cannot be incorporated into certain printouts used to analyze change over time. Therefore, do not use this strategy for long-term follow-up of a glaucoma patient. Fast threshold is indicated when a quick and immediate answer to the question of progression is needed and one is willing to sacrifice that information over time.

Printouts

Numeric printouts present the raw data from the test, the actual retinal sensitivity in decibels for each point tested. The *defect depth* printout highlights only the defective areas by presenting the differences between the actual retinal sensitivity and the expected sensitivity in decibels at each point tested. The higher the number, the more defective the point. Defective points are only identified if the difference between actual and expected is at least 6 dB. The *gray scale* printout is a graphic representation in shades of gray of the actual retinal sensitivity at each point tested. The higher the sensitivity, the lighter gray the representation. The various shades of gray are assigned to 4-dB groups of sensitivity. It should also be noted that the gray scale interpolates by shading in areas between tested points, and extrapolates by shading in edge points, making a diamond shape test pattern appear round. By looking at the gray scale plot, areas of decreased sensitivity can be quickly identified.

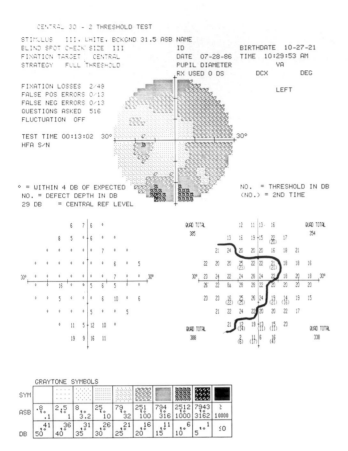

Figure 10–6. A 30-2 threshold field printout without STATPAC displays a gray scale, a defect depth table, and the threshold values. Note that the gray scale suggests a significant depression but inspection of actual threshold values reveals only a 2- to 3-dB difference between the edges of the depression.

Gray scale printouts can also be very misleading (Fig. 10–6). A change in one level of shading may be due to a 1-dB up to 9-dB difference and it is left to the clinician to decide if this is an abnormal decrease.

Point Selection

There is an infinite number of points or combination of points that can be tested in the visual field. Logic dictates that a balance between too many points causing patient fatigue and unreliable results, and too few points, resulting in missed defects, be reached. With the knowledge that glaucoma selectively affects the paracentral and nasal areas of the visual field first, time and energy can be saved by concentrating on these areas, much like Armaly did.

CATCH TRIALS

With Goldmann perimetry, the perimetrist would note on the record if the patient maintained good fixation, good cooperation, and gave consistent responses. This information would allow the doctor to judge if the test was reliable and valid. The HFA has tried to substitute this subjective appraisal with objective measurements, the catch trials (Table 10–4). Interspersed between 33 stimulus presentations will be 1 false-positive and 1 false-negative catch trial randomly presented. Fixation loss catch trials make up about one tenth of all presentations, but more are presented early in the test to insure that the patient is fixating properly, allowing the test to be stopped and the patient reinstructed if too many fixation losses occur. A score is indicated on each printout of how many times the patient improperly responded over the number of times a catch trial was conducted.

Fixation Losses

To determine the patient's ability to maintain fixation, a stimulus is presented in the blind spot. If the patient is not fixating properly, the stimulus will be seen and the response button pressed. To speed up the test, newer versions of the HFA no longer automatically plot the blind spot at the beginning of the test but rather assume an anatomically predicted location. If the patient misses the first or second fixation loss catch trial, the HFA will stop testing and plot the blind spot. If there are more than 20% fixation losses during the test, the results may be considered unreliable and are generally not used to make specific clinical decisions.

Studies indicate that the most common cause for visual field tests to be unreliable is excessive fixation losses.[15–17] It has recently been shown that the majority of fields labeled as unreliable because of increased fixation losses may be due to an avoidable artifact.[17] If

TABLE 10–4. RELIABILITY INDICES: AUTOMATED VISUAL FIELDS

If FP are flagged, discard field regardless of other indicators
Re-instruct patient and repeat field

If FL are flagged, discard field
Repeat VF and have HFA plot blindspot at beginning of test
Monitor first ten FL trials during the test

If FL and FN are both flagged, discard field
Repeat field, plot blind spot, give encouragement and rest
  periods as needed

If only FN are flagged, consider keeping field if repeated
  points in "good" area of field are within 2 dB

FP = false-positives; FL = fixation losses; FN = false-negatives; HFA = Humphrey Field Analyzer; VF = visual field.
Note: An inattentive patient who responds only to a few stimuli (or none) will *not* have any indices flagged. Therefore, the absence of "flags" does not mean the patient was reliable. Be very cautious of markedly depressed fields without clinical evidence for such a change.

during the test, the perimetrist notices that two or more fixation losses have occurred in any of the first *ten* trials, which is not enough to automatically stop the test, he or she should pause the test and ask the HFA to plot the patient's true blind spot. If the HFA still cannot find the blind spot, direct the HFA to replot it with the size I stimulus.

In addition to poor fixation and an unexpected position for the blind spot, fixation losses can result from poor occlusion of the non-tested eye and in a visual field test that shows a high number of false-positive responses.

False-Negatives

To judge if the patient's responses are consistent, a point already tested is later retested with a stimulus that is 9 dB brighter than previously seen. If more than 33% of these retested points are missed, the field is labeled unreliable. If fixation losses are also increased, there is a high probability that the patient is unreliable. False-negative responses can also occur in a normal individual if they become inattentive or fatigued, or if they change their criteria for responding to the stimuli during the test. In addition, patients with significant visual field loss, including that due to glaucoma, can give inconsistent responses.[15,16,18] If fixation losses are low, and false-negatives are high, consider accepting the field as reliable if there are other indications that disease is present. Patients with large visual field defects usually have increased false-negatives because of the nature of the testing process (Fig. 10–7). Normal visual fields can appear falsely abnormal if there is a high number of false negative responses.

An artificial "clover-leaf" pattern to the gray scale printout will appear in a normal patient that gives normal responses during the initialization of the visual field test, but becomes fatigued and less responsive as the test progresses (Fig. 10–8). Truly abnormal visual fields may show a high number of false negatives, an elevated short-term fluctuation, and an abnormal pattern standard deviation.

False-Positives

In early versions of automated projection perimeters, the servomotor that moved the stimulus made a noise while moving between presentations. Overly anxious patients would key their response to the sound of the motors and not to the visualization of the stimulus, thereby responding to stimuli that were clearly subthreshold. To catch these patients, the HFA would make a noise but not present a stimulus. If the patient responded, a false-positive response was recorded. Thirty-three percent of false-positive responses exceeds the criteria for reliability determined for the HFA. Since the newer machines have silent servomotors, the HFA will just pause and not make a presentation. Properly instructing the patient at the begin-

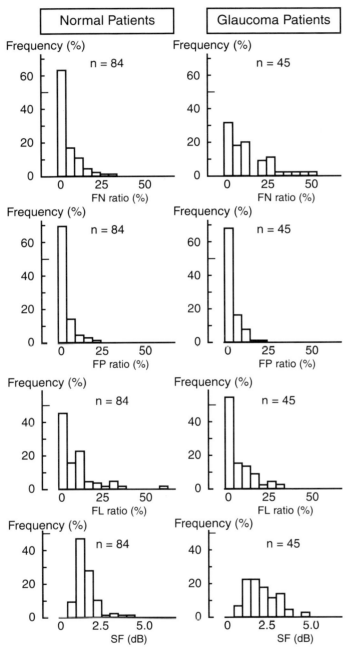

Figure 10–7. A comparison of the reliability indices for glaucoma patients versus normal controls is seen. Both groups displayed similar results for fixation losses and false-positives. However, glaucoma patients showed a considerable increase in false-negatives and short-term fluctuation. Both indices measure the amount of variability in a field, indicating that glaucoma patients have a large amount of intratest fluctuation. (*Reprinted with permission from Heijl A, Lindgren G, Olson J. Doc Ophthalmol Proc Ser. 1987;49:593–600.*[18])

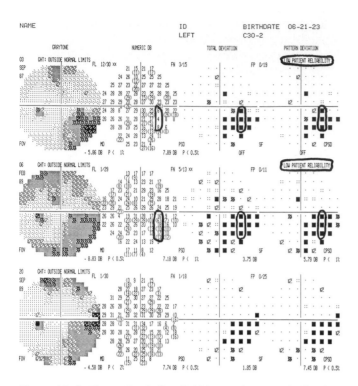

Figure 10–8. The patient's first field has an increase in fixation losses. While fixation losses improved on the second field, false-negatives are now flagged and inspection of the "good" areas confirms excessive variability. By the third field, the reliability indicators are all normal. This improvement represents a learning effect. Note that between the first and second tests, three points greatly improved, yet remained plotted with a black box since they still deviated significantly from expected values.

ning of the test that he is not expected to see all stimuli and to respond only when sure that he saw a stimulus will usually eliminate excessive false-positives.

Patients with increased false-positives will have areas of white in their gray scale, representing false supersensitivity (Fig. 10–9). These are sometimes termed white scotomas and if randomly distributed throughout the area tested can create the appearance of a "popcorn" pattern to the gray scale printout. It is not uncommon to find a high number of fixation losses in a visual field with increased false-positives because the patient is responding even when the stimulus is not seen. The reliability of a visual field with high false-positives is extremely poor. True visual field loss can be missed. The clinician should use great caution in using this type of visual field as the basis for clinical decisions.

Despite the automation of the testing procedure and the objective scoring of the patient's reliability, nothing will replace the physical presence of a perimetrist in the room during the test. The technician

should constantly monitor fixation as well as reposition the patients who start to lean. The technician can continuously encourage and correct a hesitant or poorly motivated patient. The reliability of many visual field tests is improved markedly when the technician recognizes fatigue and pauses the test when needed. While the responsibility for determining how and where to test is now automatically determined, the technician still plays a vital role by determining when to override the machine's programming.

SCREENING VERSUS THRESHOLD TESTING

Once a patient is identified as a glaucoma suspect, thorough visual field testing is warranted. Some practitioners advocate the use of a central threshold test as the initial visual field because it gives the most information for detecting glaucoma. Further, if it is felt that the patient has glaucoma, a base-line threshold visual field has already been done. While in theory this is correct, two issues suggest a full field screening test may have advantages as the initial test to perform on a glaucoma suspect.

First, the value of a threshold field is diminished when the responses are unreliable and variable. A significant number of patients display a learning curve, doing very poorly on their first threshold test if they have had no previous experience in being tested on an automated perimeter (Figs. 10–10 and 10–11). The HFA manual recommends that two threshold fields be done and averaged or merged into one base-line field.[19] Of note is the fact that the variability of responses of the first automated visual field resulted in the exclusion of first visual fields from the STAT-PAC data base of normal values.[20–22] There is an inconsistency of logic to use a "normal" data base of second and third visual field tests to analyze the first visual field of your patient. One alternative is to examine a new patient with a suprathreshold screening test. Since a screening visual field test is less rigorous, the effects of the learning curve are reduced, making it more likely to yield a reliable, valid suprathreshold test as the first visual field examination. Likewise, the patient will "learn" how to respond to an automated visual field examination on the screening test and will likely perform better on the first threshold test.

Second, only the central 30° (or less) is usually tested with a threshold test in a glaucoma suspect or patient, since it is felt that threshold testing is so sensitive that shallow paracentral scotomas will always be detected before peripheral nasal defects.[23] How-

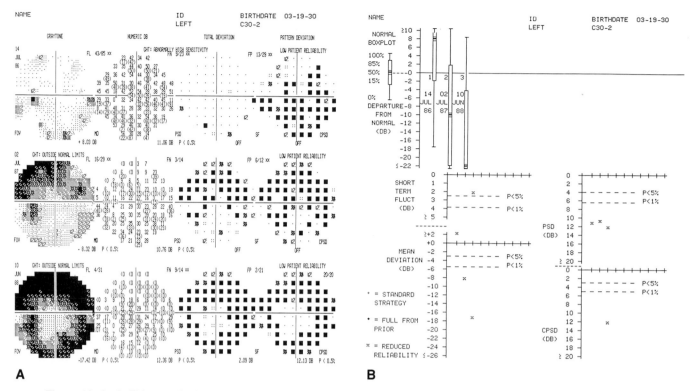

A **B**

Figure 10–9. **A.** This unreliable patient has all the reliability parameters flagged including a high number of false-positive catch trials. Note the patches of white in the first field's gray scale, indicating unrealistic supersensitivity. The false supersensitivity made the total deviation plot look "normal" while the elevator lowered all the threshold values so that the pattern deviation plot showed a severely depressed field. **B.** Utilizing a boxplot representation, this is the same patient **A.** with the first field's median (50% of points) showing 8 dB more sensitivity than expected, an unrealistic outcome. Note that by the third field, 50% of all points were now 22 dB *less* than expected. Even though the false-positive indicator looks normal, the upper tail still indicates a few "super points."

ever, some studies indicate that if properly tested, isolated peripheral nasal defects will precede shallow central scotomas in 10 to 15% of glaucoma suspects even when central threshold testing was normal.[24,25] Certainly, the peripheral visual field should be explored at least once as part of a base-line work-up and a screening test is best for this purpose.

With Goldmann perimetry, patients were first tested with the Armaly-Drance "selective perimetry,"

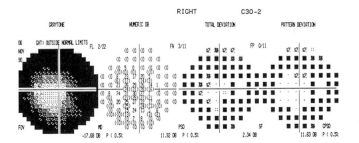

Figure 10–10. This patient was attentive for only the first portion of the test and then rapidly fatigued. A "cloverleaf" or "popcorn" configuration results since the central portion of the field is tested first. Note that the reliability indices were "normal."

a suprathreshold screening test. Only those failing the screening test were referred for detailed perimetry.[26] A similar scheme can be followed for glaucoma suspects with automated visual field testing. The first test should be a full-field screening examination. If the test is abnormal or inconsistent with other clinical findings, an immediate follow-up threshold field can be performed (Fig. 10–12). If the test is normal, the patient should return for a follow-up threshold field within 6 to 12 months.

SCREENING TESTS

The purpose of any visual field test is to separate normal patients from those with defects. The ability to correctly identify all of the eyes with visual field loss is called the sensitivity of the perimetric test. Just as important is the ability of the test to correctly identify the normal patients, the specificity of the test. There is always a trade-off and no test is 100% sensitive and 100% specific. Some tests are designed to emphasize sensitivity over specificity and vice versa.

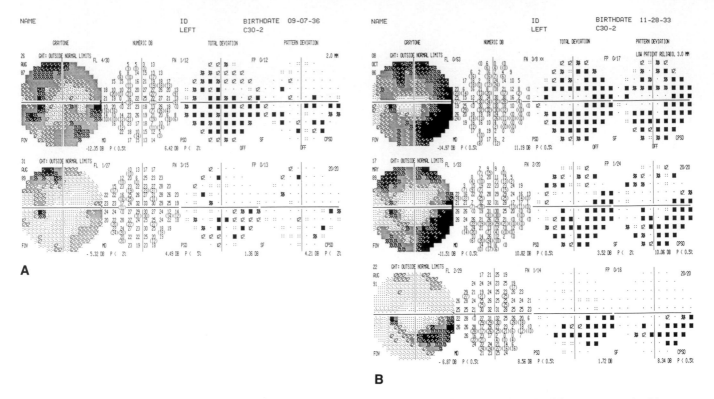

Figure 10–11. A. Even though 2 years elapsed between tests, the second field showed marked improvement in this glaucoma suspect. The patient had no prior field experience and displays the concentric depression that is typical for an inexperienced subject. Note that unlike the patient in Figure 10–8, the reliability indicators are normal for both fields. Although the overall field improved, a mild depression persists. **B.** A patient with an inferior arcuate defect who showed a marked learning curve between his first, third, and fifth field (second and fourth not shown). By the fifth field, the superior field looks normal and the inferior arcuate defect is clearly delineated.

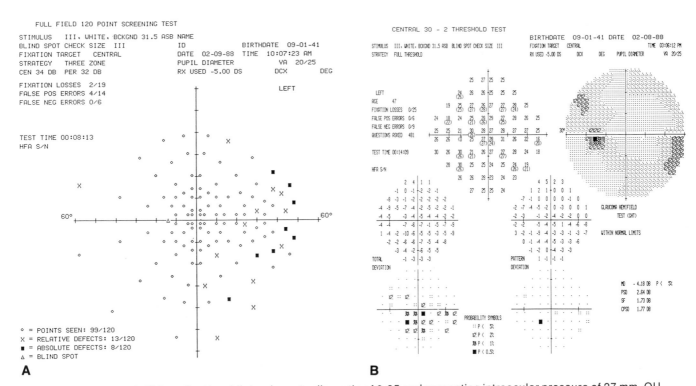

Figure 10–12. A. This patient has bilateral cup-to-disc ratio of 0.85 and presenting intraocular pressure of 27 mm, OU. An isolated, peripheral nasal defect involving both hemifields is noted on a Full Field 120 screening exam. The total number of defects exceeds Kosoko's criteria for abnormality. **B.** The same patient now tested with a Central 30-2 threshold test, which shows no indication of abnormality by STATPAC analysis when only the central field is tested. The fellow eye had a dense inferior, arcuate scotoma extending from the blind spot to the periphery.

When screening large numbers of low-risk patients, it is better to emphasize specificity. When testing patients at higher risk, such as glaucoma suspects, sensitivity should be emphasized.

The HFA has an extensive battery of screening tests to choose from, with many practitioners having individual preferences. However, to know the true value of any of these tests, one has to know its sensitivity and specificity. This can only be determined by a clinical trial, where known glaucoma patients and normal controls are tested with various patterns of points. Published clinical trials have been performed only on a few of the many screening tests available.

Central 40

With the single intensity testing strategy, this is a quick, base-line test for new patients.[27] However, since the interpretation scheme is biased towards high specificity, it is inappropriate to use on patients with risk factors for glaucoma.

Armaly

The HFA version of this test was found to have a sensitivity of only 64% in one study, but the interpretation strategy used was not published.[28]

Full 120

One hundred and twenty points, 70 nasal and 50 temporal, are distributed throughout the central and peripheral visual fields. Interpreting the test is rather simple. Kosoko and associates obtained a sensitivity of 97% and a specificity of 88% for glaucoma by labeling all fields with more than 17 missed points as abnormal (Fig. 10–13.A.).[29] The emphasis of this analysis is on correctly identifying true glaucoma patients from a high-risk group. Since in this analysis it makes no difference if the missed point is either a relative or absolute defect, the threshold-related or three-zone screening strategies can be employed.

The Baltimore Eye Survey used the Full 120 as its initial screening visual field.[30] Eight missed points in any quadrant of the visual field was considered abnormal and follow-up testing was done (Fig. 10–13.B.). It has also been suggested by others that if there is a difference of ten missed points between the right and left eye, there should be a suspicion of glaucoma, even if each eye missed less than 17 points.[31] Furthermore, if less than 17 points are missed, but there is a recognizable defect such as a nasal step or arcuate defect, the field is considered abnormal (Fig. 10–13.C.). The three-zone strategy may help in recognizing these defects.

A normal eye will take approximately 6 minutes to run this test, while a severely depressed field will take 9 to 10 minutes. This is the only HFA screening test recommended for glaucoma suspects at this time. The age–reference level option was not employed in any of the clinical studies and its use has not been clinically validated.

THRESHOLD TESTS

Numerous studies have documented the excellent sensitivity of central threshold tests for glaucoma.[32,33] Several studies have compared the sensitivity and specificity for the detection of glaucoma between Goldmann and automated perimetry. Some glaucoma suspects that were classified as normal with Goldmann perimetry were found to have repeatable defects with automated visual field testing. The automated visual field testing also showed the defects to be larger and deeper than with Goldmann perimetry (Fig. 10–14). Apparently, the Goldmann perimetry is rather insensitive and misses subtle defects. Although automated visual field testing is more sensitive, up to 20% of the optic nerve can be damaged before a defect is detected.[4] At this point automated visual field threshold examinations represent the most sensitive visual field test for glaucoma, but its limitations must be recognized.

Central 30-2

Seventy-six points are tested within 30°. The points straddle the horizontal and the vertical midlines, spaced 6° apart. For the first threshold visual field, the only strategy available is "full threshold." On follow-up, "full from prior" strategy can be employed using the stored data from the last test. Using the "full threshold" strategy, the average test time for most glaucoma patients is about 13 minutes per eye. A normal eye will take about 10 minutes while a severely disturbed field will take up to 17 minutes. STATPAC analysis and FASTPAC are available for this test. While FASTPAC will reduce the test time up to 40%, threshold tests done with this software cannot be analyzed with the glaucoma change probability analysis. Therefore, FASTPAC may not be a desirable strategy to select for some long-term glaucoma patients.

Central 24-2

The peripheral points of the Central 30-2 do not seem to contribute to the initial detection of glaucoma and add to the time of the test. Spurious defects appear more frequently outside 20°, confusing interpretation. The Central 24-2 removes these edge points except along the nasal horizontal meridian, and consists

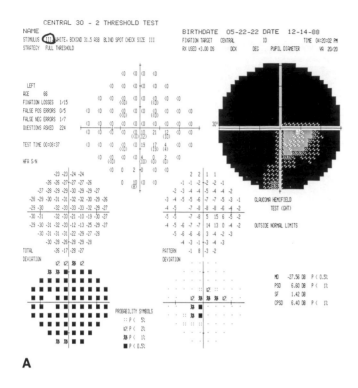

A

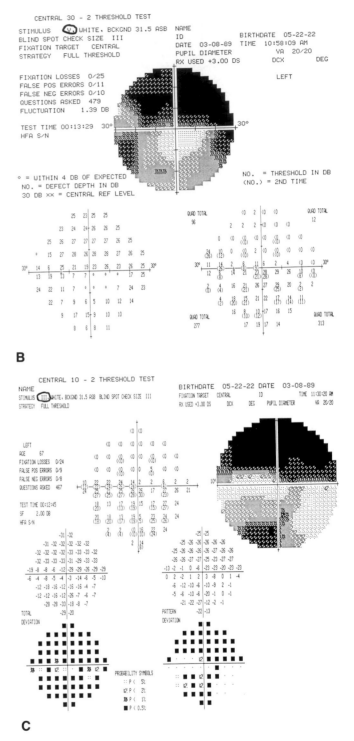

B

C

Figure 10–16. A. This patient with endstage glaucoma responded to only 10 out of 76 points and displayed splitting of fixation. **B.** Same patient retested with a size V stimulus in an attempt to obtain a readable field test. Forty-three points now responded and it appears that the inferior fixation is spared. Later testing showed this to be misleading. **C.** Same patient now tested with 10-2, size III. Note the defect in the field below fixation that was not delineated by the 30-2 size V examination. This patient is close to losing all central vision.

central vision remaining, the HOV is not circular, but rather more depressed supranasally.[34] This would suggest that the superior part of the remaining central island of vision is at greater risk for splitting fixation. Only the 10-2 pattern of points is capable of following the central island of vision in endstage glaucoma.

With very severe endstage glaucoma, even the Central 10-2 test may show a predominance of absolute defects. It may be necessary to use the size V target with the 10-2 field in order to follow the remaining visual function. Extreme caution must be exercised at this point since STATPAC analysis is available only for 10-2 fields done with the size III target, and the interpretation of a size V Central 10-2 will be based solely on the clinician's experience and intuition.

INTERPRETING THRESHOLD VISUAL FIELDS

Using Algorithms

An algorithm applies a simple rule or set of rules to interpret the results of a test. The interpretation of the Full 120 screening test is by a single rule: if 17 or more points are missed, the field is abnormal. This rule was determined empirically by adjusting the cut-off point until the sensitivity and specificity were acceptable.

The interpretation of threshold visual fields can also be accomplished by a set of rules. A simple rule of thumb is that a depression of 5 dB is abnormal.[35] Since 5-dB depressions can occur commonly in normal fields, clusters of adjacent 5-dB defects are judged to be more clinically significant than a single defective point.[36] Guidelines for judging visual field abnormality have recently been suggested. Three different sets of rules were developed, depending on how sensitive (with a decreasing specificity) you want the test to be (Table 10–5).[37]

A further refinement is the comparison of matched (mirror imaged) groups of points across the horizontal midline (Fig. 10–17). Since glaucoma seems to affect one half of the visual field before the other, mirror image analysis compares areas of the

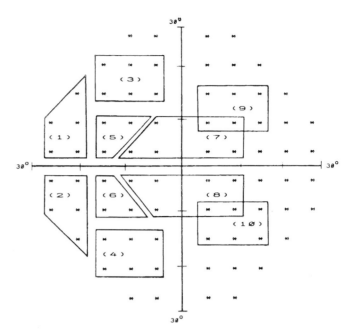

Figure 10–17. As refined by Sommer and colleagues[38], the sums of corresponding groups of threshold values from a central 30-2 are compared across the midline. If the difference between the sums of any corresponding groups exceeds the values listed in Table 10–6, the field is considered abnormal. (*Figure used by permission from Lalle PA, Fingeret M, Eiden SB. J Am Optom Assoc. 1989;60:12:900–911.*)

superior half of the field to corresponding parts in the inferior half.[32,38] The threshold values of points within a group are summed and the total is compared to the mirror image group in the opposite hemisphere (Table 10–6). If the difference between any two matched groups exceeds a predetermined value, the visual field is considered abnormal. Since a severely depressed visual field will no longer show asymmetry between the superior and inferior halves, the sum

TABLE 10–5. CRITERIA FOR ABNORMALITY WITH AUTOMATED VISUAL FIELDS (ANALYSIS WITHOUT STATPAC)

Strict (least sensitivity, best specificity)

4 or more adjacent points of $P < 5\%$ or worse

or

3 or more adjacent points of $P < 1\%$ or worse

Moderate (better sensitivity, less specificity)

3 or more adjacent points of $P < 5\%$ or worse

or

2 or more adjacent points of $P < 1\%$ or worse

Liberal (best sensitivity, least specificity)

2 or more adjacent points of $P < 5\%$ or worse

or

1 point or more of $P < 1\%$ or worse

Note: The point above and below the blind spot are excluded from analysis. If used with the Octopus perimeter, substitute 5 dB for $P < 5\%$ and 10 dB for $P < 1\%$. Mirror image analysis is suggested for comparing points across the horizontal midline. (*Modified from Caprioli J. Am J Ophthalmol. 1991;111(2):235–239.*)

TABLE 10–6. MIRROR IMAGE ANALYSIS CRITERIA FOR ABNORMALITY

Groups Compared		Criteria for Abnormal (Difference in Decibels)
Superior Field	**Inferior Field**	
1	vs 2	25
3	vs 4	35
5	vs 6	15
7	vs 8	35
9	vs 10	50

or

Sum of 1 thru 10 equals 810 or less, the field is also considered abnormal.

of all groups, top and bottom, is compared to detect an overall depression.

The unique quality of this technique is that it eliminates the need to compare the patient's visual field to some statistically "normal" HOV. Since the effects of small pupils and cataracts will be approximately the same in the superior and inferior visual fields, the technique eliminates these artifacts as well. The need for a completely reliable subject is not necessary since the patient is only being compared to himself. The mirror image analysis allows individual fields to be interpreted for normalcy but does not lend itself to analyzing for change over time. Mirror image analysis does not require STATPAC but must be computed by the perimetrist. Recognizing its clinical value, a modified version of a mirror image analysis (glaucoma hemifield test) is now incorporated into STATPAC.

Using Statistical Analysis

The major challenge every practitioner faces with interpreting visual fields is to decide if the field is abnormal. Implicit in any definition of abnormal is a knowledge of what is normal. There is rarely one criterion for normalcy, rather there is a continuous range of values with a gradual transition from common values to less common findings. Attention is paid to the ends of the spectrum, the values least likely to occur. By convention, these extreme values are assumed to be abnormal. Statistics are used to differentiate and quantify the "normal" or more common values from the "abnormal" or less common values. Many biological events are amenable to statistical analysis. Random events seem to behave in a given manner and can be described using familiar statistics such as mean, median, and standard deviation.

The basic assumption of a statistical analysis is that an uncommon value is considered abnormal. This is not necessarily true. For example, while an IOP of 24 mm Hg is an uncommon IOP it does not prove there is glaucoma, nor does an IOP of 16 mm Hg exclude the possibility of glaucoma. However, since an uncommon value is more likely to be truly abnormal, statistics are useful to differentiate a diseased state from normal.

What is seen with independent events is a symmetrical distribution of scores around the middle score, the median. This is known as a Gaussian curve and, because the distribution of values around the mid-point is symmetrical, the median value will also be the average value or mean. If the curve is high and steep on both sides, it indicates there was very little range in scores, with most values being close to the mean. If the curve is low and flat, it indicates a wide range of scores, more variability. Therefore, two curves can have the same mean and median values, but completely different shapes: one with more variability than the other (Fig. 10–18).

One way to describe the shape of a Gaussian curve is to present the median value and the range of 70% of the total scores. As an example, the average score on a test may be 80 with 35% of the results between 80 and 90. Since the curve is symmetrical, the other 35% will be between 70 and 80. In statistical terminology, that would be a distribution of scores with a mean of 80 and one *standard deviation* (SD) of 10. Two SDs from the mean would encompass 95% of all scores. A large SD indicates a high degree of variability in the test results, whereas a small SD indicates that all scores are close to the mean.

The concept of a normal range of scores has come to mean all scores within two SDs of the average. Scores outside this range (the 2.5% at each end of the curve) are considered "outside the normal limits." These are the basic statistical tools for defining "normal." In our example, the average value was 80 and a range of normal was from 60 to 100.

When a point in the visual field is tested on 100 normal individuals, the values of the threshold for

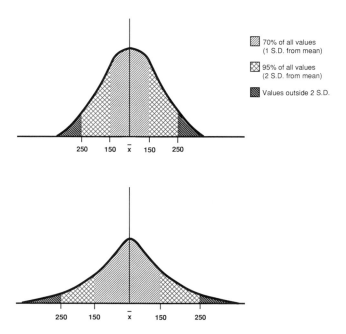

Figure 10–18. The distribution of scores from two different events are shown with both gaussian curves having the same mean and median. However, the lower curve has a greater range of values (larger standard deviation). Therefore, the range of "normal" values will be greater for the lower curve while most normal values cluster around the median in the upper curve.

that one point will fall along a curve. In a Gaussian distribution, there will be an average value and an equal number of points above and below the mean value. We could generate an average threshold value for a point in the visual field for those 100 normal individuals, and specify the range of normal values by calculating the SD. A new patient could be tested and the threshold value for the same point compared to our normal values to decide if that patient's visual field at that point is "abnormal." Each point in the visual field could be compared to a data base of normal values to determine the normalcy of the entire field. This is valid if the age of the patient is the same as the ages of the individuals comprising the normal data base.

The Octopus perimeter uses the Gaussian model to construct its internal "normal" HOV by making two assumptions. First, it assumes that each point in the visual field will have the exact same variability of 2.4 dB (1 SD).[35,39] Second, it assumes that each point will decrease in sensitivity by 0.1 dB per decade of life. This means the HOV will not change its shape with age and that each part of the HOV has the same variability.[35,39] These assumptions have not proven to be entirely accurate when tested empirically.

When groups of patients were actually tested, it was found that many points in the visual field did not generate a Gaussian curve with the same SD. Rather, the more peripheral the point, the more the distribution became non-Gaussian with an increase in the range (variability) of values.[39–41] Points close to fixa-

tion have more of a Gaussian distribution and a small SD, implying that even a small amount of variability from the expected value would be more clinically significant.[21]

Through empirical testing, Heijl[21] found that points adjacent to fixation have 98% of their normal values within 5 dB. Thus, around fixation, the 5-dB rule-of-thumb for defining a visual field defect is valid. There is an anatomical correlate to the significance of a 5-dB defect inside 10°. Quigley and colleagues found that while an *average* test point will have to lose 20% of its ganglion cells to have a 5-dB defect, those points inside 12° had to lose up to 50% for a similar decrease.[4]

However, at 15° from fixation, the distribution of threshold values is non-Gaussian with an asymmetrical distribution around the median. It was noted that 2 SD below the median (−13 dB) was much greater than 2 SD above the median (7 dB). Therefore, even at 15° from fixation, the 5-dB rule-of-thumb is losing its clinical relevance (Fig. 10–19). At a point 27° directly above fixation, the curve was even more non-Gaussian, with some points being 20 dB less than expected yet still within the definition of normal.

Empirical testing not only showed that variability increase with eccentricity, but also that different quadrants are more variable than others, with the superior field showing the most variability (Fig. 10–20).[41,42] This means that not only will a point 15° from fixation be more variable than a point 3° from fixation, but also that a point 15° *superior* to fixation

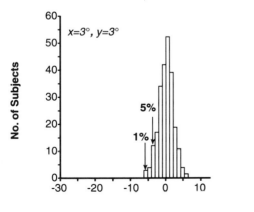
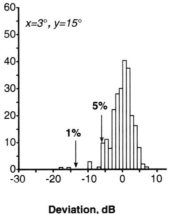
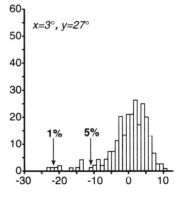

Figure 10–19. Three points in the superior nasal quadrant were measured and the spread of normal values is displayed. Arrows indicate the 95th and 99th percentiles of normal. The further the point is from fixation, the greater the range of expected normal values, invalidating the simple rule that a 5-dB defect is significant. (*Used by permission from Heijl A, Lindgren G, Olsson J, Asman P. Arch Ophthalmol. 1989;107(2):204–208.*)

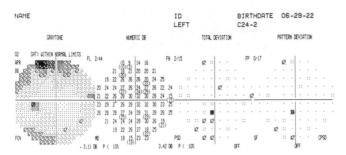

Figure 10–20. A physiological pseudodefect is seen in the superior field. This patient does not have blepharochalasis and was positioned properly. The responses from the superior visual field are the most variable and it is not uncommon for a normal patient to have a depression superiorly, especially in the first few fields. STATPAC recognizes this depression as physiological and assigns little significance to these points.

will be more variable than one 15° *inferior* to fixation. Finally, empirical data have shown that while each point decreases in sensitivity at a constant rate with age, different points will decrease at different rates. The superior field was found to steepen faster with age than the rest of the HOV. The Gaussian model assumes the same rate for each point.

In conclusion, the Gaussian model predicts a HOV that has the same shape throughout life and the same variability in each part of the HOV.[35] The empirical model, on the other hand, found that the HOV changes its shape with age and that different parts of the field are more variable than others.[40] In general, the Gaussian model of the HOV and the empirically determined model are in fair agreement inside 15°, with discrepancies increasing the farther out from fixation.

STATPAC ANALYSIS

At present, there are three versions of STATPAC, the HFA statistical program and data base for visual field interpretation. Unless otherwise noted, the word "STATPAC" will be used to refer to all three versions (original STATPAC, STATPAC Plus, and STATPAC II). FASTPAC refers to a testing option to speed up threshold testing.

The Data Base

STATPAC uses an empirically derived data base generated from the testing of normal patients ranging in age from 20 to 80 from several different clinics. To be included in the data base, a patient under the age of 65 had to have corrected 20/20 acuity and, if over 65, no worse than 20/30. For all ages, no more than 20%

fixation losses, 33% false-negatives, and 33% false-positives were allowed for a visual field to be included in the data base. The patients were tested three times and were free of ocular disease, cataracts, and miosis. Since the first threshold field is much more variable than follow-up visual fields, it made normalization of the data too difficult and was excluded from the data base.[20,21]

The STATPAC data base provides a dynamic HOV based on the empirical model. Its HOV changes its shape, allowing each patient to be tested against a HOV that is appropriate for his age. Additionally, because the empirical model recognizes that different parts of the HOV have greater variability, each point in the visual field has a specific normal mean value with a differing range of normal values.

Introducing Probability Plots

As previously described, the values at the tail ends of a normal distribution of data are considered abnormal. Non-Gaussian curves have asymmetrical tails, but the SD can still be computed. Individual point values can be assigned a "P" value, which represents the probability of normal. In STATPAC, a "P < 5%" means that the threshold value obtained from a patient for that specific point is expected to occur in less than 5% of normal patients of the same age. Similarly, a value with a P < 1% occurs in less than 1% of normal patients. A P < 0.5% means there was no such value in the data base. Clinically, the P values of <1% and <0.5% are the most significant in helping to differentiate normal from abnormal findings.[40]

A map of individual P values for each point in the visual field tested would present an awkward display of data. Schwartz first proposed using a modified gray scale to designate the clinical significance of the threshold value measured at a given point, and that idea has been incorporated in the probability plots for STATPAC.[43] An individual point is assigned a shading, based on its significance. Unlike the standard gray scale printout, there is no interpolation or extrapolation in the display. Therefore, the display will show individual points as either a dot (normal) or a small shaded box. Remembering that the normal HOV is best represented by a non-Gaussian empirical model, a 5-dB defect near fixation may be assigned a black box (most significant) while an 11-dB defect in the periphery may be represented by a dot (normal point).

While the probability plot display gives an easy, quick means of assessing the "normalcy" of each point, two caveats must be mentioned. First, while individual points are analyzed by STATPAC, it remains the clinician's task to analyze the entire field.

Second, while a probability map will aid in the analysis of a single field, it may hide progressive loss of visual fields. Once a black box is assigned to a point, any further deterioration cannot be represented (*see* Fig. 10–10). Therefore, additional schemes must be employed when using boxplots for following changes over time (see below).

Interpretation

The interpretation of visual fields is broken down into two tasks: single field analysis and change analysis. Single field analysis determines if the results of one visual field test show areas that are abnormal. Change analysis determines if there is progression or worsening of an abnormal visual field over time when compared to a base-line field. Single field analysis is employed during the diagnostic phase, while change analysis is used once the patient is under treatment.

Single Field Analysis

Single field analysis with STATPAC consists of a printout that includes the actual threshold values (numerical), a gray scale, total deviation scores and corresponding probability plot, pattern deviation scores and corresponding probability plots, global indices, and the glaucoma hemifield test (STATPAC II) (Tables 10–7 and 10–8).

Whenever a single field analysis printout is scrutinized, several parameters must be checked. Which field test was done? A 24-2 eliminates peripheral edge points and may miss a nasal step seen with other tests. Are there any artifacts due to the eyelids or to the positioning of the lens or patient (Fig. 10–21)? Which target was used? A size V target will make every point seem to be about 10 dB more sensitive, making a bad field look better. What strategy was

TABLE 10–7. COMPONENTS OF SINGLE FIELD ANALYSIS: AUTOMATED VISUAL FIELDS

Gray scale: Highlights areas of concern, limited value

Total deviation plot: Good at identifying general depressions; limited ability to show focal defects when overall depression is present; readily influenced by cataract and miosis

Pattern deviation (PD) plot: Excellent at identifying focal areas of depression, fooled by endstage disease

Glaucoma hemifield test (GHT): Most accurate single index for identifying abnormal field

Mean deviation (MD) index: Indicates overall depression; loses spatial information; readily influenced by cataract and miosis

Pattern deviation (PSD) index: Indicates irregularity of hill of vision; minimally influenced by cataract, fooled by endstage glaucoma

TABLE 10–8. TECHNIQUE OF SINGLE FIELD ANALYSIS

1. Establish that field is reliable.
2. Examine gray scale for any areas of concern (must be confirmed with PD probability plot)
3. Analyze probability plot for defects
4. Look for PSD index with $P < 5\%$
5. Look for abnormal GHT

PD = pattern deviation; PSD = pattern standard deviation; GHT = Glaucoma Hemifield Test.
Note: Random 5-dB defects occur in normal patients. For a point to be a confirmed defect, it must be abnormal in at least two consecutive fields.

used? Are the tests results reliable (Figs. 10–22 and 10–23)? What other confounding factors from the patient's history may influence the field? Vaso-occlusive events as well as optic nerve drusen can cause visual field defects identical to those caused by glaucoma. Is this the patient's first threshold visual field? Recall that STATPAC's normal data base was calculated using the second and third fields of its subjects and the variability of the first field may lead to an erroneous impression of abnormality. Unless the patient was previously tested with Goldmann or with an automated visual field screening test, caution should be exercised in interpreting the first field.

Threshold Values. The actual threshold value obtained for each point tested is printed. These raw data have not been subjected to statistical analysis and are usually of limited value. However, they are of value in two distinct circumstances. The fluctuation in "good" areas of the field can be compared to the "bad" areas to see if the visual field is reliable (see short-term fluctuation index below). They are also of value when looking for progression of a defect.

Gray Scale. The standard gray scale representation is part of the single analysis printout with STATPAC. The various shades of grade are assigned based on the actual threshold values and have not been subjected to any statistical analysis. Many clinicians who were accustomed to the isopter plots of Goldmann perimetry rely totally on the gray scale for their interpretation of automated visual fields. However, it is easily influenced by normal physiological changes. Elderly patients normally have decreased retinal sensitivity and smaller pupils. Therefore, a normal 20-year-old's gray scale will always look "better" than a 70-year-old's gray scale. Cataracts will further depress the field and darken the gray scale.

Because the gray scale is susceptible to artifact, it is of limited value in interpreting the visual field.

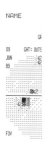

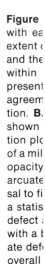

A

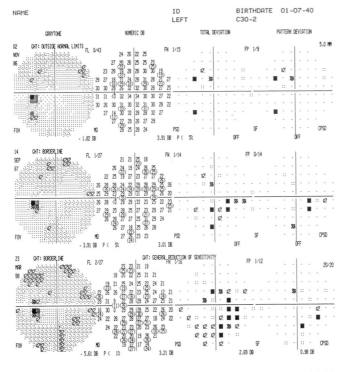

Figure 10–29. This young patient has a cup-to-disc ratio of 0.85 OU, and IOP in the low 20s with increasing general depression noted despite the absence of media opacities. A separate patho-physiological process may be responsible for this type of field loss.[56] Since older patients frequently present with physiologically induced depression, this field defect is often masked and overlooked. Note the gradual increase in the MD index while the fellow eye remained stable, exceeding a 2-dB difference between eyes.[48]

Pupil size, visual acuity, fixation loss, false-negatives, false-positives, GHT messages, and the global indices are also displayed in a compact format. Up to 16 fields can be printed on one continuous sheet.

When watching for progression, the pattern deviation plot and threshold values are the most important displays. New defects and enlarging defects will be easily spotted by observing the pattern deviation plots (Tables 10–9 and 10–10). However, it must be kept in mind that as a point loses sensitivity, the probability symbol will continue to darken, indicating a deepening scotoma. Once a black box is assigned to a point, no further reduction in sensitivity can be represented (see Fig. 10–27.A.). A point near fixation may have a black box even with a sensitivity of 24 dB remaining. The actual threshold values for all points with a $P < .5\%$ (black box) or less, must be monitored to see if the point has worsened on follow-up. Table 10–9 lists guidelines for considering if a change in threshold values is clinically significant and represents true progression of a defect.[53]

Change Analysis

The change analysis printout graphs the global indices individually for each visual field performed on a patient over time, highlighting any trends. One study has suggested that if the first visual field is mildly to moderately abnormal, a change in MD index of about 5 to 7 dB is required to represent a clinically significant change.[52] True progression of the field may occur with a smaller change in the MD, but since the visual fields of glaucoma patients are known to markedly fluctuate, only a large change can be considered as true progression. Since all the other displays will also change noticeably with a MD change of 5 dB, following the MD index is of limited value. Indeed, other studies have indicated that monitoring the change in global indices over time is only useful if the visual field was initially depressed. Global indices are best used to show trends that should direct your attention to the other displays to determine if true progression has occurred.

The change analysis printout also includes a modified bar graph of the threshold values called a boxplot (Fig. 10–31). The amount that each value deviates above (+) or below (−) the age-matched STATPAC data base is rank ordered from the best to worst points. The median value of these deviations is noted by a stripe in the box and then 1 SD of good and bad points is noted by the ends of the box. The box repre-

TABLE 10–10. ANALYZING VISUAL FIELD FOR CHANGE WITH STATPAC

1. Analyze gray scale for enlarging or deepening (gets darker) scotoma; influenced by artifact, use caution

2. Analyze pattern deviation probability plots for new, abnormal points; apply criteria from Table 10–9

3. Analyze all points with a "black box" on the pattern deviation probability plot to see if there has been a significant change in the corresponding threshold values, applying the criteria from Table 10–9.

Any suspected progression must be confirmed on two consecutive fields.

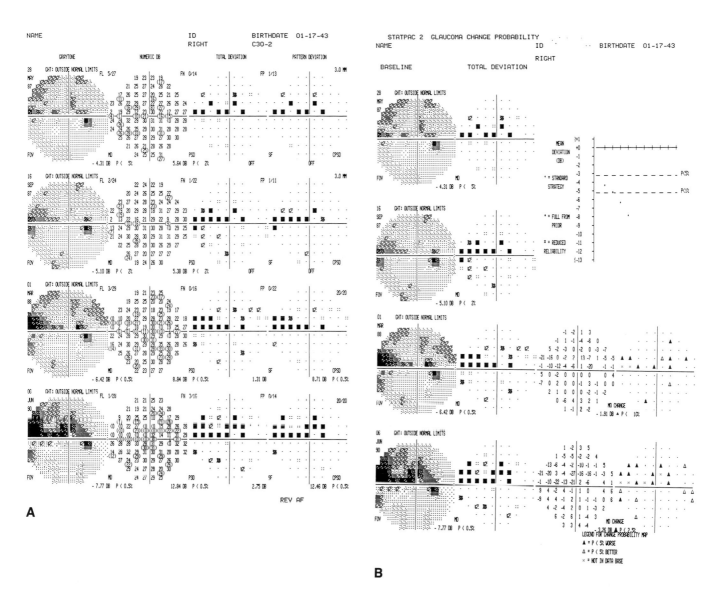

Figure 10–30. A. This patient's scotoma in the overview printout was better defined by the probability plots than the gray scale in the first two fields. Later, as the scotoma enlarged and deepened over time, the gray scale reflected the deepening by becoming darker. However, the same area on the probability plots was already marked with black boxes and further worsening could not be noted even though the points in question progressed to absolute defects. **B.** In the same patient, the glaucoma change probability now highlights those points that have progressed (scotoma deepened). Since known glaucoma patients will have much greater fluctuation than normals, a separate data base was generated for this analysis. However, because it is not as extensive as the data base for normal patients, some points lack sufficient data for analysis. This usually occurs for severely depressed points and they are marked with an "x." Two of the five points circled worsened from the base-line and are marked with a black delta. Even though the other three points worsened, they were so depressed at the time of the base-line fields that no analysis was possible on follow-up fields. The small "x" used to mark these points is difficult to discern from the dot used for normal points. Note that this analysis will also determine if the change in the MD index is significant from the base-line.

sents 70% of the deviation values. Extending from the top of the box (better points) is a tail that will stop at the value of the best point. Extending from the bottom of the box (worse points) is a tail that will stop at the value of the worst point. At the left of the display is a boxplot that represents a normal patient for that age. By comparing the height and shape of the patient's boxplot to that of the normal, valuable information can be quickly ascertained.

If the boxplot looks identical to the norm, yet continues to be graphed lower on follow-up, it indicates that the HOV is not changing shape but is becoming depressed, probably secondary to a cataract (Fig. 10–32). If the bottom of the boxplot remains about the same level, and the tail begins to extend downward, it is an indication that a scotoma may be deepening. If the bottom of the box gets lower while the median remains the same, a scotoma may be enlarging. If the bottom of the box elongates and the top shrinks while the median is getting worse, than a scotoma is getting larger and/or new scotomas are occurring. Note that once the tail or bottom of the box hits <-22 dB, no further deepening can be represented on the graph. If one visual field suggests a progression from a prior field, another test must be conducted to confirm this change.

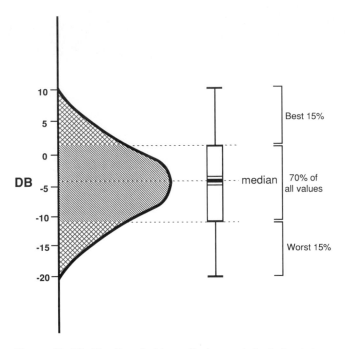

Figure 10–31. The threshold results for each tested point are subtracted from its expected values. The amount each point deviates (exceeds or is less than expected) is then ranked. The distribution of the deviation scores can be represented by a curve or by a boxplot. In this boxplot, the body represents the range of deviation for the middle 70% of points, while the tails represent the range of the 15% best and 15% worse points. A single point can markedly raise or lower the tails.

STATPAC II

While the most common progression of visual field defects in glaucoma is a deepening of existing scotomas,[13] it is difficult to detect this change with STATPAC or STATPAC Plus. For example, on the initial visual field, a central point may have a threshold value of 26 dB when 32 dB was expected. For a central point, a 6-dB defect is highly significant and will be labeled with a black box on the probability plots. However, a 26-dB point is not blind, but still relatively sensitive. It is just not sensitive enough for its location when compared to expected values. Suppose the patient's glaucoma is poorly controlled, and suffers further damage to the optic nerve, that same point now has a sensitivity of 16 dB, indicating a progression of the defect. STATPAC or STATPAC Plus would again place a black box on the probability map. This tells you that the point is significantly abnormal, but does *not* tell you the other vital piece of information, that the point got *worse*. Other parameters such as the boxplots and the graph of the global indices may point out such a trend but these parameters may lose track of small changes or can be fooled when the visual field loss is severe.

Consider one other problem when following a known glaucoma patient. The visual field of controlled glaucoma patients is not very stable and is subject to a lot of fluctuation both during a test (short-term fluctuation) and between tests (long-term fluctuation) (Fig. 10–33; *see also* Figs. 10–28.B. and 10–23).[52,54–56] Therefore, it is illogical to compare a glaucoma patient's visual field to a normal data base once you have diagnosed glaucoma. For example, whereas in a normal individual we would not expect a point to fluctuate between tests from 32 to 26 dB, that might very well be expected in a "stable" glaucoma patient.

Therefore, with glaucoma patients, there are two problems with STATPAC and STATPAC Plus: how much does a point have to change to be considered significant and indicate progress and, more importantly, how will the doctor know the point got worse? Table 10–9 is a guideline to answer these questions, but is not based on empirical data. STATPAC II attempts to solve these two problems.

STATPAC II is based on empirical data from a small group of stable glaucoma patients on which

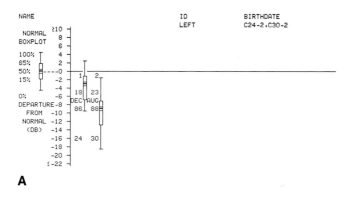

A

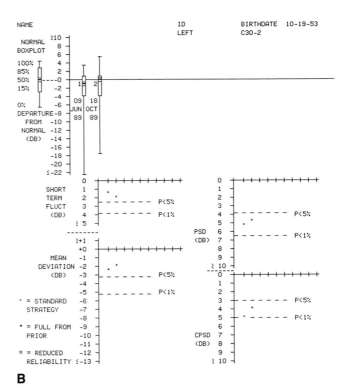

B

Figure 10–32. **A.** In the same patient as Figure 10–15, the body of the box (70% of all points) did not elongate; rather, it shifted downward indicating increasing depression. Both tails elongated, increasing the difference between the worst and best points. **B.** This is the same patient as Figure 10–13.C. and 10–24.A. Note that the better 50% of points (above the median) improved between fields, but the tail remained elongated because of several significantly depressed points. The MD index shows improvement while the PSD index remains abnormal.

visual fields were repeated four times in a month, measuring the fluctuation of the individual points tested. An assumption is made that since the data base was collected within a month while the IOP was controlled, that no visual field loss progressed. Based on this assumption, any change in the fields in the

month was due to long-term fluctuation, rather than progression.

STATPAC II is designed to determine if the change seen in a follow-up visual field or a glaucoma patient represents true progression of the disease or merely fluctuation expected in a stable glaucoma pa-

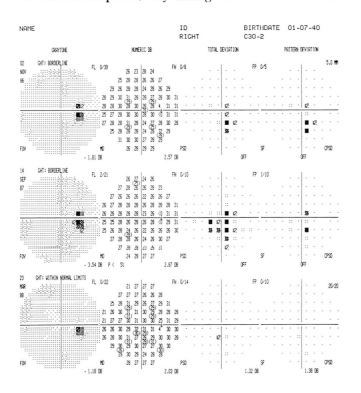

Figure 10–33. This is the fellow eye of Figure 10–29. A paracentral scotoma, present on two consecutive examinations, disappeared on the third examination. The rest of the field was stable, ruling out the learning effect as the cause of improvement. The most likely cause is a physiological fluctuation between field tests (long-term fluctuation), which can either improve or depress test points.

tient. The greater the eccentricity and depression of a point, the more it is likely to fluctuate, requiring these points to demonstrate a greater change to be considered clinically significant.

Glaucoma Change Probability

A minimum of three visual fields are necessary for this analysis. STATPAC II will combine two of the patient's threshold fields and use the average for each point as the base-line. Each subsequent visual field is then compared to the base-line. The perimetrist has the option of discarding any test, and the program will then select the two earliest visual fields remaining as the base-line. Since even a normal patient will display marked variability in the initial two fields, it is strongly recommended not to use just these two visual fields for this analysis. However, if after the patient has had several fields with an apparent flattening of the learning curve, the analysis may be performed using only the last two fields (Table 10–11).

The glaucoma change probability format will print a gray scale and a total deviation probability plot. The value that each point has changed when compared to the base-line is displayed. An additional probability plot is employed indicating that when a point has decreased significantly compared to the baseline, a black triangle will appear. If the point has improved, an open triangle will appear (*see* Fig. 10–30.B.). If there is no significant change, a circle will be shown. Because of the statistics and probability involved, a *stable* field can show a few improved points and a few progressing points each time the analysis is performed (*see* Fig. 10–28.B.). As always, only when the next field confirms that the same points have progressed can you be sure of a true change.

The STATPAC II analysis for detecting change over time in the visual fields of a glaucoma patient

TABLE 10–11. ANALYZING VISUAL FIELD FOR CHANGE WITH STATPAC II

1. Determine if base-line fields are appropriate:
   Is base-line field too depressed due to steep learning curve? (Follow-up fields show numerous open deltas)
   Is baseline too good, known progression occurred but new base-line not re-established? (Numerous black deltas are present)
2. If base-line is appropriate, remember that two to three random black deltas are expected on any given field and must be repeatable to be confirmed
3. If mean deviation index is below −15 dB, too many "X" points (data not in data base) are present, decreasing usefulness of analysis

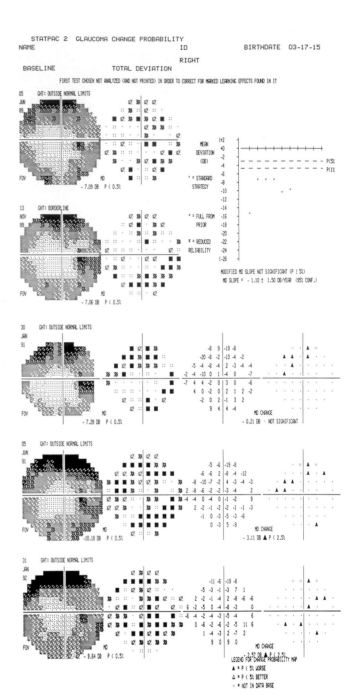

Figure 10–34. The glaucoma change probability has recognized the learning effect in this patient and has automatically discarded the first field. Since the MD index for the first field deviated significantly from the other fields, it was not included in the base-line. Note that the MD index of the first field is still shown.

has several limitations. First, there is very little information in the data base for very depressed points (a mean deviation greater than −15 dB) and STATPAC II will not be able to determine the significance of change over time in these points. These points are

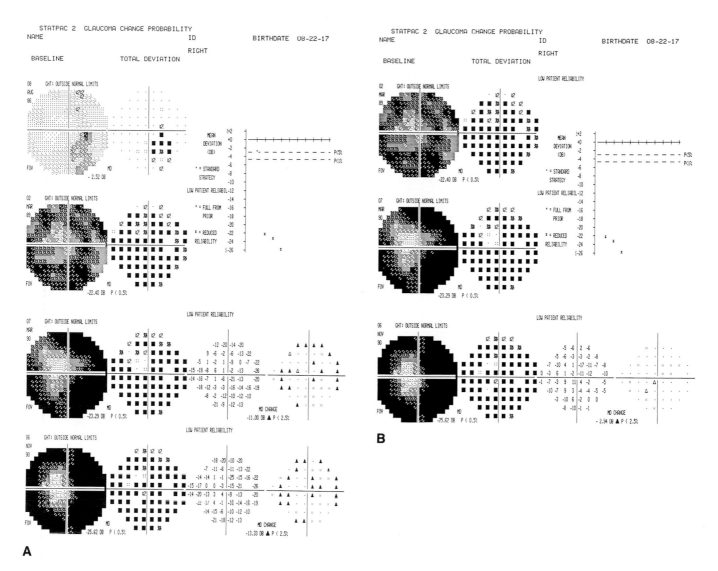

A

B

Figure 10–35. A. In analyzing the glaucoma change probability plot, it is noted that the patient's field deteriorated markedly from 1986 to 1989. However, since subsequent fields continued to deteriorate, the slope of the MD indices failed to discard the first field. The inclusion of this field's high threshold values causes the base-line (average of first and second fields) to be too high. When the March and November 1990 fields are compared to this base-line, they appear to have worsened considerably. By including a "good" field from several years prior, the base-line does not reflect the current depressed status of the patient's field. **B.** The same patient, **A.** with the inappropriate 1986 field deleted manually. Compare the change probability plot of the November 1990 field to the same data in **A.** Since the base-line is now more consistent with the present status, there are no points identified as having worsened. However, because these fields are now severely depressed, there are a large number of "**xs,**" meaning no further analysis of these points is available in the data base. The reliability indices are not displayed in this analysis and the MD index graph and a "low patient reliability" message do not indicate which catch trial was elevated. Note that when a field is deleted manually, the MD index is no longer graphed.

marked with an "x." This is unfortunate since these areas are the ones closest to blindness.

Second, the software will automatically use the first two visual fields as the base-line and will throw out the first test only if it is *way off* compared to the others (Fig. 10–34). Thus, it may appear the patient is getting better or staying stable simply because subsequent visual fields are being compared to an inappro-

priate base-line, contaminated by an artificially depressed initial visual field.

Third, the patient may truly get worse between his or her third and fourth tests and then stabilize. If you keep comparing the fifth, sixth, and so forth, visual fields to the old, base-line, which is relatively better, you will be fooled into thinking that his or her visual field is continuing to progress (Fig. 10–35).

Likewise, the glaucoma change probability display does not take into account any change in sensitivity from cataracts or miosis. Therefore, a new base-line must be established each time there is a significant improvement or progression of the visual field. Remember, current tests are compared to a base-line that may be many years old and not compared to the most recent visual field.

CONCLUSION

Visual fields are critical to the diagnosis and management of glaucoma. The presence of a defect confirms the diagnosis of glaucoma even in the absence of a detectable elevation of IOP. Progressive visual field loss despite IOP "control" is also common and, therefore, perimetry provides the best monitor for the disease. Today's state-of-the-art instruments allow automated static threshold perimetry to be performed in an accurate reproducible fashion in any office. Automated perimetry represents the greatest advancement in glaucoma management in the past 30 years (Table 10–12).

The deficiencies of the instrument must also be recognized. While automated perimetry is a very sensitive test of visual function, up to 20% of the optic nerve may still be lost before a defect is detectable.[4] The absence of a visual field defect does not prevent the diagnosis of glaucoma in the presence of other compelling clinical findings. Some patients give

**TABLE 10–12. SUGGESTED VISUAL FIELD
TESTING SCHEME**

Glaucoma Suspect

1. Full 120 Screening
   If positive, repeat with threshold field 1–3 mo
   If negative, do threshold field 6–12 mo
      or
2. C-24-2/30-2 Threshold with FASTPAC
   If positive, do threshold field without FASTPAC 1–3 mo
   If negative, do threshold field with FASTPAC 6–12 mo

Glaucoma change probability analysis cannot be used with FASTPAC. Do not use this test strategy if you want to follow glaucoma patient with this analysis.

Known Glaucoma Patient

1. 24-2 or 30-2 Test without FASTPAC every 6 mo until stable; then every year if IOP, cup-to-disc, and nerve fiber layer are stable
2. If progression noted, repeat field 1–3 mo later to confirm
3. Follow endstage glaucoma patients with 10-2 every 4–6 mo if stable or every 1–3 mo if IOP is not controlled

IOP = intraocular pressure.

unreliable visual fields some of the time, while others give unreliable results all of the time. Multiple attempts may be necessary before you are convinced that the patient is incapable of performing an automated visual field examination and manual techniques will still be needed for some patients. The automation of the testing procedure has not eliminated the need for a skilled technician to be present with the patient during the test. The greater the technician's skills, the more likely he or she will be to recognize an artifact or patient fatigue and intercede to modify the test. The skilled technician will eliminate the need to discard many "unreliable" fields.

Perhaps the greatest challenge confronting the clinician is mastering the interpretation of the results. Statistics provide a useful tool for organizing data and identifying those values that differ from a representative group of normals. However, it is incumbent on the clinician to always remember that statistics deal with numerical events while the clinician deals with patients and their disease.

REFERENCES

1. Sommer A. Intraocular pressure and glaucoma. *Am J Ophthalmol.* 1989;107:186–188.
2. Kolker AE. Visual prognosis in advanced glaucoma: A comparison of medical and surgical therapy for retention of vision. *Trans Am Ophthalmol Soc.* 1977;75:539–555.
3. Bickler-Bluth M, Trick G, Kolker AE, Cooper DG. Assessing the utility of reliability indices for automated visual fields. *Ophthalmology.* 1989;96(5):616–619.
4. Quigley HA, Dunkelgerger BS, Green WR. Retinal ganglion cell atrophy correlated with automated perimetry in human eyes with glaucoma. *Am J Ophthalmol.* 1989;107(5):453–464.
5. Quigley HA, Addicks EM, Green WR. Optic nerve damage in human glaucoma. III. Quantitative correlation of nerve fiber loss and visual field defect in glaucoma, ischemic optic neuropathy, disc edema, and toxic neuropathy. *Am J Ophthalmol.* 1983;95:673–679.
6. Drance SM. The disc and the field in glaucoma. *Ophthalmology.* 1978;85:209–214.
7. Drance SM. Disc hemorrhages in the glaucomas. *Surv Ophthalmol.* 1989;33:331–337.
8. Sommer A, Katz J, Quigley HA, et al. Clinically detectable nerve fiber atrophy precedes the onset of glaucomatous field loss. *Arch Ophthalmol.* 1991;109(1):77–83.
9. Armaly M. Visual field defects in early open angle glaucoma. *Trans Am Ophthalmol Soc.* 1971;69:147–162.
10. Rock WJ, Drance SM, Morgan RW. A modification of the Armaly visual field screening technique for glaucoma. *Can J Ophthalmol.* 1971;6:283–292.

11. Aulhorn E, Harms H. Early visual field defects in glaucoma. In: Leydecker W, ed. *Glaucoma: Tutzig Symposium*. Basel: Karger;1967:151–186.

12. Hart WM, Becker B. The onset and evaluation of glaucomatous visual field defects. *Ophthalmology*. 1982;89: 268–279.

13. Mikelberg FS, Drance SM. The mode of progression of visual field defects in glaucoma. *Am J Ophthalmol*. 1984; 98(4):443–445.

14. Trobe JD, Acosta PC, Shuster JJ, Krischer JP. An evaluation of the accuracy of community-based perimetry. *Am J Ophthalmol*. 1980;90:654–660.

15. Katz J, Sommer A. Reliability indices of automated perimetric tests. *Arch Ophthalmol*. 1988;106(9):1252–1254.

16. Katz J, Sommer A, Witt K. Reliability of visual field results over repeated testing. *Ophthalmology*. 1991; 98(1):70–75.

17. Sanabria O, Feuer WJ, Anderson DR. Pseudo-fixation loss in automated perimetry. *Ophthalmology*. 1991;98(1): 76–78.

18. Heijl A, Lindgren G, Olsson J. Reliability parameters in computerized perimetry. *Doc Ophthalmol Proc Ser*. 1987; 49:593–600.

19. *Field Analyzer Owners Manual*. San Leandro, California: Humphrey Instruments Co;1983.

20. Heijl A, Lindgren G, Olsson J. The effect of perimetric experience in normal subjects. *Arch Ophthalmol*. 1989; 107(1):81–86.

21. Heijl A, Lindgren G, Olsson J, Asman P. Visual field interpretation with empiric probability maps. *Arch Ophthalmol*. 1989;107(2):204–208.

22. Heijl A, Lindgren G. Normal variability of static threshold values across the central visual field. *Arch Ophthalmol*. 1987;105(11):1544–1549.

23. Seamone C, LeBlanc R, Rubillowics M, et al. The value of indices in the central and peripheral visual fields for the detection of glaucoma. *Am J Ophthalmol*. 1988;106: 180–185.

24. Caprioli J, Spaeth GL. Static threshold examination of the peripheral nasal visual field in glaucoma. *Arch Ophthalmol*. 1985;103:1150–1154.

25. LeBlanc RP, Lee A, Baxter M. Peripheral nasal field defects. In: Heijl A, Greve EL, eds. 6th International Visual Field Symposium, Santa Margherita Ligure. *Doc Ophthalmol Proc Ser*. 1985;42:377–381.

26. Armaly MF. Selective perimetry for glaucomatous defects in ocular hypertension. *Arch Ophthalmol*. 1972;87: 515–524.

27. Comer G, Tassinari J, Sherlock L. Clinical comparison of the threshold-related and single-intensity strategies of the Humphrey Field Analyser. *J Am Optom Assoc*. 1988;59(8):605–609.

28. Marraffa M, Marchini G, Albertini R, Bonomi L. Comparison of different screening methods for the detection of visual field defects in early glaucoma. *Int Ophthalmol*. 1989;13:43–45.

29. Kosoko O, Sommer A, Auer C. Screening with automated periphery using a threshold-related three level algorithm. *Ophthalmology*. 1986;93(7):882–886.

30. Tielsch JM, Sommer A, Katz J, et al. Racial variations in the prevalence of primary open-angle glaucoma. The Baltimore Eye Survey. *JAMA*. 1991;266(3):369–374.

31. Lalle PA, Fingeret M, Eiden SB. Automated perimetry in the management of glaucoma. *J Am Optom Assoc*. 1989;60(12):900–911.

32. Duggan C, Sommer A, Auer C, Burkhard K. Automated differential threshold perimetry for detecting glaucomatous visual field loss. *Am J Ophthalmol*. 1985; 100(9):420–423.

33. Heijl A. Automatic perimetry in glaucoma visual field screening. A clinical study. *Graefe's Arch Clin Exp Ophthalmol*. 1976;200:21–27.

34. Weber J, Schultze T, Ulrich H. The visual field in advanced glaucoma. *Int Ophthalmol*. 1989;13:47–50.

35. Bebie H. Computerized techniques of visual field analysis. In: Drance SM, Anderson DR, eds. *Automatic Perimetry in Glaucoma. A Practical Guide*. Orlando, FL: Grune & Stratton; 1985:148–185.

36. Sommer A, Duggan C, Auer C, Abbey H. Analytic approaches to the interpretation of automated threshold perimetric data for the diagnosis of early glaucoma. *Trans Am Ophthalmol Soc*. 1985;83:250–267.

37. Caprioli J. Automated perimetry in glaucoma. *Am J Ophthalmol*. 1991;111(2):235–239.

38. Sommer A, Enger C, Witt K. Screening for glaucomatous visual field loss with automated threshold perimetry. *Am J Ophthalmol*. 1987;103(5):681–684.

39. Heijl A, Asman P. A clinical study of perimetric probability maps. *Arch Ophthalmol*. 1989;107(2):199–203.

40. Heijl A, Lindgren G, Olsson J. A package for the statistical analysis of visual fields. *Doc Ophthalmol Proc Ser*. 1987;49:153–168.

41. Katz J, Sommer A. Asymmetry and variation in the normal hill of vision. *Arch Ophthalmol*. 1986;104(1):65–68.

42. Young WO, Stewart WC, Hunt H, Crosswell H. Static threshold variability in the peripheral visual field in normal subjects. *Graefe's Arch Clin Exp Ophthalmol*. 1990;228:454–457.

43. Schwartz B, Nagin P. Probability maps for evaluating automated visual fields. *Doc Ophthalmol Proc Ser*. 1985; 42:39–48.

44. Guthauser U, Flammer J. Quantifying visual field damage caused by cataract. *Am J Ophthalmol*. 1988;106(10): 480–484.

45. Wood JM, Wild JM, Smerdon DL, Crews SJ. Alterations in the shape of the automated perimetric profile arising from cataract. *Graefe's Arch Clin Exp Ophthalmol*. 1989;227:157–161.

46. Lam BL, Alward WLM, Kolder HE. Effect of cataract on automated perimetry. *Ophthalmology*. 1991;98(7):1066–1070.

47. Enger C, Sommer A. Recognizing glaucomatous field loss with the Humphrey STATPAC. *Arch Ophthalmol*. 1987;106(10):1355–1357.

COLOR PERCEPTION

Lakowski, Drance, and others have shown that color vision defects occur early in glaucoma patients and suspects. These defects tend to be centered about the blue or blue-yellow axis.[4] Yamazaki and colleagues demonstrated a selective reduction of blue chromatic and achromatic (luminance) sensitivities in glaucoma suspects and glaucoma patients. Low-tension glaucoma patients showed mostly normal chromatic and luminance sensitivities when compared to high-tension glaucoma patients.[5]

Hamill and co-workers found a two- to threefold increase in color discrimination defects among patients with ocular hypertension compared to normal individuals. However, no direct correlation was seen between the acquired color defects and the extent of optic disc damage in glaucoma patients.[6] Another study did find a correlation between diffuse retinal nerve fiber layer loss and yellow-blue and green-blue color matching defects, but not with focal nerve fiber layer loss.[7]

The opponent cell theory of color processing gives us some help in understanding why selective color defects may occur in glaucoma. If ganglion cells are grouped according to the red-green and blue-yellow channels, then their cell axons, which comprise the optic nerve, would also be similarly grouped and could be selectively damaged in glaucoma.[8] Moreover, there are physiological and anatomical differences between the blue and red-green cones. Blue cones make up approximately 13% of the total cone population and are less sensitive to light than red or green cones.[9] Also, blue chromatic and luminance signals are carried in larger diameter axons than those axons that carry red-green signals.[10] Quigley and associates[11] have demonstrated in animal models that larger diameter axons are more susceptible to damage from increased intraocular pressure than smaller fibers. These factors may account for the reason why yellow-blue defects often occur early in glaucoma.

Similar color vision defects can appear in normal individuals with age. This may be due to a decrease in the number of ganglion cell axons with advancing age.[12] Pupil size, refractive error, and clarity of media may also affect color perception. Because of these factors, there is an overlap in the responses when comparing groups of glaucoma patients, glaucoma suspects, and normal age-matched patients. Therefore, the clinical value of color vision testing for the detection of early glaucomatous damage is considered by some to be limited.[5] Moreover, foveally mediated color vision defects have not been demonstrated in all glaucoma patients who exhibit definite visual field loss. Further investigation into this area is needed to expand our knowledge of how color discrimination and glaucoma are related.

Methods of Color Vision Testing

The Nagle anomaloscope is the standard by which all color vision tests are compared. The patient is asked to match two monochromatic lights to a monochromatic test color. It is of limited clinical use because of its expense and the expertise required to analyze the results.[13]

The most commonly used color vision test in glaucoma research is the Farnsworth-Munsell 100 hue test (Fig. 11–1). The patient must sort 85 desaturated colored discs into a logical color sequence. The results are plotted on a polar coordinate graph. The colors are desaturated so that even patients with normal color vision make a small number of mistakes. This test is easy to administer and to score, but is time consuming, limiting its routine use clinically.

A modified version of the Farnsworth-Munsell 100 hue test is the D-15 test (Fig. 11–2). The patient sorts 15 color samples into a logical color sequence. The test is scored on a polar coordinate plot similar to the 100 hue test. The D-15 is easily administered and less time consuming than the 100 hue test. However, the color differences between the samples are quite large and therefore not as sensitive as the 100 hue test. The D-15 was designed by Farnsworth as a pass-fail test for congenital color anomalies. It does not provide enough quantitative data to make it useful for detection of color vision defects early in the glaucomatous process.

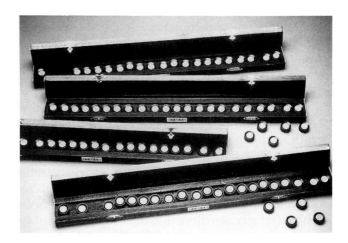

Figure 11–1. The Farnsworth-Munsell 100 Hue Test. (*Courtesy of Macbeth, Division of Kollmorgen Instruments Corporation. Newburgh, New York.*)

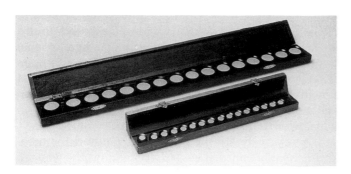

Figure 11–2. The Farnsworth Panel D-15 Test is available with two different size color pegs. The larger size is shown in the background. (*Courtesy of Michael Fischer, OD.*)

Adams and colleagues[14] recognized the need for a simple color vision test for routine clinical use in glaucoma. The authors modified the D-15 test to increase its sensitivity to subtle color discrimination anomalies. The D-15 standard scoring criterion requires that in order to fail, the subject must make two errors where colors are placed adjacent that are actually on opposite sides of the color circle. Adams and colleagues[14] modified the scoring criterion so that only one single place error or any error greater than a single place resulted in failure. Using this method, the authors found a significant loss of color discrimination in glaucoma patients as compared to an age-matched normal population.

The authors also developed a desaturated version of the D-15. When applying their pass-fail criterion to the D-15 desaturated test, 78% of the glaucoma patients and 58% of the glaucoma suspects failed while only 11% of the normal group failed.[14] This modified method of the D-15 test provides the practitioner with a simple method for determining color discrimination loss and appears to be more sensitive than the traditional D-15 test (Fig. 11–3).

CONTRAST SENSITIVITY

Many investigators have studied the relationship between glaucoma and contrast sensitivity, examining each of the three types: spatial, temporal, and combined spatiotemporal modulation. To test contrast sensitivity, the frequency of the stimulus is varied either spatially or temporally at different levels of contrast. The threshold at which the stimulus can be perceived is determined. A contrast sensitivity function, also called a modulation transfer function, can be generated for each variety of contrast sensitivity.

Spatial Contrast Sensitivity
Spatial contrast sensitivity can be considered a variation of traditional visual acuity assessment. Classically, visual acuity can be defined as the ability to see two separate objects as separate at 100% contrast. Spatial contrast sensitivity is the minimum separation

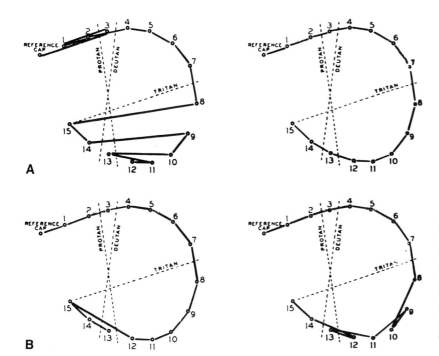

Figure 11–3. Farnsworth dichotomous D-15 panel test. **A.** Left side, example of a failure with two crossings across the circle. Right side, an example of a test with no errors. **B.** Examples of test failures using the criterion in the Adams and associates study. (*From Adams AJ, Rodic R, Husted R, Stamper R. Spectral sensitivity and color discrimination changes in glaucoma and glaucoma-suspect patients.* Invest Ophthalmol Vis Sci. *1982;23:518.*)

tivity in glaucoma patients under the age of 50 in all four quadrants of the retina. The largest decrease in sensitivity was found in the lower nasal quadrant, while the upper temporal quadrant had the smallest loss. When the subjects' visual fields were tested, they exhibited loss in these same areas. Therefore, there appeared to be some positive correlation between peripheral spatiotemporal contrast sensitivity loss and visual field defects.

In summary, spatial and temporal contrast sensitivity testing, particularly when done in the periphery, give the practitioner useful information about a patient's level of visual function. There is promise that in the future these functional tests may enable clinicians to detect glaucomatous damage earlier than traditional visual field testing, especially when there is a greater understanding of the effect of age on the test results.

Peripheral Color Contrast

A new screening test for early glaucomatous visual loss has been described by Yu and associates,[28] using a color monitor driven by a personal computer to vary the color contrast between a 25° annulus and the background. A gap in the annulus is randomly removed from one of four quadrants, and the patient has to identify the position of the gap. The minimum color contrast at which the gap can be identified is determined.

Yu and associates[28] found all patients with glaucoma had thresholds greater than two standard deviations above the normal mean. Moreover, 97% of glaucoma patients tested had thresholds greater than four standard deviations above the mean. Ocular hypertensive patients with low-to-medium risk of developing glaucoma had thresholds within the upper limit of normal. Ocular hypertensives with a high risk of developing glaucoma showed a bimodal distribution, with one group showing normal thresholds, and the other noticeably elevated thresholds. The threshold values were not affected by age, refractive error, or pupil size. The authors suggest that testing peripheral color contrast is a reliable and sensitive method to discriminate between glaucomatous patients and normals. However, they recommend a larger randomized trial and longitudinal studies be performed to confirm their data.

ELECTROPHYSIOLOGY

Electrophysiological tests give objective information about visual function, as compared to psychophysical tests that rely on the patient's cooperation and responses to obtain the test results. Electrophysiological testing directly assesses the patient's visual system integrity by measuring the electrical response from a specific structure to a stimulus. These tests are minimally invasive, requiring electrodes to be placed on the skin or scalp or a contact lens placed on the eye to capture the electrical response. The VEP and the ERG are two electrophysiological tests which may be of value in the diagnosis and management of glaucoma.

Visual Evoked Potential (VEP)

The VEP provides information about the pattern processing ability of the visual system, as compared to the visual field that reflects luminance processing. The VEP measures the response in the occipital cortex to stimulation of the retina. The stimulus may either be a pattern of reversing black and white checks presented on a TV monitor or a flash stimulus, using a bright light source such as a strobe. Two electrodes are needed to capture the response: one is placed on the scalp above the inion and the other, a ground electrode, on the earlobe (Fig. 11–7).

The VEP response amplitude is quite small compared to the intrinsic activity of the brain: therefore, it is normally masked by the overall noise from the brain. To unmask the VEP response, the stimulus is repeated a number of times. Each time the stimulus is presented, a response occurs at a specific time interval. Using a computer, the intrinsic brain activity (noise) gets averaged out since it is not time linked to the stimulus as is the VEP response[29] (Fig. 11–8).

Early studies of the VEP did not uncover abnormalities in glaucoma patients.[30] More recent investigations found evidence to the contrary. Atkin and colleagues[31] found 75% of open-angle glaucoma patients had abnormal VEP latencies, as compared to less than 50% of ocular hypertensives when measuring the VEP to pattern stimuli. Other authors have observed delayed latencies in 15 to 50% of ocular hypertensive eyes.[32–34]

A prospective study by Bray and co-workers[35] using the pattern VEP found 7 out of 22 ocular hypertensive patients with VEP abnormalities developed glaucomatous field defects during the follow-up period of 3.2 years. None of the ocular hypertensive patients with normal VEPs developed glaucomatous visual field defects. Further prospective studies are needed to clarify the prognostic role of the pattern VEP for the detection of early glaucomatous damage (Fig. 11–9).

The flash VEP is not only objective, but also fast, accurate, easy to interpret, and repeatable. Using the flash instead of a pattern stimuli decreases the effects of refractive error, pupil size, and media opacities.[36]

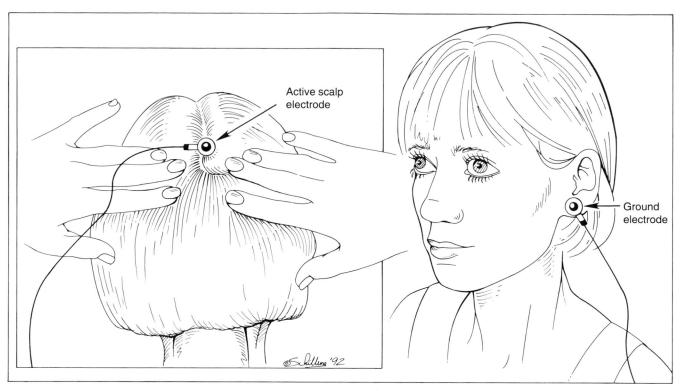

Figure 11–7. Placement of electrodes for recording of the VEP.

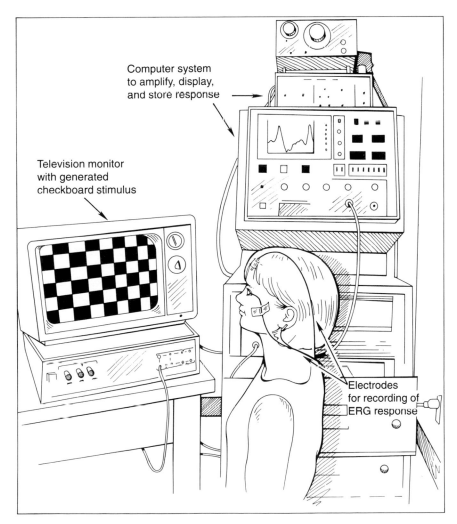

Computer system to amplify, display, and store response

Television monitor with generated checkboard stimulus

Electrodes for recording of ERG response

Figure 11–8. Schematic diagram of the recording of a pattern VEP.

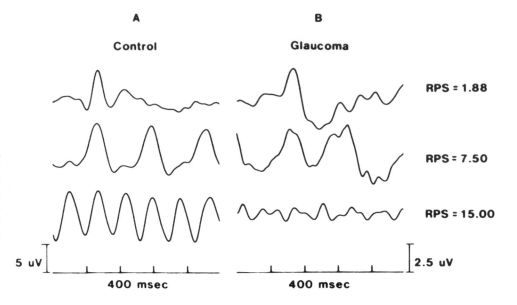

	A	B
	Control	**Glaucoma**

RPS = 1.88

RPS = 7.50

RPS = 15.00

5 uV

400 msec

2.5 uV

400 msec

Figure 11–9. Example of pattern VEPs. Control: subjects with no ocular pathology and 20/20 visual acuity. Glaucoma: subjects with moderate-to-severe primary open-angle glaucoma. Note the irregularly shaped waveforms and the failure of periodicity. (*From Sutija VG, Eiden SB, Wicker D, et al. Electrophysiological assessment of visual deficit in glaucoma. Appl Optics. 1987;26:1424.*)

A decreased amplitude and increased latency of the early flash VEP response has been found in patients with glaucoma.[36,37] Early VEP abnormalities lend support to the theory that the earliest glaucomatous damage is in the magnocellular pathways, which relay pattern processing information.[38,39]

Watts, Good, and O'Neill[40] believe the flash VEP may be of value as part of a continuous monitoring program for glaucoma patients and suspects. They showed a positive correlation between decreased

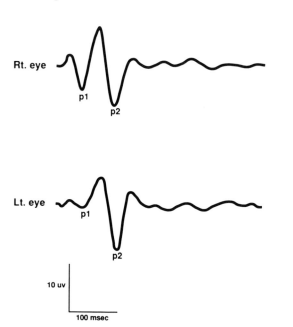

Rt. eye

p1

p2

Lt. eye

p1

p2

10 uv

100 msec

Figure 11–10. Example of a flash VEP from a patient with unilateral (left eye) POAG. Note the decrease in amplitude of the P1 peak. (*From Watts MT, Good PA, O'Neill EC. The flash VEP in the diagnosis of glaucoma. Eye. 1989;3:734.*)

early amplitudes of flash VEPs, visual field loss, and increased cup-to-disc ratios, suggesting the early response peak of the flash VEP may have its origins in the ganglion cell nerve fibers (Fig. 11–10).

The stimulus intensity arriving at the retina affects the VEP amplitude. Media opacities for one may decrease the stimulus intensity leading to a decrease in the VEP, clouding its use in diagnosing early glaucoma. Also, there is a large variability of flash VEP amplitudes in the normal population, creating overlap in amplitudes between normal and glaucomatous eyes, which limits the usefulness of the test in detecting the early pathological changes in glaucoma.[35]

Both the pattern and flash VEP furnish information about the functional ability of the visual system. It appears that measuring the VEP in glaucoma suspects can complement visual field testing. The pattern VEP gives objective data on pattern processing, while the flash VEP gives data on luminance processing.[35] Further prospective studies are needed before the prognostic significance of the flash and pattern VEP for the glaucoma patient is established.

Electroretinogram (ERG)

The ERG represents the electrical response of the retina to a light stimulus. Similar to the VEP, the ERG is recorded using a minimally invasive technique by placing a contact lens with an electrode on the eye (Figs. 11–11 and 11–12). The amplified response is transmitted to a computer for display and storage.

Two types of stimuli, flash and pattern, can be used to elicit the ERG response. The flash ERG depicts activity from the photoreceptors, bipolar cells, and Müller cells. The ganglion cell activity is not rep-

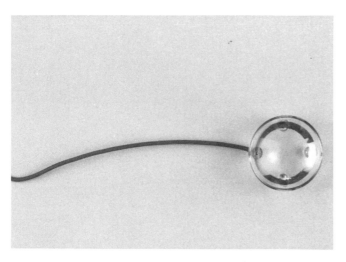

Figure 11–11. A contact lens electrode used in the recording of the ERG.

resented in the flash ERG. Therefore, the flash ERG amplitude is not usually altered in glaucoma patients even with severe optic nerve damage.[41] The pattern ERG is tested with a checkerboard pattern of alternating black and white squares (Fig. 11–13). It may reflect the activity of the proximal retinal layers, and

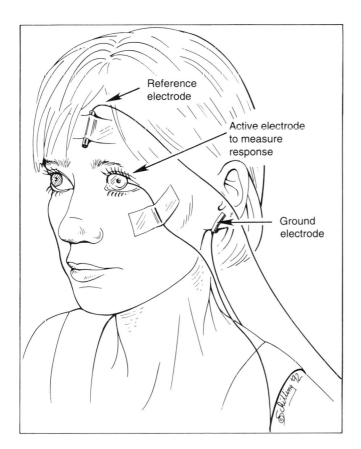

Reference electrode

Active electrode to measure response

Ground electrode

Figure 11–12. Placement of electrodes for recording the ERG.

therefore provide information about ganglion cell activity.[42] Sutija and associates believe the decrease in pattern ERG amplitude in glaucoma may reflect compromised amacrine-ganglion cell synapses in the proximal retina, rather than a loss of strictly ganglion cell function.[43]

Investigators have found the reduction in the pattern ERG amplitude in glaucoma correlates with cup-to-disc ratios, neural retinal rim area, and visual field defects.[44] Trick and colleagues[45] also found a decreased amplitude and an increased latency of the pattern ERG in glaucoma, but did not find a correlation with cup-to-disc ratio, neuroretinal rim area, and visual field loss. This may be due to patient selection and data collection methods since, in an earlier study, Trick[46] did find a correlation between the decreased pattern ERG amplitude and the aforementioned indices.

There are two component waves of the pattern ERG. The first wave (P_1) does not appear to be affected by optic nerve damage, while the second wave (N_2) is reduced[47] (Fig. 11–14). Weinstein and coworkers[48] uncovered a bimodal distribution disturbance of the N_2 wave in ocular hypertension. One group had amplitudes that were indistinguishable from the normal group while the other group showed findings similar to the glaucoma patients. The authors suggest that the N_2 amplitude may be used to determine which ocular hypertensives are at high risk for development of glaucomatous visual field loss.

The difficulty with the use of the pattern ERG as an early predictor of glaucomatous damage stems from the large interindividual variation in the ERG amplitude, causing overlap between the normal and glaucoma populations. In order to decrease this overlap, investigators are examining new variations of ERG measurement. By using large and small check sizes modulated at a high temporal frequency, Bach and Speidel-Fiaux[49] found little overlap between the glaucoma and normal groups with a multivariate discriminant analysis. A larger reduction of pattern ERG amplitude was found at higher rather than lower temporal frequencies. This lends support to other studies that conclude that the retinal mechanisms, which relay high temporal frequency information, are damaged early on in glaucoma.[26,50]

Watanabe and associates[51] described a new method of pattern ERG evaluation. Two targets were used as stimuli: one target covered the whole central retinal area within an 18° radius; the other, which included the Bjerrum area, covered a paracentral ring between 10 and 18°. The authors used a ratio of full-field stimulus response to Bjerrum ring stimulus response to cancel out various factors that cause the

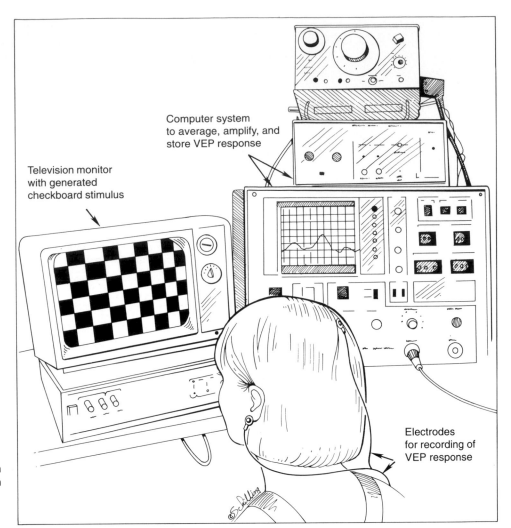

Figure 11–13. Schematic diagram of the recording of the pattern ERG.

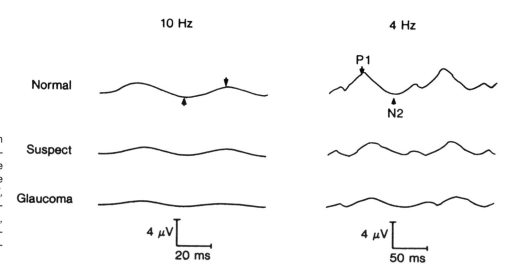

Figure 11–14. Example of pattern ERG recordings from normal, suspect, and glaucoma patients. Note the decrease in amplitude for the P$_1$ and N$_2$ waves. (*From Odom JV, Feghali JG, Jin J, Weinstein GW. Visual function deficits in glaucoma, electroretinogram pattern and luminance nonlinearities.* Arch Ophthalmol. *1990;108:222–227.*)

large interindividual variation in ERG amplitudes. These factors include pupil size, eye movements, and unstable fixation. This method produced a narrower range of normal ERG amplitude values and decreased the overlap between the glaucoma and control groups. These new concepts in pattern ERG evaluation may hold great promise in separating true glaucoma patients from the normal population. First, studies need to be directed towards finding the origin of the pattern ERG in the human retina before its value as a diagnostic tool can accurately be assessed.

In conclusion, psychophysical and electrophysiological tests may allow earlier detection of glaucomatous damage; however, much research is still needed. The ERG, VEP, color, and contrast sensitivity testing methods are plagued with sensitivity and specificity problems. Furthermore, longitudinal studies are needed to ascertain how well abnormalities detected by these methods determine which glaucoma suspects will go on to develop glaucoma. In the case of the electrophysiological tests, the VEP and pattern ERG tests need to be further developed to enable them to be practical for routine clinical use.

REFERENCES

1. Quigley HA, Addicks EM, Green WR. Optic nerve damage in human glaucoma. III. Quantitative correlation of nerve fiber loss and visual field defect in glaucoma, ischemic neuropathy, papilledema and toxic neuropathy. *Arch Ophthalmol.* 1982;100:135–146.

2. Drance SM. Correlation of optic nerve and visual field defects in simple glaucoma. *Trans Ophthalmol Soc UK.* 1975;95:288–296.

3. Hichings RA, Spaeth GL. The optic disc in glaucoma. II. Correlation of the appearance of the optic disc with the visual field. *Br J Ophthalmol.* 1977;61:107–113.

4. Lakowski R, Drance SM. Acquired dyschromatopsia: The earliest functional losses in glaucoma. *Doc Ophthalmol.* 1979;19:159–165.

5. Yamazaki MD, Drance SM, Lakowski R, Schulzer MD. Correlation between color vision and highest intraocular pressure in glaucoma patients. *Am J Ophthalmol.* 1988;106:397–399.

6. Hamill TR, Post RB, Johnson CA, Kelter JL. Correlation of color vision deficits and observable changes in the optic disc in a population of ocular hypertensives. *Arch Ophthalmol.* 1984;102:1637–1639.

7. Airaksinen PJ, Lakowski R, Drance SM, Price M. Color vision and retinal nerve fiber layer in early glaucoma. *Am J Ophthalmol.* 1986;101:208–213.

8. Breton ME, Drum BA. Functional testing in glaucoma, visual psychophysics and electrophysiology. In: Rich R, Shields MB, Kaplan T, eds. *The Glaucomas.* St. Louis, MO: C.V. Mosby; 1989.

9. Drance SM, Lakowski R, Schulzer M, Douglas GR. Acquired color vision changes in glaucoma. *Arch Ophthalmol.* 1981;99:829–831.

10. De Monasterio FM. Asymmetry of on- and off-pathways of blue sensitivity cone of the retina of macaques. *Brain Res.* 1979;166:39–48.

11. Quigley HA, Sanchez RM, Dunkelberg GR, L'Hernault NL, Baginski TA. Chronic glaucoma selectively damages large optic nerve fibers. *Invest Ophthalmol.* 1987;28:913–920.

12. Balazsi AG, Rootman J, Drance SM, Schulzer M, Douglas GR. The effect of age on the nerve fiber population of the human optic nerve. *Am J Ophthalmol.* 1984;97:761–766.

13. Lakowski R, Bryett J, Drance SM. A study of colour in ocular hypertensives. *Can J Ophthalmol.* 1972;7:86–95.

14. Adams AJ, Rodic R, Husted R, Stamper R. Spectral sensitivity and color discrimination changes in glaucoma and glaucoma-suspect patients. *Invest Ophthalmol Vis Sci.* 1982;23:516–524.

15. Ross JE, Bron AJ, Clarke DD. Contrast sensitivity and visual disability in chronic simple glaucoma. *Br J Ophthalmol.* 1984;68:821–827.

16. Arundale K. An investigation into the variation of human contrast sensitivity with age and ocular pathology. *Br J Ophthalmol.* 1978;62:213–215.

17. Sekuler R, Hutman LP. Spatial vision and aging. I. Contrast sensitivity. *J Gerontol.* 1980;35:692–699.

18. Arden GB, Jacobson JJ. A simple grating test for contrast sensitivity: Preliminary results indicate value in screening for glaucoma. *Invest Ophthalmol Vis Sci.* 1978;17:23–32.

19. Stamper RL, Hsu-Winges C, Sopher M. Arden contrast sensitivity testing in glaucoma. *Arch Ophthalmol.* 1982;100:947–950.

20. Skalka HW. Effect of age on Arden grating acuity. *Br J Ophthalmol.* 1980;64:21–23.

21. Adams AJ, Heron G, Husted R. Clinical measures of central vision function in glaucoma and ocular hypertension. *Arch Ophthalmol.* 1987;107:782–787.

22. Sponsel WE, DePaul KL, Martone JF, et al. Association of Vistech contrast sensitivity and visual field findings in glaucoma. *Br J Ophthalmol.* 1991;75:558–560.

23. Korth M, Horn F, Storck B, Jonas JB. Spatial and spatiotemporal contrast sensitivity of normal and glaucoma eyes. *Graefe's Arch Clin Exp Ophthalmol.* 1989;227:428–435.

24. Falcao-Reis F, O'Donoghue E, Buceti R, Hitchings RA, Arden G. Peripheral contrast sensitivity in glaucoma and ocular hypertension. *Br J Ophthalmol.* 1990;74:712–716.

25. Tyler CW. Specific deficits of flicker sensitivity in glaucoma and hypertension. *Invest Ophthalmol Vis Sci.* 1981;20:204–212.

26. Breton ME, Wilson TW, Wilson R, Spaeth GL, Krupin T. Temporal contrast sensitivity loss in primary open-angle glaucoma and glaucoma suspects. *Invest Ophthalmol Vis Sci.* 1991;32:2931–2941.

27. Atkin A, Bodis-Wolner I, Wokstein M, Moss A, Podos S. Abnormalities of central contrast sensitivity in glaucoma. *Am J Ophthalmol.* 1979;88:205–211.

28. Yu TC, Falcao-Reis F, Spileers W, Arden GB. Peripheral color contrast. *Invest Ophthalmol Vis Sci.* 1991;32:2779–2789.

29. Sherman J. Visual evoked potential. In: Terry JE, ed. *Ocular Disease.* Springfield, IL: Charles C. Thomas; 1984.

30. Cappin JM, Nissim S: Visual evoked responses in the assessment of field defects in glaucoma. *Arch Ophthalmol.* 1975;93:9–18.

31. Atkin A, Bodis-Wollner I, Podos SM, et al. Flicker threshold and pattern VEP latency in ocular hypertension and glaucoma. *Invest Ophthalmol Vis Sci.* 1983;24:1524–1528.

32. Howe JW, Mitchell KW. Visual evoked cortical potential to paracentral retinal stimulation in chronic glaucoma, ocular hypertension and an age-matched group of normals. *Doc Ophthalmol.* 1985;63:37–44.

33. Towle VL, Moskovitz A, Schwarz B. The visual evoked potential in glaucoma and ocular hypertension. Effects of check size, field size and stimulation rate. *Invest Ophthalmol Vis Sci.* 1983;24:175–183.

34. Rouland JF, Hache JC: Visual-evoked potentials in glaucoma and ocular hypertension. *Glaucoma.* 1990;12:77–78.

35. Bray LC, Mitchell KW, Howe JW. Prognostic significance of the pattern visual evoked potential in ocular hypertension. *Br J Ophthalmol.* 1991;75:79–83.

36. Nykanen H, Raitta C. The correlation of visual evoked potentials (VEP) and visual field indices (Octopus G1) in glaucoma and ocular hypertension. *Acta Ophthalmol.* 1989;67:393–395.

37. Good PA, Masters JB, Mortimer MJ. Flash stimulation evoked potentials in diagnosis of chronic glaucoma. *Lancet.* 1987;1:1259–1260.

38. Marx MS, Podos SM, Bodis-Wollner I, et al. Sign of early damage in glaucomatous monkey eyes: Low spatial frequency losses in the pattern ERG and VEP. *Exp Eye Res.* 1988;46:173–184.

39. Neima D, Le Blanc R, Regan D. Visual field defects in ocular hypertension and glaucoma. *Arch Ophthalmol.* 1984;102:1042–1045.

40. Watts MT, Good PA, O'Neill EC. The flash VEP in the diagnosis of glaucoma. *Eye.* 1989;3:732–737.

41. Alvis DL. Electroretinographic changes in controlled chronic open-angle glaucoma. *Am J Ophthalmol.* 1966;61:121–131.

42. Maffei L, Fiorentini A. Electroretinographic responses to alternating gratings before and after section of the optic nerve. *Science.* 1981;211:953–955.

43. Sutija VG, Eiden SB, Wicker D, et al. Electrophysiological assessment of visual deficit in glaucoma. *Appl Optics.* 1987;26:1421–1431.

44. Korth M, Horn F, Stork B, Jonas J. The pattern-evoked electroretinogram (PERG): Age-related alterations and changes in glaucoma. *Graefe's Arch Clin Exp Ophthalmol.* 1989;227:123–130.

45. Trick GL, Bickler-Bluth M, Cooper DG, Kolker AE, Nesher R. Pattern reversal electroretinogram (PRERG) abnormalities in ocular hypertension: Correlation with glaucoma risk factors. *Curr Eye Res.* 1988;7:201–206.

46. Trick GL. PRRP abnormalities in glaucoma and ocular hypertension. *Invest Ophthalmol Vis Sci.* 1986;27:1730–1736.

47. Holder GE. Significance of abnormal pattern electroretinography in anterior visual pathway disfunction. *Br J Ophthalmol.* 1987;71:166–171.

48. Weinstein GW, Arden GB, Hitchings RA, et al. The pattern electroretinogram (PERG) in ocular hypertension and glaucoma. *Arch Ophthalmol.* 1988;106:923–928.

49. Bach M, Speidel-Fiaux A. Pattern electroretinogram in glaucoma and ocular hypertension. *Doc Ophthalmol.* 1989;73:173–181.

50. Trick GL. Retinal potentials in patients with primary open-angle glaucoma: Physiological evidence for temporal frequency tuning deficits. *Invest Ophthalmol.* 1985;26:1750–1758.

51. Watanabe I, Iijima H, Tsukahara S. The pattern electroretinogram in glaucoma: An evaluation by relative amplitude from the Bjerrum area. *Br J Ophthalmol.* 1989;73:131–135.

Chapter 12

AN APPROACH TO DIAGNOSING GLAUCOMA

Thomas L. Lewis

Reaching an early and accurate differential diagnosis may be the most important step in the management of a patient with glaucoma. An early diagnosis permits timely intervention of treatment that has the best prognosis for long-term control of the disease.[1-3] The greatest clinical challenge, therefore, is timing the initiation of treatment so as to start as early as possible in patients with true glaucoma, without overtreating. The clinician must be as sure as possible that the clinical evidence is sufficient to warrant committing patients to a lifetime of treatment for their disease.[4]

The timing of when you label a patient as having some form of glaucoma is critical for several reasons. On the one hand, making this decision too hastily can result in the treatment of patients presenting with normal fluctuation in clinical parameters or who are simply glaucoma suspects. Prior to the 1970s, it was a common practice to treat all patients with elevated intraocular pressures, even though the majority of these patients never develop glaucoma.[5,6] The side effects from the treatment of glaucoma are significant, making the overdiagnosis and treatment of the disease inappropriate.

Conversely, waiting until a glaucoma patient has absolute, reproducible visual function loss from the disease before a diagnosis is made and treatment begun, dramatically reduces the potential benefit of the therapeutic regimen.[1,7,8] In some glaucoma patients, as much as 50% of the ganglion cell axons may be destroyed in the optic nerve, with the patient presenting clinically with normal visual fields.[9] There is a narrow window of opportunity in which an early yet not premature diagnosis of glaucoma can be made and treatment initiated prior to excessive amount of tissue damage from the glaucomatous process.

Making a timely differential diagnosis in a patient with a subtle presentation of glaucoma is difficult. This is especially true in patients that you are examining for the first time. Having the advantage of prior clinical information to establish baseline parameters is of great value in detecting the disease. This is because the most important clinical observation to be made in the early diagnosis of a glaucoma patient is *change* in any of the key clinical parameters that are typically altered by the disease, i.e., intraocular pressure, the anterior chamber angle, the optic nerve, the nerve fiber layer, and visual function.[10,11] The only possible way to observe change is through multiple examination. Change over time beyond the point of normal variation or fluctuation confirms the diagnosis and allows treatment to begin.

There are times, however, when it is not possible nor appropriate to allow enough time to pass to observe changes in these parameters. You may find on a single visit that the potential risk of damage to the optic nerve is such that treatment must be strongly considered.

RELATIVE RISK

The most effective way of assuring the proper differential diagnosis of glaucoma is by collecting a complete matrix of clinical information and determining the probability of whether or not the patient will develop the disease. It is only through proper testing that the true relative risk of the patient for glaucoma will surface. Unfortunately, there is no single clinical test with a 100% specificity and sensitivity for glaucoma.[3] Therefore, a combination of tests, analyzed collectively, is necessary for the proper diagnosis.

Years of clinical studies have uncovered different risk factors for glaucoma. It is clear that the prevalence of the disease is greater in patients with certain clinical characteristics as opposed to others. For example, patients with elevated intraocular pressures have a greater prevalence for glaucoma than individuals with pressures below 21 mm Hg.[12,13] Ocular hypertensive patients, therefore, are at greater risk of developing glaucoma than ocular normotensive patients. It is important to understand what this really means from a clinical perspective.

Simply because one clinical finding or characteristic places a patient at greater risk of developing glaucoma does not mean that all individuals with this finding or characteristic will get the disease. Using ocular hypertension as an example, a study that followed patients for an average of 16 years, one group with ocular hypertension and the other normotensive, found that 5.5% of the ocular hypertensive patients developed glaucoma whereas 0.25% of the normotensive patients were diagnosed with the disease.[14] This clearly points out that the risk of glaucoma is greater with ocular hypertension (more than 20 times in the study) but that not everyone with ocular hypertension developed the disease. In fact, the vast majority (94.5%) did not over a 16-year period. Similar data exist for other risk factors for glaucoma.

It is, therefore, the relative risk for the development of glaucoma that is important to determine in a timely manner when dealing with a glaucoma suspect. A complete analysis of the patient will permit the clinician to assess this risk.

PATIENT PROFILE

An effective way to determine the probability of a patient developing glaucoma is to create a profile that identifies his or her risk factors for the disease. Initially, it may be valuable to display this profile on a clinical form (Table 12–1), which helps you analyze all the appropriate risk factors and visualize the profile of the patient. With experience, you will be able to develop the same perspective mentally without committing it to paper.

The patient profile form forces the clinician to develop an appropriate clinical examination regimen for the early, differential diagnosis of glaucoma. It assures that all the necessary clinical tests are completed and properly analyzed. With incomplete clini-

TABLE 12–1. PATIENT PROFILE

Factors	Low Risk	Moderate Risk	High Risk
Age	_____	_____	_____
Gender	_____	_____	_____
Race	_____	_____	_____
Family history	_____	_____	_____
High blood pressure	_____	_____	_____
Low blood pressure	_____	_____	_____
Heart disease	_____	_____	_____
Atherosclerosis	_____	_____	_____
Local vasospasms	_____	_____	_____
Migraine headache	_____	_____	_____
Corticosteroid use	_____	_____	_____
Refractive error	_____	_____	_____
Intraocular pressure	_____	_____	_____
Anterior chamber angle	_____	_____	_____
Optic nerve	_____	_____	_____
Nerve fiber layer	_____	_____	_____
Visual fields	_____	_____	_____
Color vision	_____	_____	_____
Afferent pupillary defect	_____	_____	_____
Retinal vein occlusion	_____	_____	_____
Ocular trauma	_____	_____	_____
Exfoliation syndrome	_____	_____	_____
Pigmentary dispersion syndrome	_____	_____	_____
Rubeosis irides	_____	_____	_____
Ocular inflammation	_____	_____	_____

cal data, the clinician is not able to effectively diagnose the more difficult presentations of glaucoma.

DIAGNOSTIC PUZZLE

Each patient presents a diagnostic challenge for the clinician. Subconsciously, the clinician handles each new patient as a "puzzle," needing to collect all the pieces of the puzzle in order to solve the diagnostic dilemma. Glaucomas are a group of diseases in which the concept of a diagnostic puzzle is very relevant to their early differential diagnosis. If all the pieces of the puzzle are collected, it is much easier to determine the relative risk of that patient for developing glaucoma, to feel comfortable in making an early definitive diagnosis, and to properly follow the patient once treatment has been initiated.

The following clinical findings or patient characteristics are important pieces of the puzzle for glaucoma (Fig. 12–1).

Risk Factors

There are a variety of risk factors, which are general, systemic, and ocular in nature, that apply to glaucoma. These risk factors vary for the different types of glaucoma. Risk factors can be causal or noncausal for the disease. This distinction is important in planning treatment for the patient. In reality, the most important risk factors clinically are those which are treatable.[15]

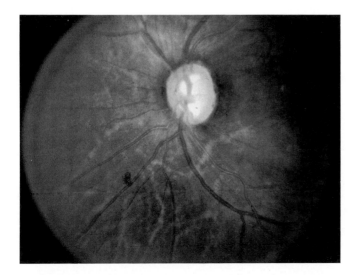

Figure 12–1. Focal damage to the neuroretinal rim. Left eye of a glaucoma patient with a notch at the inferior rim at 6 o'clock, and thinning of the neuroretinal rim. Narrow wedge of nerve fiber layer dropout are present at 1 and 6 o'clock.

In primary open-angle glaucoma, the general risk factors include a family history,[16,17] an elderly age,[12] and being black.[18] Systemic risk factors are high[19] or low blood pressure[20] and diabetes mellitus.[21] Ocular risk factors include elevated intraocular pressure,[22] the presence of nerve fiber layer dropout,[23] large physiological cups,[24] high myopia,[25] glaucoma in one eye,[8,26] and retinal vein occlusions.[27]

The risk factors for low-tension glaucoma are primarily vascular in nature, related to either a poor perfusion of blood to the optic nerve or local vasospastic events.[28,29] In addition to age and being a woman,[30] systemic risk factors for low-tension glaucoma are low blood pressure,[31] occlusive vascular diseases,[31] and a history of migraine headaches.[32] Ocularly, one might observe flame-shaped hemorrhages[33] on or near the optic nerve as well as a significant difference in intraocular pressure when compared from the erect to the supine position.[34]

In narrow angle glaucoma, the major risk factor clearly is an anatomically narrow angle. This type of angle is influenced by familial factors,[35] increasing age,[36] moderate-to-high hyperopia,[36] and gender and racial issues. Women are three times more likely to have narrow angles than men.[37] Orientals[38] and Eskimos[39] are predisposed to narrow angles.

Finally, certain ocular conditions are risk factors for the secondary development of glaucoma. A few of the more important ones may include pigmentary dispersion syndrome,[40] exfoliation syndrome,[41] ocular trauma,[42] retinal neovascular diseases,[43] uveitis,[44] and a history of systemic or ocular use of steroids.[45]

The presence of one or more of these risk factors would increase the probability of a patient developing one of the various forms of glaucoma. The more risk factors, the greater the probability.

Intraocular Pressure

Measuring intraocular pressure through tonometry is an essential step in collecting information for the proper diagnosis of glaucoma. However, relying too heavily on a single tonometric reading can cause overdiagnosis and treatment and, even more important, can result in missing glaucoma patients with large diurnal variations in intraocular pressure or low-tension glaucoma.[46]

The clinical interpretation of tonometry is complicated by two problems. First is the issue of what is "normal" intraocular pressure for a specific patient. The second problem is that intraocular pressure is constantly fluctuating by several mm Hg on a moment-to-moment basis[47] and by as much as 10 or more mm Hg in certain glaucoma patients from day-to-day.[48] Because of this, a single tonometric reading may represent such a small sample that it gives a very misleading representation of the patient's true pressure.

It is clear that intraocular pressure, which is statistically abnormal (above 21 mm Hg), increases the risk (7 to 22 times) for the development of glaucoma.[49] The higher the pressure, the greater the risk of damage.[46] However, the vast majority of ocular hypertensive individuals will never develop glaucoma.[50–53] The incidence of glaucoma in patients with ocular hypertension is about 0.5 to 1% per year.[51] Most clinicians will attempt to lower intraocular pressure if it exceeds 30 mm Hg because of the risk of a secondary retinal vein occlusion[54] and because of the probability (33.3%) of damage to the optic nerve with pressures this high.[55]

Unfortunately, the only way to determine whether or not a certain level of intraocular pressure has exceeded that which is normal for a given patient is to look for tissue damage in the optic nerve. The level of pressure that causes damage varies significantly from individual to individual and even in the same person as they get older.[8,47] With age, there seems to be an increased susceptibility to optic nerve damage from levels of intraocular pressure that were previously well tolerated.[12,53] There is no single level of intraocular pressure above which all patients develop glaucoma and below which all patients are free of the disease.[22] Pressures below 21 mm Hg do not make an individual immune from glaucoma.[56]

The fact that intraocular pressure is constantly fluctuating is an important concept in understanding the clinical value of tonometry. Fluctuation of intraocular pressure is due to a multitude of factors, some of which are occurring normally inside the body every day,[57–59] and other external influences such as temperature,[60] exercise,[61] and fluid intake.[62] The short-term fluctuation in intraocular pressure that occurs diurnally can be problematic for the early diagnosis of glaucoma. The highest intraocular pressure can be reached at any time of the day, not necessarily just in the early morning.[48] It is essential, therefore, to record the time of day that tonometry is performed. Diurnal pressure changes of more than 10 to 15 mm Hg have been observed in glaucoma patients.[63] In fact, normal individuals have shown fluctuations as much as 10 mm Hg. Any diurnal pressure swing of more than 6 mm Hg should be considered suspicious. In a glaucoma suspect with suspicious optic nerves or visual fields but yet a low intraocular pressure on a single tonometric reading, a large diurnal fluctuation should be considered and assessed clinically. Even after treatment has begun, periodic evaluation of di-

urnal fluctuation in intraocular pressure is important.[64,65]

Long-term fluctuation can also occur in intraocular pressure. Several studies have indicated that a gradual increase in pressure over time may be more important in causing damage to the optic nerve than the absolute level of pressure at any given moment.[66] The presence of change over time in intraocular pressure is an important risk factor for glaucoma regardless of the baseline intraocular pressure for that patient.

Asymmetry in intraocular pressure between the eyes is another significant risk factor for glaucoma,[67] especially if the difference in pressures is more than 5 mm Hg.[68] Asymmetry in intraocular pressure can cause asymmetrical damage even in low-tension glaucoma,[69] and should also alert the clinician to a possible secondary cause for the glaucoma, i.e., trauma, exfoliation, inflammation.[70]

All things considered, the clinician should not rely too heavily on a single tonometric reading since, by itself, it is a very poor indicator for glaucoma.[15,71] It is not possible to develop a magical cut-off point for intraocular pressure that differentiates normal from abnormal patients.[51] In fact, the sensitivity (50 to 70%) and specificity (90%) for tonometry[72] at a cut-off pressure of 21 mm Hg related to glaucoma is not impressive.[46] Because of the significant variation in intraocular pressure, one third to one half of all glaucoma patients show intraocular pressure below 21 mm Hg on a single pressure reading.[73] Therefore, if you rely too heavily on tonometry for the detection of glaucoma, you will miss a significant number of patients with the disease.

Using tonometry to develop baseline pressure levels, to monitor long-term and short-term fluctuation, and to look for symmetry between the two eyes makes evaluating intraocular pressure a useful *component* in the clinical work-up for the diagnosis and management of glaucoma (Table 12–2). The current status of understanding of the role of intraocular pressure in the etiology of glaucoma indicates that it is a major, but not decisive, risk factor in the early disease process.[74] The chance of developing glaucoma in an individual eye is additionally modified by other risk factors, some of which are not yet validated

TABLE 12–2. VALUE OF TONOMETRY IN DIAGNOSING GLAUCOMA

Developing a base-line
Monitoring short-term fluctuation
Monitoring long-term fluctuation
Asymmetry

on a prospective basis of epidemiological proof. Intraocular pressure alone cannot be relied on for the diagnosis of glaucoma and it is not the sole determinant of visual field survival in patients receiving therapy.[75] However, intraocular pressure is one of the few, if not the only, risk factors amenable to treatment, and therefore remains the focus of patient management.

Biomicroscopy

Assessing the anterior portion of the eye and the anterior chamber angle is essential for the diagnosis and treatment of glaucoma. Biomicroscopy, in combination with gonioscopy, through both a dilated and non-dilated pupil, allows the clinician to differentiate open from closed angles and also in many instances primary from secondary glaucomas. This information is critical in designing an appropriate management plan for a glaucoma patient.

With the biomicroscope, the clinician should assess the cornea for the presence of edema or pigment on the back surface; the anterior chamber for pigment, cells, flare, keratic precipitates, and hyphema; the iris for pigment, defects in the pupillary ruff, exfoliation flakes, transillumination defects, rubeosis irides, iris atrophy, and posterior synechiae; and the crystalline lens for thickening, pigmentation, or exfoliation flakes.

Gonioscopy may reveal a narrow or closed angle, pigmentation, exfoliation, anterior synechiae, angle recession, or neovascularization. The openness of the angle, the curvature of the iris, the degree of pigmentation in the angle, and the presence of abnormal material or anatomy should be recorded.[76] If a closed angle is observed, compression gonioscopy should be performed to determine whether the closure is synechial or appositional. This will influence the treatment of the patient.

There is debate whether provocative testing is of any value in identifying those patients with narrow angles that are most likely to close. The provocative tests currently available are hampered by high false-positive and false-negative results.[77] If you wish to perform a provocative test, the choice might be a combined dark room-prone test with a rise of pressure of 8 mm Hg or more considered positive.[78]

Biomicroscopy and gonioscopy should be performed frequently on patients with a history of ocular trauma and with diabetic retinopathy, retinal vein occlusions, and other diseases that can lead to neovascularization of the retina.

Clinical Assessment of the Optic Nerve

A stereoscopic, magnified view of the optic nerve through a dilated pupil is critical for the early diagnosis of glaucoma. This can be achieved through a variety of techniques that include the biomicroscope in association with a Hruby lens, goniolenses, fundus contact lenses, and high plus lenses (i.e., 60 D, 78 D, 90 D). Stereophotography is critical for documentation of the appearance of the optic nerve for two reasons. One obvious reason is medicolegal. The other is that the permanent record created by ocular photography allows the best opportunity for the observation of subtle changes in the optic nerve tissue over time. Without photography, these changes are difficult to document clinically. Over the past 20 years, glaucoma specialists have moved from a detailed drawing or description, or both, of the optic nerve head to photography, stereophotography, red-free photography, and, currently, computer-aided video analysis and laser tomography.[79]

Stereoscopic assessment of the optic nerve should stress four points: the integrity of the neuroretinal rim, with respect to thickness and color; the size and shape of the cup; the symmetry of the optic nerves between the two eyes; and the integrity of the surrounding retinal nerve fiber layer (Table 12–3). It is critical for the clinician to direct his or her attention on changes in the neuroretinal rim tissue and not solely on the cup portion of the optic nerve.[80] The cup-to-disc ratio is dependent on the overall size of the disc and has a wide normal range.[81] The earliest disc changes in glaucoma cannot be adequately identified by estimates of cup-to-disc ratio.[82,83]

The majority of glaucoma patients incur some degree of both focal and diffuse damage to the optic nerve during the course of the disease (Table 12–4).[83] The most specific optic nerve findings (87%) for glaucoma include focal changes in the neuroretinal rim usually in the form of a notch (see Fig. 12–1).[84] Notches occur most frequently on the inferior rim followed by the superior rim.[85] Temporal rim pallor is seen infrequently.[85] Vertical elongation of the cup

TABLE 12–3. EARLY CHANGES IN THE OPTIC NERVE AND NERVE FIBER LAYER IN GLAUCOMA

Optic Nerve
Enlargement of cup
Narrowing of rim
Asymmetry of cupping between the two eyes
Notching of the neuroretinal rim
Disc hemorrhages
Acquired peripapillary atrophy
Baring of the circumlinear vessel

Nerve Fiber Layer
Diffuse loss
Focal loss: wedges, slits

TABLE 12–4. CORRELATION OF STRUCTURAL DAMAGE AND FUNCTIONAL CHANGES IN GLAUCOMA

Diffuse Glaucomatous Damage	Focal Glaucomatous Damage
Optic Nerve	
Concentric enlargement of the cup	Vertical elongation of cup
Diffuse nerve fiber loss	Notching of rim
	Wedge or slit defects in nerve fiber layer
	Hemorrhages
Visual Function	
Generalized depression of threshold	Paracentral scotoma
Generalized contraction of isopter	Nasal steps
Color vision defects	
Decreased latency and amplitude of pattern electroretinograms	
Decrease in spatial and temporal contrast sensitivity	

also occurs from focal damage to the optic nerve.[83,85–87]

Even though focal damage is specific for glaucoma, more commonly one sees a generalized thinning of the neuroretinal rim due to diffuse damage to the optic nerve (Fig. 12–2).[80,83,88] In some cases, this can be reflected through baring of the circumlinear vessels on the surface of the nerve.[89] In low-tension glaucoma, the neuroretinal rim may be significantly thinner.[90] In more advanced glaucoma cases, bean-pot enlargement of the cup can result in bayoneting

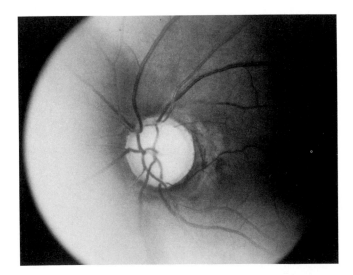

Figure 12–2. Generalized damage to neuroretinal rim. Left eye of glaucoma patient with symmetrical thinning and pallor of the neuroretinal rim. Peripapillary atrophy is present around the entire optic nerve head but more extensive temporally.

of the large blood vessels as they cross the inner edge of the neuroretinal rim.[85] Asymmetrical cup-to-disc ratios between the two eyes of more than 0.2 is highly significant for the diagnosis of glaucoma.[24]

Pallor of the neuroretinal rim, although not specific for glaucoma, is quite commonly found and indicative of the death of ganglion cell axons.[91,92] The color of the neuroretinal rim can be misleading since it is influenced by the technique used to examine the optic nerve and by media changes.[93] Peripapillary atrophy is present in many individuals with glaucoma, especially low-tension glaucoma.[94] As neuroretinal rim damage approaches the edge of the disc, peripapillary atrophy becomes more prevalent.[95]

Associated findings in glaucoma may include the presence of large, elongated laminar dots in the center of the optic nerve[96] as well as splinter or flame-shaped hemorrhages on or near the disc.[97,98] These hemorrhages, which are more commonly found in low-tension glaucoma,[33] may represent infarction of the blood supply to the optic nerve and, therefore, could be a clinical sign of impending nerve damage and visual field loss.[98–100] They have been shown to precede clinical changes in the optic nerve fiber layer and visual fields in some glaucoma patients.[100,101]

Proper assessment of the optic nerve is very sensitive (70 to 90%)[102,103] and specific (80 to 97%)[102,103] for the early diagnosis of glaucoma. There are a few glaucoma patients who will show visual function loss prior to presenting with clinically observable damage to the optic nerve, especially individuals with a large physiological cup prior to the onset of the glaucoma.[11,103] Early intervention to lower intraocular pressure may actually reverse optic nerve changes in some patients.[104]

Clinical Assessment of the Nerve Fiber Layer

Evaluation of the retinal nerve fiber layer within two disc diameters of the optic nerve is essential for the proper diagnosis and management of glaucomas. Various techniques can be used to perform this evaluation including indirect ophthalmoscopy and procedures similar to those used to evaluate the optic nerve. Detection of subtle nerve fiber layer loss is difficult and clinically challenging. The use of red-free light for both the evaluation and photographing of the retinal nerve fiber layer is helpful in accentuating the reflection of light off of this tissue and in observing any defects that might exist.[105] Nerve fiber defects can occur focally in the form of slits or wedges (Fig. 12–3) or diffusely around the optic nerve (see Table 12–4).[106] The predominant pattern of nerve fiber damage distinguishing glaucomatous field loss is dif-

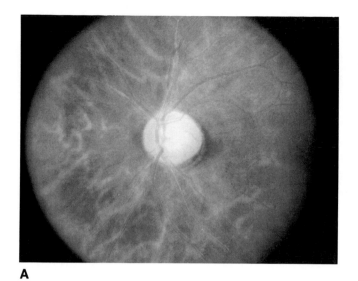

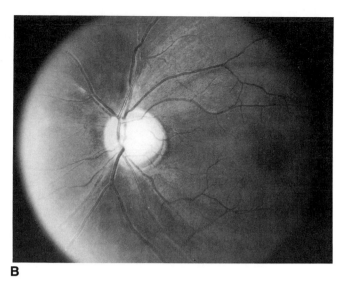

A   **B**

Figure 12–3. Focal nerve fiber layer dropout. Color and companion red-free photography of the left eye of a glaucoma patient with several slit-like defects in the nerve fiber layer between 12 and 2 o'clock and a large wedge defect between 5 and 7 o'clock. (*See also* Color Plate 12–3.)

fuse rather than focal. The presence of nerve fiber layer defects is highly specific (80 to 90%) and sensitive (85 to 97%) for glaucoma,[106–109] if you realize that slit-like defects are found in normal people and are neither common nor reliable for glaucoma.[110]

The clinical importance of nerve fiber layer dropout is that it seems to occur early in the disease in many glaucoma patients, usually preceding visual field loss.[107–109,111] In fact, it may be the earliest recognizable sign of glaucoma.[112] When approximately 50% of axons in a given area have been destroyed at the level of the lamina cribrosa, the retrograde degeneration appears clinically on the surface of the retina.[113] Studies have shown nerve fiber defects to be present up to 5 years before detectable visual field loss occurred clinically.[108,114] In addition, there is a very strong correlation between the type of nerve fiber layer defect (focal or diffuse) and the type and location of subsequent visual field loss.[115] Therefore, there appears to be great value in assessing the nerve fiber layer for the presence of glaucomatous damage and for the progression of this damage once it has begun.

Evaluation of Visual Function

Assessment of visual function can be accomplished through a variety of psychophysical and electrophysiological tests.[116,117] These include evaluation of visual fields, color vision, contrast sensitivity, pattern electroretinograms, and visual evoked potentials. Color vision and visual field testing are the most practical to perform clinically in a private practice setting.

There continues to be concern regarding the specificity of the changes seen in psychophysical and electrophysiological testing as it relates to glaucoma. This is due to the significant overlap between the findings in normal patients, glaucoma suspects, and glaucoma patients. In addition, changes similar to those seen in glaucoma can also be found in a variety of other conditions including aging, cataracts, and other media changes.[118] One clear result of data from psychophysical testing is that nerve fibers mediating central visual function are adversely affected in glaucoma, even early in the disease process.[119]

Glaucoma can produce morphologic damage to the optic nerve focally, diffusely, or in combination. Diffuse changes such as concentric enlargement of the cup and generalized thinning of the neuroretinal rim and nerve fiber layer are often difficult to distinguish from normal patients, as well as to quantify. Functionally, this type of damage manifests itself by general depression of the visual field, color vision defects, changes in contrast sensitivity, and altered electrodiagnostic tests (*see* Table 12–4). The value of psychophysical and electrodiagnostic testing may rest in improving the specificity and diagnostic value of evaluating diffuse damage.

Yellow-blue and blue-green color vision defects have been identified in certain glaucoma patients, indicating a loss of macular function.[120–122] As high as 20% of glaucoma suspects[123] may have color vision defects, yet 25% of advanced glaucoma patients may not.[124,125] Color vision loss is often associated more with glaucoma patients who have higher levels of intraocular pressure.[126,127]

The most practical procedure to perform clinically, which is sensitive for acquired color vision defects, is a desaturated D-15 test done monocularly under proper illumination.[128] Two or more cross-over defects with this test indicate failure. Color vision tests should be conducted on all glaucoma suspects as the results represent an additional piece of information to assess their risk of developing the disease. Color vision defects, if they occur, usually correlate well with the extent of the visual field loss.[129] Color vision abnormalities may be present before changes in the visual field and assist the clinician in making an earlier diagnosis of visual function loss.[121,123,125]

Visual field testing has been the standard method of assessing visual function loss in glaucoma. Automated perimetry has become a practical form of visual field testing within the last 10 years and shows its greatest value clinically in the diagnosis and management of glaucoma.[130,131] Changes in retinal sensitivity are uncovered at an earlier stage with automated than with manual perimetry.[132] Threshold visual fields in the central 30° should be performed on all glaucoma suspects. Threshold perimetry, with a statistical analysis of the data, has a 93% sensitivity and 84% specificity for glaucoma.[133] Screening tests with automated perimeters may have some value in detecting the presence of field abnormalities in those patients who otherwise present with minimal risks for glaucoma.[134]

The location of the earliest visual field loss will depend on the type of glaucoma. Individuals with very high intraocular pressures may present primarily with diffuse damage to the optic nerve and a general depression of sensitivity of the visual field.[126,135] This may be difficult to differentiate from similar changes occurring in otherwise normal individuals from small pupils, uncorrected refractive error, media changes,[136] or age.[137] If the damage to the optic nerve is primarily focal in nature, the glaucoma patient would present with the classical field defects of increased fluctuation in isolated areas of the visual field,[138] paracentral scotomas 5 to 20° from fixation, and either central or peripheral nasal steps (Fig. 12–4).[136,139] These defects occur more frequently in a superior than inferior hemisphere of the visual field.[3,140] Between 75 and 90% of the earliest visual field defects appear in the central 30° of the visual field.[139] Visual field defects, such as generalized constriction, enlargement of the blind spot, and baring of the blind spot, which have traditionally been associated with glaucoma, are in reality not specific for the disease and should not be used as criteria for a definitive diagnosis or on-going management.[136]

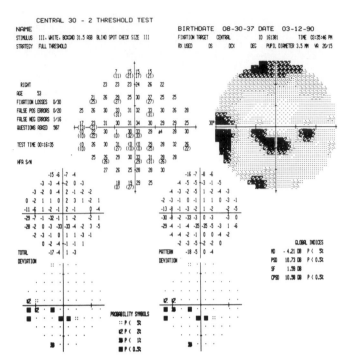

Figure 12–4. Visual field defects. Automated visual field printout of the right eye of a glaucoma patient showing an extensive inferior arcuate scotoma and a nasal field defect in the central visual field.

It is not uncommon in early glaucoma for the nasal hemisphere to show incongruity between the superior and inferior quadrants (*see* Fig. 12–4).[3,141,142] Visual field defects in glaucoma are often limited to a single altitudinal hemifield, with the corresponding hemifield possibly remaining unaffected for up to 10 years.[3] Low-tension glaucoma usually causes focal types of field defects that are somewhat unique in being closer to fixation and denser.[143] Asymmetry in the sensitivity between the two eyes of more than a few decibels on repeated testing may be clinically significant.[144] Glaucoma patients with asymmetrical nerve damage and/or visual field loss may show an afferent pupillary defect.[145]

The most important aspect of visual field testing in glaucoma is to detect the field loss as early as possible. This has been aided by the introduction of automated perimetry.[146] Quigley's studies have shown that a significant portion of the optic nerve is already destroyed before traditional methods of assessing visual function become abnormal.[9] Once damage has reached this level, progression of visual field loss occurs more rapidly since there is less of a buffer or redundancy in the number of ganglion cells and their receptive fields.[6]

If glaucoma can be identified prior to visual field defects through observation of the optic nerve changes, treatment of the disease has the best chance of slowing down or preventing any further damage.[3,147] If glaucoma is not treated until the patient has absolute reproducible visual field defects, damage to the optic nerve may be so significant that even with a dramatic reduction of intraocular pressure the disease continues to progress.[148]

Summary

Collecting all the pieces of the puzzle (clinical data, patient characteristics) makes the diagnosis become clear. With the data available from a complete work-up, the clinician is able to analyze the information and assess the probability of the patient developing glaucoma. If the patient does have several risk factors, it is important to determine whether or not damage from glaucoma has already occurred in the eye. If it has, treatment must be initiated.

An analysis of each piece of clinical data in isolation from another does not give complete insight into the relative risk of the patient for glaucoma.[10,149] The simultaneous analysis of multiple pieces of the puzzle has shown to be much more effective in predicting which patients will eventually develop the disease.[150–152] As an example, if you were to examine 1000 patients over the age of 40, you may find 7 to 8% with intraocular pressures over 21 mm Hg, 5 to 6% with cup-to-disc ratios of greater than 0.5, 2 to 5% with visual field loss, but only 0.5 to 1% with glaucoma. Even though each of these findings is a risk factor for glaucoma, their prevalence in the general population exceeded the prevalence of glaucoma. This is true for all of the risk factors discussed. By analyzing multiple risk factors in an individual, the probability of identifying those patients with the greatest chance of progressing to glaucoma increases dramatically.[12,148,149,152–154]

MANAGEMENT OF THE PATIENT

The reason for making as early a definitive diagnosis of glaucoma as possible is to initiate an appropriate treatment. The process used to reach the decision to treat or not is complex and varies among clinicians. Many factors must be weighed before committing a patient to a life of drugs and/or surgery. These would include the cumulative risk of the patient to develop some type of glaucoma, the patient's age, the patient's level of anxiety about the disease, the doctor's level of concern, the likelihood of patient compliance with treatment, and the ability of the patient to be able to afford the care on a long-term basis.[151] Ultimately, the decision to treat will be made by weighing the benefits versus the risk to the patient.

CONCLUSION

The early differential diagnosis of glaucoma is the most critical step in the proper management of the disease. Early diagnosis is possible if the clinician collects all the appropriate clinical data and properly analyzes the patient's characteristics. This allows a determination of the relative risk or probability of the patient developing glaucoma.

REFERENCES

1. Fruhauf A, Muller F, Sismuth M. Untersuchungen zur Prognose des Glaukoms. *Klin Monatsbi Augenheilkd.* 1967;151:477–485.
2. Graham PA. The definition of pre-glaucoma. A prospective study. *Trans Ophthalmol Soc UK.* 1968;88:153–165.
3. Hart WM, Becker B. The onset and evolution of glaucomatous visual field defects. *Ophthalmology.* 1982;89:268–279.
4. Phelps CD. The "no treatment" approach to ocular hypertension. *Surv Ophthalmol.* 1980;25:175–182.
5. Drance SM. Review: The medical management of open angle glaucoma. *Can J Ophthalmol.* 1978;13:123–127.
6. Quigley HA. Glaucoma's optic nerve damage: Changing clinical perspectives. *Ann Ophthalmol.* 1982;14:611–612.
7. Chandler PA. Long-term results in glaucoma therapy. *Am J Ophthalmol.* 1975;80:62–69.
8. Grant WM, Burke JF. Why do some people go blind from glaucoma? *Am J Ophthalmol.* 1982;89:991–998.
9. Quigley HA, Addicks EM, Green WR. Optic nerve damage in human glaucoma. III. Quantitative correlation of nerve fiber loss and visual field defects in glaucoma, ischemic optic neuropathy, papilledema, and toxic optic neuropathy. *Arch Ophthalmol.* 1982;100:135–146.
10. Krupin T, Rosenberg LF, Ruderman JM. Update: Diagnostic concept in open-angle glaucoma. *Curr Opin Ophthalmol.* 1991;2:120–127.
11. Motolko M, Drance SM. Features of the optic disc in pre-glaucomatous eyes. *Arch Ophthalmol.* 1981;99:1992–1994.
12. Armaly MF, Krueger DE, Maunder L, et al. Biostatistical analysis of the collaborative glaucoma study. I. Summary report of the risk factors for glaucomatous visual field defects. *Arch Ophthalmol.* 1980;98:2163–2172.

13. Hoskins HD. The management of elevated intraocular pressure with normal optic discs and visual fields. II. An approach to early therapy. *Surv Opthalmol.* 1977; 21:479–493.

14. Jenson JE. Glaucoma screening. A 16-year follow-up of ocular normotensives. *Acta Ophthalmol.* 1984;62: 203–209.

15. Anderson DR. Glaucoma: The damage caused by pressure. XLVI Edward Jackson Memorial Lecture. *Am J Ophthalmol.* 1989;108:485–495.

16. Paterson G. A nine-year follow-up of studies on first-degree relatives of patients with glaucoma simplex. *Trans Ophthalmol Soc UK.* 1970;90:515–525.

17. Rosenthal AR, Perkins ES. Family studies in glaucoma. *Br J Ophthalmol.* 1985;69:664–667.

18. Martin MJ, Sommer A, Gold EB, et al. Race and primary open-angle glaucoma. *Am J Ophthalmol.* 1985;99: 383–387.

19. Leske MC, Podgor MJ. Intraocular pressure, cardiovascular risk variables and visual field defects. *Am J Epidemiol.* 1983;118:280–287.

20. Francois J, Neetens A. The deterioration of the visual field in glaucoma and the blood pressure. *Doc Ophthalmol.* 1970;28:70–132.

21. Becker B. Diabetes mellitus and primary open-angle glaucoma. *Am J Ophthalmol.* 1971;70:1–16.

22. Sommer A. Intraocular pressure and glaucoma. *Am J Ophthalmol.* 1989;107:186–188.

23. Hoyt WF, Frisen L, Newman NW. Fundoscopy of the nerve fiber layer defects in glaucoma. *Invest Ophthalmol.* 1973;12:814–829.

24. Yablonski ME, Zimmerman TJ, Kass MA, Becker B. Prognostic significance of optic disc cupping in ocular hypertensive patients. *Am J Ophthalmol.* 1980;89:585–590.

25. Perkins ES, Phelps CD. Open-angle glaucoma, ocular hypertension, low tension glaucoma and refraction. *Arch Ophthalmol.* 1982;100:1464–1467.

26. Kass MA, Kolker AE, Becker B. Prognostic factors in glaucomatous visual field loss. *Arch Ophthalmol.* 1976; 94:1274–1276.

27. David R, Zangwill L, Badarna M, Yassur Y. Epidemiology of retinal vein occlusion and its association with glaucoma and increased intraocular pressure. *Ophthalmologica.* 1988;197:69–74.

28. Drance SM, Douglas GR, Wijsmank K, et al. Response of blood flow to warm and cold in normal and low-tension glaucoma patients. *Am J Ophthalmol.* 1988;105: 35–39.

29. Gasser P. Ocular vasospasm. A risk factor in the pathogenesis of low-tension glaucoma. *Int Ophthalmol.* 1989;13:281–290.

30. Levene R. Low tension glaucoma: A critical review and new material. *Surv Ophthalmol.* 1980;24:621–664.

31. Drance SM, Sweeney VP, Morgan RW, Feldman F. Studies of factors involved in the production of low tension glaucoma. *Arch Ophthalmol.* 1973;89:457–465.

32. Phelps CD, Corbett JJ. Migraine and low-tension glaucoma. *Invest Ophthalmol Vis Sci.* 1985;26:1105–1108.

33. Kitazawa Y, Shirato S, Yamamoto T. Optic disc hemorrhage in low-tension glaucoma. *Ophthalmology.* 1986;93:853–857.

34. Hyams SW, Frankel A, Keroub C, Antal J. Postural changes in intraocular pressure with particular reference to low tension glaucoma. *Glaucoma.* 1984;6:178–181.

35. Low, RF. Primary angle-closure glaucoma: Inheritance and environment. *Br J Ophthalmol.* 1972;56:13–20.

36. Fontana SC, Brubaker RF. Volume and depth of the anterior chamber in the normal aging human eye. *Arch Ophthalmol.* 1980;98:1803–1808.

37. Alsbirk PH. Corneal diameter in Greenland Eskimos: Anthropometric and genetic studies with special reference to primary angle-closure glaucoma. *Acta Ophthalmol.* 1975;53:635–646.

38. Fujita K, Negishi C, Fujikik, et al. Epidemiology of primary angle closure glaucoma. Report 1. *Jpn J Clin Ophthalmol.* 1983;37:625–629.

39. Alsbirk PH. Angle-closure glaucoma surveys in Greenland Eskimos. *Can J Ophthalmol.* 1973;8:260–264.

40. Sugar HS. Pigmentary glaucoma: A 25-year review. *Am J Ophthalmol.* 1966;62:499–507.

41. Sugar HS. The pseudoexfoliation syndrome. *Met Pediatr Syst Ophthalmol.* 1982;6:227–236.

42. Jones WL. Post-traumatic glaucoma. *J Am Optom Assoc.* 1987;58:708–715.

43. Brown GC, Magargal L, Schachat A, Shah H. Neovascular glaucoma: Etiologic considerations. *Ophthalmology.* 1984;91:315–319.

44. Posner A, Schlossman A. Syndrome of unilateral recurrent attacks of glaucoma with cyclitic symptoms. *Arch Ophthalmol.* 1948;39:517–535.

45. Schwartz B. The response of ocular pressure to corticosteroids. *Int Ophthalmol Clin.* 1966;6:929–987.

46. Sommer A. Glaucoma screening: Too little, too late? *J Gen Intern Med.* 1990;5(suppl):533–537.

47. Leydhecker W. The intraocular pressure: Clinical aspects. *Ann Ophthalmol.* 1976;8:389–399.

48. Katavisto M. The diurnal variations of ocular tension in glaucoma. *Acta Ophthalmol (Copenh).* 1964; 78(suppl):3–130.

49. Sponsel WE. Tonometry in question: Can visual screening tests play a more decisive role in glaucoma diagnosis and management? *Surv Ophthalmol.* 1989; 33(suppl):291–300.

50. Armaly MF. Ocular pressure and visual fields. A 10-year follow-up study. *Arch Ophthalmol.* 1969;81:25–40.

51. Kitazawa Y, Horie T, Aoki S, et al. Untreated ocular hypertension. A long-term prospective study. *Arch Ophthalmol.* 1977;95:1180–1184.

52. Linner E. Ocular hypertension: The clinical course during ten years without therapy: Aqueous humor dynamics. *Acta Ophthalmol.* 1976;54:707–720.

53. Perkins ES. The Bedford glaucoma survey. II. Rescreening of normal population. *Br J Ophthalmol.* 1973; 57:186–192.

54. Ellenberg G, Freedman J. Retinal vein occlusion and

ocular hypertension. *Ann Ophthalmol.* 1982;14:920–922.

55. Schappert-Kemmijser J. A five-year follow-up of subject with IOP of 20–30 mm Hg without anomalies of optic nerve and visual field typical for glaucoma at first investigation. *Ophthalmologica.* 1971;162:289–295.

56. Cotton T, Ederer F. The distribution of intraocular pressures in the general population. *Surv Ophthalmol.* 1980;25:123–129.

57. Kass MA, Sears ML. Hormonal regulation of intraocular pressure. *Surv Ophthalmol.* 1977;22:153–176.

58. Shiose Y. The aging effect on intraocular pressure in an apparently normal population. *Arch Ophthalmol.* 1984;102:883–887.

59. Shiose Y. Statistical analysis of systemic effect on intraocular pressure. *Glaucoma.* 1984;6:231–235.

60. Blumenthal M, Blumenthal R, Peritz E, et al. Seasonal variation in intraocular pressure. *Am J Ophthalmol.* 1970;69:608–610.

61. Marcus DF, Krupin T, Podos SM. The effect of exercise on intraocular pressure. I. Human beings. *Invest Ophthalmol.* 1970;9:749–752.

62. Galin MA, Davidson R, Pasmanik S. An osmotic comparison of urea and mannitol. *Am J Ophthalmol.* 1963;55:244–247.

63. Kitazawa Y, Horie T. Diurnal variation of intraocular pressure and its significance in the medical treatment of primary open-angle glaucoma. In: Krieglstein GK, Leydhecker W, eds. *Glaucoma Update.* New York: Springer; 1979:169–176.

64. Horie T, Kitazawa Y. The clinical significance of diurnal pressure variation in primary open-angle glaucoma. *Jpn J Ophthalmol.* 1979;23:310–333.

65. Loewenthal LM. Glaucoma: The value of a diurnal curve and Goldmann visual fields. *Ann Ophthalmol.* 1977;9:75–77.

66. Schwartz B, Talusan AG. Spontaneous trends in ocular pressure in untreated ocular hypertension. *Arch Ophthalmol.* 1980;98:105–111.

67. Davanger M. The difference in ocular pressure in the two eyes of the same person. In individuals with healthy eyes and in patients with glaucoma simplex. *Acta Ophthalmol.* 1965;43:299–313.

68. Crichton A, Drance SM, Douglas GR, Schulzer M. Unequal intraocular pressure and its relation to asymmetric visual field defects in low-tension glaucoma. *Ophthalmology.* 1989;96:1312–1314.

69. Cartwright MJ, Anderson DR. Correlation of asymmetric damage with asymmetric intraocular pressure in normal-tension glaucoma (low-tension glaucoma). *Arch Ophthalmol.* 1988;106:898–900.

70. Alexander LJ. Diagnosis and management of primary open-angle glaucoma. In: Classe JG, ed. *Optometry Clinics: Glaucoma.* Norwalk, CT: Appleton & Lange; 1991:19–102.

71. Leske MC, Rosenthal J. Epidemiologic aspect of open-angle glaucoma. *Am J Epidemiol.* 1979;109:250–272.

72. Hollows FC, Graham PA. Intraocular pressure, glau-coma and glaucoma suspects in a defined population. *Br J Ophthalmol.* 1966;50:570–586.

73. Kahn HA, Milton RC. Alternative definitions for open-angle glaucoma: Effect on prevalence and association in the Framingham Eye Study. *Arch Ophthalmol.* 1980;98:2172–2177.

74. Krieglstein GK. Glaucoma editorial overview. *Curr Opin Ophthalmol.* 1990;1:103–104.

75. Sonsel WE. Quantification and monitoring of visual field defects and a prospective, randomized comparison of pilocarpine and timolol using computerized perimetry (summary). *Surv Ophthalmol.* 1989;33(suppl):427–428.

76. Greenidge KC. Angle-closure glaucoma. *Int Ophthalmol Clin.* 1990;30:177–185.

77. Wand M. Provocative tests in angle-closure glaucoma: A brief review with commentary. *Ophthalmic Surg.* 1974;5:32–37.

78. Harris LS, Galin MA. Prone provocative testing for narrow-angle glaucoma. *Arch Ophthalmol.* 1972;87:493–496.

79. Caprioli J, Miller JM. Videographic measurements of optic nerve topography in glaucoma. *Invest Ophthalmol Vis Sci.* 1988;29:1294–1298.

80. Airaksinen PJ, Drance SM, Schulzer M. Neuroretinal rim area in early glaucoma. *Am J Ophthalmol.* 1985;99:1–4.

81. Bengtsson B. The variation and covariation of cup and disc diameters. *Acta Ophthalmol.* 1976;54:804–818.

82. Lichter PR. Variability of expert observers in evaluating the optic disc. *Trans Am Ophthalmol Soc.* 1976;74:532–572.

83. Pederson JE, Anderson DR. The mode of progressive disc cupping in ocular hypertension and glaucoma. *Arch Ophthalmol.* 1980;98:490–495.

84. Trobe JD, Glaser JS, Cassady J, et al. Nonglaucomatous excavation of the optic disc. *Arch Ophthalmol.* 1980;98:1046–1050.

85. Read RM, Spaeth GL. The practical clinical appraisal of the optic disc in glaucoma: The natural history of cup progression and some specific disc-field correlations. *Trans Am Acad Ophthalmol Otolaryng.* 1974;78:255–274.

86. Kirsch R, Anderson DR. Clinical recognition of glaucomatous cupping. *Am J Ophthalmol.* 1973;75:442–454.

87. Sommer A, Pollack I, Maumenee AE. Optic disc parameters and onset of glaucomatous field loss. I. Methods and progressive change in disc morphology. *Arch Ophthalmol.* 1979;97:1444–1448.

88. Balazsi AG, Drance SM, Schulzer M, Douglas GR. Neuroretinal rim area in suspected glaucoma and early chronic open-angle glaucoma. *Arch Ophthalmol.* 1984;102:1011–1014.

89. Herschler J, Osher R. Baring of the circumlinear vessels. An early sign of optic nerve damage. *Arch Ophthalmol.* 1980;98:865–869.

90. Caprioli J, Spaeth G. Comparison of the optic nerve in high- and low-tension glaucoma. *Arch Ophthalmol.* 1985;103:1145–1149.

91. Schwartz B. Cupping and pallor of the optic disc. *Arch Ophthalmol.* 89;1973:272–277.

92. Schwartz B. Optic disc changes in ocular hypertension. *Surv Ophthalmol.* 1980;25:148–154.

93. Sorenson PN. The colour of the optic disc variation with location of illumination. *Acta Ophthalmol.* 1980; 58:1005–1010.

94. Buus DR, Anderson DR. Peripapillary crescents and halos in normal-tension glaucoma and ocular hypertension. *Ophthalmology.* 1989;96:17–19.

95. Jonas JB, Naumann COH. Parapapillary chorioretinal atrophy in normal and glaucoma eyes. II. Correlations. *Invest Ophthalmol Vis Sci.* 1989;30:919–926.

96. Miller KM, Quigley HA. The clinical appearance of the lamina cribrosa as a function of the extent of glaucomatous optic nerve damage. *Ophthalmology.* 1988; 95:135–138.

97. Kottler MS, Drance SM. Studies on hemorrhages on the optic disc. *Can J Ophthalmol.* 1976;11:102–105.

98. Shihab ZM, Lee PF, Hay P. The significance of disc hemorrhage in open-angle glaucoma. *Ophthalmology.* 1982;89:211–213.

99. Diehl DLC, Quigley HA, Miller NR, et al. Prevalence and significance of optic disc hemorrhage in a longitudinal study of glaucoma. *Arch Ophthalmol.* 1990;108: 545–550.

100. Drance SM. Disc hemorrhages in glaucomas. *Surv Ophthalmol.* 1989;33:331–337.

101. Airaksinen PJ, Mustonen E, Alanko HI. Optic disc hemorrhages precede retinal nerve fiber layer defects in ocular hypertension. *Acta Ophthalmol (Copenh).* 1981;59:627–641.

102. Drance SM. Correlation between optic disc changes and visual field defects in chronic open-angle glaucoma. *Trans Am Acad Ophthalmol Otolaryng.* 1976;81: 224–225.

103. Hoskins HD, Gelber EC. Optic disc topography and visual field defects in patients with increased intraocular pressure. *Am J Ophthalmol.* 1975;80:284–290.

104. Schwartz B, Takamoto T, Nagin P. Measurements of reversibility of optic disc cupping and pallor in ocular hypertension and glaucoma. *Ophthalmology.* 1985;92: 1396–1407.

105. Miller NR, George TW. Monochromatic (red free) photography and ophthalmoscopy of the peripapillary retinal nerve fiber layer. *Invest Ophthalmol Vis Sci.* 1978;17:1121–1124.

106. Airaksinen PJ, Drance SM, Douglas GR, et al. Diffuse and localized nerve fiber loss in glaucoma. *Am J Ophthalmol.* 1984;98:566–571.

107. Sommer A, Quigley HA, Robin AL, et al. Evaluation of nerve fiber layer assessment. *Arch Ophthalmol.* 1984; 102:1766–1771.

108. Sommer A, Katz J, Quigley HA, et al. Clinically detectable nerve fiber atrophy precedes the onset of glaucomatous field loss. *Arch Ophthalmol.* 1991;109:77–83.

109. Quigley HA, Miller NR, George T. Clinical evaluation of nerve fiber layer atrophy as an indicator of glau-

comatous optic nerve damage. *Arch Ophthalmol.* 1980; 98:1564–1568.

110. Quigley HA. Examination of the retinal nerve fiber layer in the recognition of early glaucoma damage. *Trans Am Ophthalmol Soc.* 1986;84:920–966.

111. Caprioli J. Correlation of visual function with optic nerve and nerve fiber layer structure in glaucoma. *Surv Ophthalmol.* 1989;33(suppl):319–330.

112. Drance SM, Airaksinen PJ. Signs of early damage in open-angle glaucoma. In: Weinstein GW, ed. *Open Angle Glaucoma.* New York: Churchill Livingston; 1986:17–29.

113. Quigley HA, Addicks EM. Quantitative studies of retinal nerve fiber layer defects. *Arch Ophthalmol.* 1982; 100:807–814.

114. Sommer A, Miller NR, Pollack I, et al. The nerve fiber layer in the diagnosis of glaucoma. *Arch Ophthalmol.* 1977;95:2149–2156.

115. Airaksinen PK, Drance SM, Douglas GR, et al. Visual field and retinal nerve fiber layer comparison in glaucoma. *Arch Ophthalmol.* 1985;103:205–207.

116. Flammer J, Drance SM. Correlation between color vision scores and quantitative perimetry in suspected glaucoma. *Arch Ophthalmol.* 1984;102:38–39.

117. Stamper RL. Psychophysical changes in glaucoma. *Surv Ophthalmol.* 1989;33(suppl):309–318.

118. Balazsi AG, Rootman J, France SM, et al. The effect of age on the nerve fiber population in human optic nerve. *Am J Ophthalmol.* 1984;97:760–766.

119. Marx MS, Bodis-Wollner I, Lustgarten JS, et al. Electrophysiological evidence that early glaucoma affects foveal vision. *Doc Ophthalmol.* 1988;67:281–301.

120. Adams AJ, Heron G, Husted R. Clinical measures of central vision function in glaucoma and ocular hypertension. *Arch Ophthalmol.* 1987;105:782–787.

121. Drance SM, Lakowski R, Schulzer M, Douglas GR. Acquired color vision changes in glaucoma. Use of 100-hue test and Pickford anomaloscope as predictors of glaucomatous field change. *Arch Ophthalmol.* 1981; 99:829–831.

122. Sample PA, Weinreb RN, Boynton RM. Acquired dyschromatopsia in glaucoma. *Surv Ophthalmol.* 1986;31: 54–64.

123. Lakowski R, Drance SM. Acquired dyschromatopsias: The earliest functional losses in glaucoma. *Doc Ophthalmol Proc Ser.* 1979;19:159–165.

124. Airaksinen PJ, Lakowski R, Dance SM, Prince M. Color vision and retinal nerve fiber layer in early glaucoma. *Am J Ophthalmol.* 1986;101:208–213.

125. Lakowski R, Bryett J, Drance SM. A study of colour vision in ocular hypertensives. *Can J Ophthalmol.* 1972; 7:86–95.

126. Flammer J. Psychophysics in glaucoma. A modified concept of disease. In: Greve EL, Leydhecker W, eds. *2nd European Glaucoma Symposium.* The Hague: W. Junk Publishers; 1985:11–17.

127. Yamazaki Y, Drance SM, Lakowski R, Schulzer M. Correlation between color vision and highest intraoc-

ular pressure in glaucoma patients. *Am J Ophthalmol.* 1988;106:397–399.

128. Adams AJ, Rodic R, Husted R, Stampler RL. Spectral sensitivity and color discrimination changes in glaucoma and glaucoma-suspect patients. *Invest Ophthalmol Vis Sci.* 1982;23:516–524.

129. Flammer J, Drance SM. Correlation between color vision scores and quantitative perimetry in suspected glaucoma. *Arch Ophthalmol.* 1984;102:38–39.

130. Keltner JL, Johnson CA. Screening for visual field abnormalities with automated perimetry. *Surv Ophthalmol.* 1983;28:175–183.

131. Keltner JL, Johnson CA. Effectiveness of automated perimetry in following glaucomatous visual field progression. *Ophthalmology.* 1982;87:247–254.

132. Heijl A, Drance SM. A clinical comparison of three computerized automatic perimeters in the detection of glaucoma defects. *Arch Ophthalmol.* 1981;99:832–836.

133. Enger C, Sommer A. Recognizing glaucomatous field loss with the Humphrey STATPAC. *Arch Ophthalmol.* 1987;105:1355–1357.

134. Kosok O, Sommer A, Auer C. Screening with automated perimetry using a threshold-related three-level algorithm. *Ophthalmology.* 1986;93:882–886.

135. Drance SM, Douglas GR, Airaksinen PJ, et al. Diffuse visual field loss in chronic open-angle and low-tension glaucoma. *Am J Ophthalmol.* 1987;104:577–580.

136. Aulhorn E, Harms H. Early visual field defects in glaucoma. In: Leydhecker W, ed. *Glaucoma Symposium, Tutzig Castle, 1966.* Basel, Switzerland: S. Karger; 1967:151–186.

137. Jaffe GJ, Alvarado JA, Juster RP. Age-related changes of the normal visual field. *Arch Ophthalmol.* 1986;104: 1021–1025.

138. Werner EB, Drance SM. Early visual field disturbances in glaucoma. *Arch Ophthalmol.* 1977;95:1173–1176.

139. Bryars JH, Cowan EC, Linton D. The earliest visual field changes in glaucoma simplex. *Trans Ophthalmol Soc UK.* 1974;97:1050–1051.

140. Nicholas SP, Werner EB. Location of early glaucomatous visual field defects. *Can J Ophthalmol.* 1980;15: 131–133.

141. Duggan C, Sommer A, Auer C, Burkhard K. Automated differential threshold perimetry for detecting glaucomatous visual field loss. *Am J Ophthalmol.* 1985; 100:420–423.

142. Mikelberg FS, Schulzer M, Drance SM, Lau N. The rate of progression of scotomas in glaucoma. *Am J Ophthalmol.* 1986;101:1–6.

143. Caprioli J, Spaeth GL. Comparison of visual field defects in the low-tension glaucomas with those in the high-tension glaucomas. *Am J Ophthalmol.* 1984;97: 730–737.

144. Feuer WJ, Anderson DR. Static threshold asymmetry in early glaucomatous field loss. *Ophthalmology.* 1989; 96:1285–1297.

145. Kohn AN, Moss AP, Podos SM. Relative afferent pupillary defects in glaucoma without characteristic field loss. *Arch Ophthalmol.* 1979;97:294–296.

146. Heijl A, Drance SM, Douglas GR. Automated perimetry (Competer). Ability to detect early glaucomatous field defects. *Arch Ophthalmol.* 1980;98:1560–1563.

147. Chandler PA, Grant MW. Ocular hypertension versus open-angle glaucoma. *Arch Ophthalmol.* 1977;95:585–586.

148. Wilson R, Walker AM, Ducker DF, Crick RP. Risk factors for rate of progression of glaucomatous visual field loss. *Arch Ophthalmol.* 1982;100:737–741.

149. Hart WM, Yablonski M, Kass MA, Becker B. Multivariate analysis of the risk of glaucomatous visual field loss. *Arch Ophthalmol.* 1979;97:1455–1458.

150. Ford VJ, Zimmerman TJ. How to follow "ocular hypertension." *Ann Ophthalmol.* 1982;14.309–310.

151. Kass MA. When to treat ocular hypertension. *Surv Ophthalmol.* 1983;28(suppl):229–232.

152. Drance SM, Schulzer M, Douglas GR, Sweeney VP. Use of discriminant analysis. II. Identification of persons with glaucomatous visual field defects. *Arch Ophthalmol.* 1981;99:1019–1022.

153. Wilensky JT, Podos SM, Becker B. Prognostic indicators in ocular hypertension. *Arch Ophthalmol.* 1974;91: 200–202.

154. Wilson MR, Hertzmark E, Walker AM, et al. A case-control study of risk factors in open-angle glaucoma. *Arch Ophthalmol.* 1987;105:1066–1071.

TREATMENT AND MANAGEMENT OF THE GLAUCOMAS

Chapter 13

PHARMACOLOGY OF
ANTIGLAUCOMA MEDICATIONS

Wolfgang H. Vogel
Carla U. Vogel

Intraocular pressure (IOP) is regulated by the proper balance between the inflow and outflow of aqueous fluid. Both are controlled by a variety of receptors located on different intraocular structures as well as by specific metabolic processes (Fig. 13–1). Drugs can be used to reduce the inflow or increase the outflow of aqueous and lower the IOP and, thus, potentially prevent or reduce the pathological and clinical consequences of elevated IOP.

The response to any drug therapy depends on the triad of the drug, the patient, and the clinician. The structure of the drug determines its pharmacokinetic and pharmacodynamic profile. Absorption, penetration through membranes in the body, and reaching specific sites of action in tissues is best achieved by drugs that can exist both in the charged and uncharged forms. The interaction of specific drug molecules with specific receptors causes pharmacological responses resulting in therapeutic effects and adverse reactions. The structure of the drug also determines its efficacy (maximal effect produced), potency (the dose necessary to achieve such effects), and the duration of action (half-life). Different routes of administration, whether topical, oral, or injection, or forms of preparations, in a solution, ointment, or gel, can modulate the onset, intensity, and duration

of drug action. For example, a solution of a drug is easily applied to the eye but does not remain there for long, and delivery of the drug into the eye is short lived. An ointment stays on the eye longer, delivers more drug over time, but may interfere with vision. Therapeutic and adverse effects are sometimes overlapping. Pilocarpine reduces IOP in open-angle glaucoma and causes miosis as an unwanted adverse reaction, while miosis is its intended effect in treating an acute angle closure glaucoma attack.

Drug actions are similar among patients but may vary. Certain patients do not respond as well as anticipated or show greater adverse reactions. The constitution of an individual is determined by genetic factors (family history) and environmental conditions. For example, higher doses of atropine are needed to produce mydriasis and cycloplegia in eyes with dark irides as compared to those with light irides. A genetically determined sensitivity to a drug can result in unforseen adverse reactions (e.g., allergic reactions, idiosyncratic reactions). In a patient with glaucoma, a concomitant disease, such as severe asthma, will determine the choice of drug and prohibit the use of any antiglaucoma drug that constricts the bronchi. Age is a major factor in the therapeutic response and occurrence of adverse reactions. The best therapeutic re-

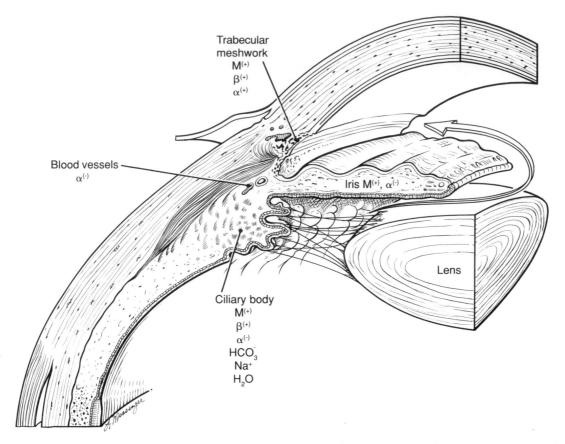

Trabecular
meshwork
$M^{(+)}$
$\beta^{(+)}$
$\alpha^{(+)}$

Blood vessels
$\alpha^{(-)}$

Iris $M^{(+)}$, $\alpha^{(-)}$

Lens

Ciliary body
$M^{(+)}$
$\beta^{(+)}$
$\alpha^{(-)}$
HCO_3^-
Na^+
H_2O

Figure 13–1. Schematic representation of the factors controlling IOP. The level of IOP is governed by an interplay between the production of aqueous and its outflow. These processes are regulated by receptors on different intraocular structures as well as by metabolic processes and may be modified by pathological processes or medications. $M^{(+)}$ = muscarinic receptors.

sponses can usually be expected in young and middle-aged individuals, whereas more serious adverse reactions will occur in the very young (up to 5 years) or old (above 60 to 65 years). Previous drug experience of the patient or close blood relatives is often a good indicator of the expected therapeutic and/or adverse drug responses. Simultaneous drug therapy for other health problems must also be carefully evaluated to avoid drug interactions (e.g, MAO inhibitors and sympathometic drugs).

The clinician plays a major role in the outcome of drug therapy. A thorough knowledge of the pharmacology of a drug and its specific indications, contraindications, and drug interactions are essential in choosing the "right" drug. Patient instructions delivered in an assuring and encouraging attitude can markedly enhance compliance, increase the therapeutic response (placebo effect), and reduce the severity or unpleasantness of adverse reactions. In glaucoma, patient compliance is often poor since the patient has no visual symptoms and therefore does not experience noticeable clinical improvement dur-

ing therapy, but might be bothered by adverse reactions. The clinician must educate and assure the patient, "tailor" the drug regimen to the patient's needs, reinforce applications, answer questions, communicate with other clinicians, and improve the clinician-patient relationship to achieve the best results.[1]

ANTIGLAUCOMA DRUGS

Direct Acting Cholinergic or Muscarinic Drugs

Site of Action. Acetylcholine, released from autonomic nerve fibers, interacts with cholinergic receptors. If these receptors are located on the surface of cells in various tissues next to synapses of the parasympathetic nervous system, they are classified as muscarinic receptors. If these receptors are located in ganglia, the adrenal medulla, or the neuromuscular junction, they are classified as nicotinic (Fig. 13–2). In

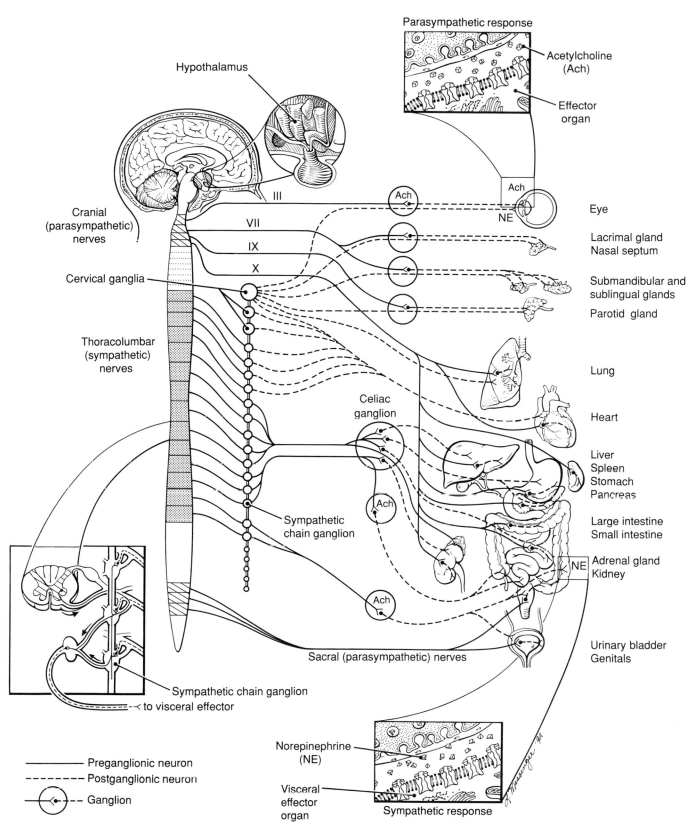

Figure 13–2. Schematic representation of the autonomic nervous system. Drugs may alter the response of a particular system.

Parasympathetic response

Acetylcholine (Ach)

Effector organ

Hypothalamus

Cranial (parasympathetic) nerves

Cervical ganglia

Thoracolumbar (sympathetic) nerves

Celiac ganglion

Sympathetic chain ganglion

Sympathetic chain ganglion
-----< to visceral effector

Sacral (parasympathetic) nerves

—————— Preganglionic neuron
- - - - - Postganglionic neuron
Ganglion

Eye
Lacrimal gland
Nasal septum
Submandibular and sublingual glands
Parotid gland
Lung
Heart
Liver
Spleen
Stomach
Pancreas
Large intestine
Small intestine
Adrenal gland
Kidney
Urinary bladder
Genitals

Norepinephrine (NE)

Visceral effector organ

Sympathetic response

227

in IOP is dose dependent. A 0.7% solution lowers IOP by about 8 mm Hg whereas a 3.4% solution reduces IOP by about 10 mm Hg. Interestingly, the drug vehicle alone can cause a slight reduction of 3 mm Hg[2]. If pilocarpine is administered via Ocuserts, the therapeutic effect may last for 1 week or longer.[3] Ocuserts are plastic drug delivery devices containing pilocarpine. They are placed into the eye of the patient with the drug released at a relatively constant rate.

Carbachol is a synthetic drug that does not penetrate the eye as readily as pilocarpine though penetration may be enhanced by the presence of a wetting agent. Its effects, while similar to those seen with pilocarpine, are prolonged leading to its three times per day dosage.

The chemical structures of the muscarinic drugs, pilocarpine and carbachol, is found in Figure 13–4.

Clinical Usage and Dosage. In open-angle glaucoma, the desired effects are on the ciliary body to increase aqueous outflow and lower IOP. In addition, stimulation of muscarinic receptors on the trabecular meshwork may contribute to this increase in outflow. Miosis does *not* contribute to the therapeutic action in open-angle glaucoma.

In angle closure glaucoma, miosis is the important therapeutic feature. The effects on the ciliary body play no significant role. As the sphincter muscle of the iris constricts, it allows for better flow from the posterior to the anterior chamber and "uncrowds" the angle. In eyes with very high IOP causing iris ischemia, these drugs may not be effective until the pressure is sufficiently lowered by the use of other medications.

It has been claimed that the pilocarpine-phenylephrine provocative test can identify individuals suffering from or at risk of developing acute angle closure glaucoma. However, an extensive study has shown that this test lacks sensitivity to detect eyes at risk and that a positive result was usually associated with damaged outflow that did not respond to peripheral iridectomy.[4]

Among muscarinic drugs, pilocarpine is the drug of first choice. Due to greater adverse reactions, the

TABLE 13–2. DIFFERENT MUSCARINIC DRUGS

	Percentage (%)
Isopto Carpine	0.25, 0.5, 1, 2, 3, 4, 5, 6, 8, 10
Pilocar	0.5, 1, 2, 3, 4, 6
Ocu-Carpine	0.5, 1, 2, 3, 4, 5, 6
Akarpine	1, 2, 4
Pilostat	0.5, 1, 2, 3, 4, 6
Pilagan	1, 2, 4
Pilopine HS Gel	4
Isopto Carbachol	0.75, 1.5, 2.25, 3
Ocuserts	20 or 40 microgram/hr/wk

use of carbachol is usually limited to patients who have become refractory or allergic to pilocarpine.

Some preparations and dosages of pilocarpine and carbachol follow (see also Table 13–2).

Isopto Carpine (pilocarpine HCl) is manufactured by Alcon Laboratories, Inc., and is available in 15- and 30-mL dispensers. Solutions contain 0.25, 0.5, 1, 2, 3, 4, 5, 6, 8, or 10% pilocarpine hydrochloride. It is administered by instilling one drop into the eye up to four times daily.

Pilocar (pilocarpine HCl) is manufactured by IOLAB, and is available as a 15-mL dispenser or 1-mL dropperettes. Solutions contain 0.5, 1, 2, 3, 4, or 6% pilocarpine hydrochloride. It is administered by instilling one drop into the eye up to four times daily in open-angle glaucoma and according to need in angle closure glaucoma.

Pilagan (pilocarpine nitrate) is manufactured by Allergan Pharmaceuticals, Inc., and is available in a 15-mL dispensers. Solutions contain 1, 2, or 4% pilocarpine nitrate. It is administered by instilling one drop four times daily.

Pilostat (pilocarpine HCl) is manufactured by Bausch and Lomb Pharmaceuticals, Inc., and is available in a 15-mL dispenser. Solutions contain 0.5, 1, 2, 3, 4, or 6% pilocarpine hydrochloride. It is administered by instilling one drop into the affected eye four times daily.

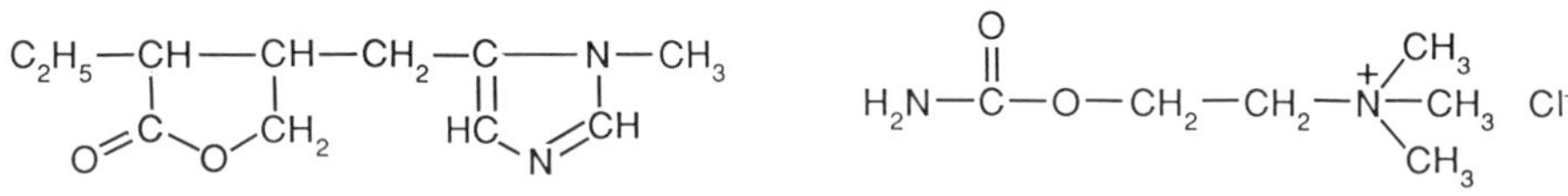

Figure 13–4. The chemical structures of muscarinic drugs.

PILOCARPINE

CARBACHOL

Akarpine (pilocarpine HCl) is manufactured by Akorn, Inc., and is available in 15-mL dispensers. Solutions contain 1, 2, and 4% pilocarpine hydrochloride. One drop is applied four times a day.

Ocu-Carpine (pilocarpine HCl) is manufactured by Ocumed, Inc., and is available in 15-mL bottles. Solutions contain 0.5, 1, 2, 3, 4, 5, or 6% pilocarpine hydrochloride.

Pilopine HS Gel (pilocarpine HCl) is manufactured by Alcon Laboratories, Inc., and is available as a 4% gel preparation in a 5-gram tube. It is administered by applying a ½-inch ribbon into the lower conjunctival sac once a day at bedtime.

Ocuserts are time-release wafers that are placed into the cul-de-sac of the eye and deliver a specified amount of pilocarpine into the eye for 1 week. Ocuserts are manufactured by Alza Corporation, as Pilo-20 (20 μg/hour/week) and Pilo-40 (40 μg/hour/week). The unit contains a core reservoir of pilocarpine and alginic acid. The core is surrounded by a hydrophobic ethylene/vinyl acetate (EVA) copolymer membrane, which allows for a constant diffusion of the stored drug from the unit into the eye. The release rate is somewhat higher during the first 6 hours after placement and usually is not influenced by concomitant use of other glaucoma drugs, but the simultaneous use of epinephrine might increase its absorption into the body.

Isopto Carbachol (carbachol) is manufactured by Alcon Laboratories, Inc., and is available in 15- and 30-mL dispensers. Solutions contain 0.75, 1.5, 2.25, and 3% carbachol. It is administered by instilling one drop into the eye three times daily.

E-pilo is a combination of epinephrine and pilocarpine and is described under adrenergic agonists.

Adverse Reactions and Contraindications. Topical application of direct acting cholinergic drugs to the eye can cause stinging and irritation (Table 13–3). Allergic reactions to the drug, or to an inactive ingredient, are rare. Persistent miosis with visual impairment or ciliary spasm causing myopia and pain in the form of browaches or headaches is infrequent. If these reactions occur initially, they may subside or disappear with time. In certain eyes, angle closure glaucoma can develop because of the formation of a relative pupillary block. While cataracts may result from drug therapy, the occurrence of floaters and ret-

TABLE 13–3. MAJOR OCULAR ADVERSE REACTIONS OF AND CONTRAINDICATIONS TO MUSCARINIC DRUGS

Adverse Reactions	Contraindications
Ocular	
Stinging	Neovascular, malignant or uveitic glaucoma
Miosis (vision)	
Myopia	Ocular infections and inflammation
Corneal haze	
Cataracts	History of retinal detachment
Allergic reactions (rare)	
"Browache," headache	
	Aphakic eyes
Angle closure glaucoma (rare)	
Systemic	
Sweating, salivation	Asthma
Bradycardia	Diarrhea, ulcer, bladder dysfunction
Dyspnea	Parkinson's disease
Gastrointestinal and genitourinary disorders	Certain heart disorders

inal detachment has not been firmly established. The use of gel, but not drops, has been reported to cause a long-lasting, subtle, diffuse superficial corneal haze.[5] Pilocarpine does not cause an increased incident of optic nerve hemorrhages.[6]

Potential systemic adverse reactions include sweating, salivation, bradycardia, arrhythmia, dyspnea, gastrointestinal disturbances, (cramps, diarrhea), and involuntary micturition.

In cases of severe side effects or overdose reactions, atropine is the recommended antidote since it binds to muscarinic receptors. However, atropine does not cause an effect per se but "shields" and blocks these receptors from the excessive stimulation caused by the high amount of cholinergic drug molecules.

Contraindications to the use of cholinergic drugs include the presence of neovascular glaucoma, uveitic glaucoma, or malignant glaucoma; ocular inflammations or acute ocular infections; cataracts; a history of retinal detachments; corneal abrasions; and aphakic or severe myopia. Asthma, ulcer, other gastrointestinal problems, bladder dysfunction, Parkinson's disease, and cardiac irregularities constitute systemic contraindications.

ter 20 minutes. Miosis disappears slowly over a period of 1 week. The IOP drops within 1 to 4 hours of application and the hypotensive effects disappear after 8 to 72 hours.

Echothiophate iodide (or Phospholine Iodide) is a synthetic preparation that is also an irreversible inhibitor of acetylcholinesterase. Miosis starts after 10 minutes, with maximal miosis after 30 minutes, and the effects wearing off during the next 7 days. IOP falls within 1 to 4 hours and returns to pretreatment values after 6 to 60 hours.

The chemical structures of anticholinesterase drugs are found in Figure 13–6.

Clinical Usage and Dosage. Anticholinesterases contract the longitudinal muscle fibers of the ciliary body that pull on the scleral spur and in turn the trabecular meshwork. This opens the channels and increases aqueous outflow. In normal eyes and those with open-angle glaucoma, IOP is lowered. Paradoxically, in a few eyes a rise in IOP can be observed. Thus, tonometric measurements should be made hourly for at least 4 hours after first application of the drugs. If a rise occurs, mydriatic drugs can alleviate this problem. The use of the anticholinesterases in open-angle glaucoma has declined in recent years, mostly due to the advent of laser therapy and the fact that these drugs can cause cataracts. Presently, they are more often employed in aphakic eyes when other drugs do not provide adequate reduction in IOP.

In angle closure glaucoma, they potentially could be used since they do cause miosis. However, they often produce such a marked miosis and shallowing

TABLE 13–5. DIFFERENT ANTICHOLINESTERASE MEDICATIONS

	Percentage (%)
Floropryl	0.025
Humorsol	0.125 or 0.250
Phospholine	0.030, 0.060, 0.125, or 0.250

of the anterior chamber that they actually worsen a pupillary block.

Some preparations and dosages of anticholinesterase drugs follow (see also Table 13–5).

Isoflurophate (Floropryl) is manufactured by Merck, Sharp & Dohme. It is available in a 3.5-gram tube of ointment containing 0.025% of isoflurophate. It is administered by applying a quarter inch strip of ointment into the inferior cul-de-sac every 8 to 72 hours. Gradually, intervals between applications can be increased.

Demecarium bromide (Humorsol) is manufactured by Merck, Sharp & Dohme, and is available in a 5-mL dispenser (Ocumeter with a controlled drop tip). Solutions contain 0.125 or 0.25% demecarium bromide. It is administered by instilling one drop twice a day to twice a week.

Echothiophate iodide (Phospholine Iodide) is manufactured by Wyeth-Ayerst Laboratories, and is available in a 5-mL dispenser. Solutions contain 0.03, 0.06, 0.125, and 0.25% echothiophate iodide. It is administered by instilling one drop twice a day.

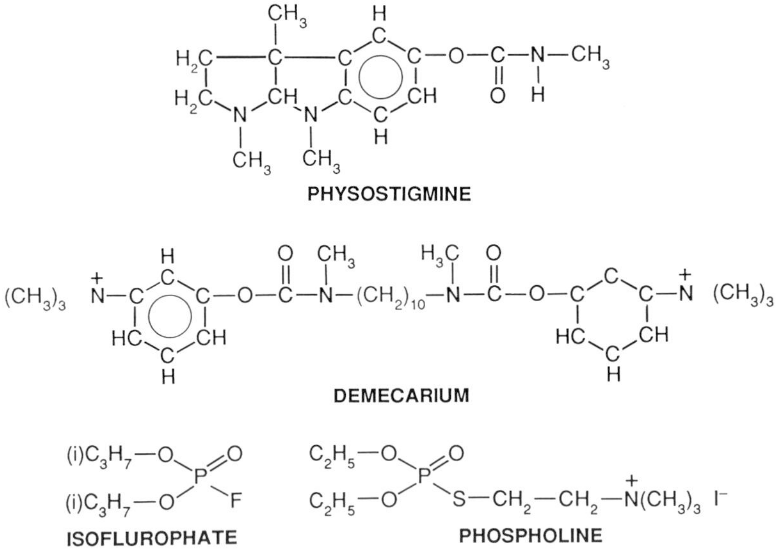

Figure 13–6. The chemical structures of anticholinesterase drugs.

Adverse Reactions and Contraindications. Adverse reactions are usually an extension of the pharmacological effects and are quite similar though sometimes more intense than those seen with the muscarinic agonists (Table 13–6).

In the eye, stinging and burning can occur. Miosis can interfere with vision, particularly in dim light. Contraction and spasm of the ciliary body can lead to impaired accommodation and pain. The latter may force the discontinuation of the drug, but may subside and disappear over time. The drugs, or preservatives, can cause allergic reactions including an allergic conjunctivitis or contact dermatitis. After long-term use, lenticular changes can develop in some patients, ranging from the presence of small vacuoles and haze to frank cataracts. Such changes are seen more frequently in older individuals. Iris cysts can occur, but can be prevented or suppressed by the concomitant use of phenylephrine. It is still uncertain whether these drugs cause floaters or retinal tears; the latter might be of particular importance with the use of echothiophate. A rare complication is the depigmentation of skin of the eyelid in black patients. Inflammation of some ocular structures, in particular the iris, can occur. Due to their stimulatory effects on skeletal muscles, eyelid twitching can be observed.

Systemically, abdominal cramps or diarrhea and an urgency to urinate or involuntary micturition may occur. Constriction of bronchi can cause dyspnea or asthmatic attacks in asthmatic patients. Increased glandular activity may lead to sweating, increased salivation, and tearing. Cardiac rate can also be slowed.

In cases of an overdose, pralidoxime, an acetylcholinesterase reactivator, and atropine, a muscarinic blocker, can be used.

Many contraindications are then obvious from the pharmacological actions and adverse effects described above. These drugs should not be used if an ocular inflammation is present, such as glaucoma associated with iridocyclitis, or if there is a history of retinal detachment or high myopia. Bradycardia, hypotension, recent myocardial infarction, asthma, ulcers, epilepsy, or spastic colon conditions are general contraindications. In pregnancy, the benefit to the patient must be weighed against the potential danger to the fetus.

In patients with myasthenia gravis who are already treated with systemic anticholinesterases, ocular anticholinesterase therapy should be used with caution and in reduced doses.

Farm workers or individuals working with pesticides of the carbamate or organophosphate type, which are also anticholinesterases, should be warned about the danger of an additive effect with the use of ocular anticholinesterases. Anticholinesterases should be discontinued before a patient has general surgery if succinylcholine will be used for anesthesia since their combined effect can lead to prolonged respiratory paralysis.

Direct Acting Adrenergic Drugs

Site of Action. In the sympathetic nervous system, an impulse releases norepinephrine from the terminals of the postganglionic neurons. The released norepinephrine diffuses through the synaptic cleft and binds to postsynaptic receptors on the cells of various organs. This interaction causes a specific physiological response. Immediately after stimulation of the receptors, most of the neurotransmitter molecules are taken back into the neuron, an "active reuptake mechanism," and re-stored for subsequent release. In addition to the receptors on the synaptic site of the effector organ, receptors have also been found on the nerve terminal (presynaptic site). These "autoreceptors" also respond to norepinephrine and either promote release (excitatory) or stop release (inhibitory) of this neurotransmitter.

All the postsynaptic adrenergic receptors bind with and respond to norepinephrine. However, certain drugs have been found to stimulate these receptors selectively. For instance, phenylephrine stimulates the adrenergic receptors in the iris but does not

TABLE 13–6. MAJOR ADVERSE REACTIONS OF AND CONTRAINDICATIONS TO ANTICHOLINESTERASES

Adverse Reactions	Contraindications
Ocular	
Stinging, burning	Ocular inflammation
Miosis	History of retinal detachment
Ciliary spasm (pain)	
Blurred vision	
Lenticular changes	
Iris cysts	
Depigmentation	
Eyelid twitching	
Allergic reaction (rare)	
Systemic	
Diarrhea	Cardiac problems (MI)
Involuntary micturition	Asthma
Dyspnea, asthma	Ulcer
Sweating, salivation	Epilepsy
Cardiac problems	Drug therapy for myasthenia gravis
	Pesticides

Epinephrine HCl (epinephrine HCl) is manufactured by IOLAB Corporation, and is available in 1-mL dropperettes. Solution contains 2% epinephrine HCl. It is administered by instilling one drop in the eye once or twice daily.

Glaucon (epinephrine HCl) is manufactured by Alcon Laboratories, Inc., and is available in 10- and 15-mL dispensers. Solutions contain 1 or 2% epinephrine HCl. It is administered by instilling one drop in the eyes one to two times daily.

Eppy/N (epinephryl borate) is manufactured by Sola/Barnes-Hind, and is available in a 7.5-mL dispenser. Solutions contain 0.5, 1, or 2% epinephryl borate. It is administered by instilling one drop in each eye twice daily.

Propine (dipivefrin HCl) is manufactured by Allergan Pharmaceuticals, Inc., and is available in 5-, 10-, and 15-mL dispensers. Solution contains 0.1% dipivefrin HCl. It is administered by instilling one drop twice a day.

E-Pilo-1 (or 2, 3, 4, 6) is a combination drug consisting of pilocarpine HCl and epinephrine bitartrate. It is manufactured by IOLAB Corporation, and is available in 10-mL dispensers. The solutions contain 10 mg/mL or 1% epinephrine bitartrate and 10, 20, 30, 40, or 60 mg/mL pilocarpine HCl. It is administered by instilling one drop twice a day.

Iopidine (apraclonidine) is manufactured by Alcon Laboratories, Inc., and is available as a 1% solution in 0.25-mL dispensers. One drop is administered 1 hour before and immediately after anterior segment laser surgery.

TABLE 13–8. DIFFERENT ADRENERGIC MEDICATIONS

Product			Epinephrine Concentration (%)
Epitrate			2.0
Epifrin			0.25, 0.5, 1, 2.0
Epinephrine			2.00
Glaucon			1.0, 2.0
Eppy/N			0.5, 1.0, 2.0
Propine			0.1
E-Pilo-1	pilocarine	(1% pilocarpine)	1.0
-2	pilocarine	(2% pilocarpine)	1.0
-3	pilocarine	(3% pilocarpine)	1.0
-4	pilocarine	(4% pilocarpine)	1.0
-6	pilocarine	(6% pilocarpine)	1.0
Iodipine			1.0

TABLE 13–9. EPINEPHRINE EQUIVALENCY

Product	Labeled Strength (%)	Equivalent Epinephrine Base (Activity) (%)
Epinephrine borate		
Epinal	0.25	0.25
	0.5	0.5
	1	1
Eppy/Eppy-N	0.5	0.5
	1	1
	2	2
Epinephrine hydrochloride		
Glaucon	0.5	0.5
	1	1
	2	2
Epifrin	0.25	0.25
	0.5	0.5
	1	1
	2	2
Epinephrine bitartrate		
Epitrate	2	1.1

The above solutions contain epinephrine in the form of different salts. Since the anionic portions differ in weight, the amount of epinephrine in a 1% epinephrine-borate solution does not equal that of a 1% epinephrine-hydrochloride solution. A conversion chart is shown in Table 13–9, which compares labeled strength to epinephrine base.

Adverse Reactions and Contraindications. In the eye, mydriasis is a potential adverse reaction of epinephrine (Table 13–10). While it may be desired in patients with cataracts or those on concomitant cholinergic drug therapy, it prevents the eye from properly adjusting to different light conditions and may cause photophobia. Also, preparations can sting or irritate the eye. Some patients develop an allergic conjunctivitis or contact dermatitis that necessitates cessation of a particular drug. Prolonged epinephrine therapy may cause adrenochrome or pigment deposits in the conjunctiva and cornea or stain soft contact lenses. Macular edema with reduced vision in aphakic or pseudophakic eyes occurs in about one third of patients who are treated with epinephrine. Fortunately, this reaction seems to be reversible after discontinuation of therapy.

Systemically, epinephrine can increase heart rate or blood pressure. These changes are usually of no consequence unless the patient has cardiovascular problems such as hypertension, arrhythmias, or a recent myocardial infarction.

TABLE 13–10. MAJOR ADVERSE REACTIONS OF AND CONTRAINDICATIONS TO ADRENERGIC DRUGS

Adverse Reactions	Contraindications
Ocular	
Irritation	Narrow angle
Mydriasis, photophobia	Aphakia
Pigment deposits	
Allergic reactions	
Macular edema in aphakic eyes	
Systemic Hypertension	
Arrhythmias, tachycardia	Cardiovascular diseases
Gastrointestinal discomfort[a]	Diabetes mellitus
Taste abnormalities[a]	Hyperthyroidism
Medications	
	MAO inhibitors
	Tricyclic antidepressants
	Indomethacin
	General anesthetics

[a] Apraclonidine only.

Contraindications to the use of epinephrine may include a narrow angle, aphakia or pseudophakia, cardiovascular diseases, diabetes mellitus, and hyperthyroidism. The concurrent use of MAO inhibitors and to a lesser extent tricyclic antidepressants can enhance the systemic effects of adrenergic drugs. Such a drug interaction can even occur if MAO inhibitor therapy had been discontinued 3 weeks prior to initiation of epinephrine. Adrenergic agonists must be discontinued before use of general anesthetics since some of these agents can sensitize the heart to catecholamines. Dipivefrin causes less ocular or systemic adverse reactions than epinephrine, and contraindications are somewhat less stringent.

Apraclonidine shows few ocular (minor mydriasis, itching, dryness, allergic reactions) and systemic (bradycardia, orthostatic hypotension, gastrointestinal discomfort, taste abnormalities) reactions. Contraindications include severe cardiac problems and MAO inhibitor therapy.

Beta Antagonists

Site of Action. Norepinephrine released from sympathetic nerve terminals stimulates adrenergic receptors. This interaction produces specific physiological responses depending on the tissue. Interference with this interaction reduces or abolishes the physiological response. One of the ways this can be achieved by drugs that block the released norepinephrine from interacting with the receptor. Blockade can be selective for alpha or beta receptors. After blockade, all structures containing these specific receptors show reduced sympathetic responses and increased parasympathetic reactivity.

Pharmacological Actions. Beta antagonists or blockers "block" or "shield" selectively beta, but not alpha, receptors located at specific end organs opposite the terminals of sympathetic postganglionic fibers. These antagonists do not cause a response, but bind selectively to the receptors and prevent the action of norepinephrine with the receptor (Fig. 13–8). Depending on the type of drug used, it can either block both beta receptors or more selectively the beta 1 receptors, a beta 1 blocker. However, this distinction between beta 1 and beta 2 blockade disappears if higher doses are used.

In the eye, beta receptors are located on structures that control aqueous inflow and outflow. However, the beta blockers appear to mainly block beta receptors, probably beta 1, responsible for inflow. This blockade causes a reduction in IOP. Since instillation of a beta blocker into one eye may also reduce the IOP in the other, untreated eye, the mechanism of action may point to an additional, perhaps central hypotensive effect. In addition, they may affect the dopaminergic system.[11,12] No other significant ocular effects are seen since the iris contains alpha receptors and the muscles of the ciliary body use practically no adrenergic receptors.

Systemically, nonselective beta blockers reduce heart rate and contractility (beta 1), which can also lead to a decrease in blood pressure. They block the beta receptors on the bronchial muscle (beta 2) resulting in a constriction of bronchioles and a decrease in airflow. Beta 1 blockers are more selective for the heart with less effects on the lung. Effects on other organs in the body occur as expected but are less pronounced.

Timolol is a beta 1 and beta 2 blocker. This chemical exists in an L- and D-form with timolol being the L-form. After topical application, IOP falls markedly within 1 hour, reaches a minimum at about 3 hours, with pressure beginning to increase again after about 6 hours. The maximum decrease in IOP is about 20 to 30%. While timolol can be therapeutically effective for many years, some patients cease to respond to the medication after a few days or 1 week, known as short-term escape, and others after a few months or years, long-term drift. This is probably the result of an adjustment of ocular tissue receptors. Blockade

Adverse Effects and Contraindications. Few adverse reactions are seen in the eye (Table 13–14). Transient myopia occurs in a few patients but this usually subsides if the dose is reduced. However, systemic adverse reactions are more frequent and severe and often necessitate discontinuation of drug therapy. About 50% of all the patients will not tolerate these drugs, in particular older individuals. All adverse reactions must be carefully monitored.[23] They include numbness and tingling in extremities, metallic taste, nausea, abdominal cramps and diarrhea, weight loss, renal stone formation (in particular with acetazolamide), libido reduction in males, malaise, drowsiness, fatigue, confusion, and depression. Adverse gastrointestinal signs can be reduced if the drug is taken with food. Since some of these adverse reactions are caused by the metabolic acidosis, supplementation with sodium bicarbonate has been reported to reduce their intensity. Electrolyte disturbances can occur, in particular hypokalemia. Aplastic anemia and Stevens-Johnson syndrome are rare occurrences; the former necessitates frequent blood counts in the beginning of therapy to detect a developing agranulocytosis.

Ocular contraindications include use in patients immediately after filtering operations. Systemic contraindications include cardiac problems (hypokalemia), Addison's disease (loss of sodium and potassium), liver disease, and a sensitivity to sulfonamides.

Osmotic Agents

Site of Action. Osmotic agents increase the osmolarity of blood creating an osmotic gradient between the plasma and the surrounding tissue. In addition to specific physiological and metabolic processes, osmosis also plays a role in the movement of water molecules into or out of the eyes. Changes in the osmotic equilibrium, therefore, can increase or decrease these flows and affect IOP.

Pharmacological Actions. Osmotic agents modulate the osmotic equilibrium. They are generally hydrophilic non-electrolytes that remain in the blood and do not penetrate through cellular barriers into tissues or organs. Thus, they increase the osmolality of the plasma. As a result, water moves from tissues into the plasma to dilute and restore normal osmolality. For the eye, if plasma osmolality increases, water leaves the globe and moves into the plasma. This reduces the volume of fluid and reduces IOP. As plasma volume increases, urine formation is en-

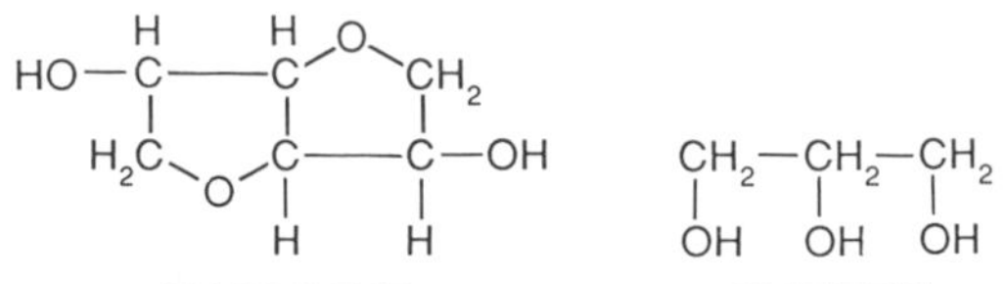

Figure 13–11. The chemical structures of osmotic agents.

hanced and diuresis occurs. In cases of ocular inflammation, the efficiency of the cellular barriers is reduced and a certain amount of the osmotic agent will enter the eye. This results in a smaller osmotic gradient between the intraocular fluid and plasma and less of a reduction in IOP.

Isosorbide and **glycerin** are osmotic agents. They are given orally. Onset of action is very rapid and a significant drop in IOP can be seen within 15 minutes. Within 1 to 2 hours IOP can decrease by 50% and the effect may last for 4 to 6 hours.[24] These drugs are not intended for chronic use.

The chemical structures of isosorbide and glycerin are given in Figure 13–11.

Clinical Usage and Dosage. Indications for these drugs are acute angle closure glaucoma and rises in IOP secondary to traumatic hyphema. They are also used in intraocular surgery to prevent rises in IOP during or after surgery, and also to shrink the vitreous and prevent its loss during intraocular surgery.

Some preparations and dosages follow.

Ismotic (isosorbide) is manufactured by Alcon Laboratories, Inc., and is available as a 45% solution in a 220-mL bottle. The initial dose is 1.5 g/kg body weight. The dose range is 1 to 3 g/kg body weight and it is given orally two to four times daily. The preparation is tolerated better if given with crushed ice.

Osmoglyn (glycerin) is manufactured by Alcon Laboratories, Inc., and is available as a 50% solution in a 220-mL bottle. Dose range is 2 to 3 mL per kg of body weight given orally 1.5 hours prior to surgery.

Adverse Reactions and Contraindications. Table 13–15 gives major adverse reactions and contraindications to osmotic agents. Oral consumption may cause nausea due to excessive sweetness of the prep-

TABLE 13–15. MAJOR ADVERSE REACTIONS OF AND CONTRAINDICATIONS TO OSMOTIC AGENTS

Adverse Reactions	Contraindications
Nausea	Dehydration
Cardiac problems (severe dehydration)	
	Cardiac decompensation
	Renal problems
	Diabetes mellitus[a]

[a] Osmoglyn only.

aration. Since these agents cause fluid loss from the body or diuresis, dehydration and thirst will occur. However, no fluid should be given during the brief treatment periods since this would reduce the therapeutic effects of the drugs.

Glycerin is metabolized in the body similar to carbohydrates and should be administered with caution to diabetic patients. This is not the case for isosorbide. The drugs are contraindicated in patients with severe cardiac or renal problems.

Combination of Antiglaucoma Drugs

The application of one drug to glaucomatous eyes often does not lower IOP sufficiently. The addition of a second or even third drug is often required. When drugs are combined, drugs of the same class are not additive in their effects. Additive reductions in IOP are usually found only with combinations of drugs from different classes involving different modes of action. On a molecular level, stimulation of different types of receptors or activation of different metabolic processes is required for additive effects to occur. For example, the combination of pilocarpine with carbachol does not cause additive effects since both stimulate the same cholinergic receptors. However, additive effects can be expected when pilocarpine (stimulation of muscarinic receptors) is combined with sympathomimetic drugs (stimulation of adrenergic receptors), beta blockers (blockade of beta receptors), or carbonic anhydrase inhibitors (inhibition of carbonic acid formation).

The combination of pilocarpine and timolol lowers IOP more effectively than pilocarpine alone. Airaksinen and associates found that pilocarpine 4% given four times a day lowered IOP on an average of 5.3 mm Hg or 19%, whereas timolol 0.5%-pilocarpine 2% given two times a day lowered IOP 7.2 mm Hg or 25% and timolol 0.5%-pilocarpine 4% given two times a day lowered IOP 10.7 mm Hg or 37%.[25] Similar results were obtained in a more recent study.[26] A

newly developed solution containing both timolol and pilocarpine gave a better reduction in IOP than timolol alone with a longer duration of action and a decreased frequency of pressure peaks.[27]

Addition of apraclonidine to non-selective beta blockers caused a further decrease in IOP from 20 to 15 mm Hg without significantly affecting the cardiovascular system.[28]

The combination of betaxolol and acetazolamide was more hypotensive than either drug alone. Betaxolol lowered IOP by 4.4 mm Hg or 27% and acetazolamide lowered IOP by 6.5 mm Hg or 42%. The combination lowered IOP by 8.3 mm Hg or 54%.[29]

Betaxolol reduced IOP from 27 to 22 mm Hg. The addition of epinephrine reduced IOP to 19 mm Hg. Interestingly, the combination of timolol, a beta 1 and beta 2 blocker, and epinephrine was ineffective. These findings suggest that epinephrine might also work partially through beta 2 receptors that are blocked by timolol but not betaxolol.[30] However, the combination of timolol and dipivefrin showed additive effects in spite of the fact that the latter works through the formation and action of epinephrine.

The addition of the prostaglandin P6F2 alpha-1-isopropyl ester was studied in patients who responded poorly to timolol. The IOP before timolol was 39 mm Hg, after timolol 31 mm Hg, and after P6F2 alpha/timolol 22 mm Hg.[31]

In general, proper combinations produce enhanced reductions in IOP and often cause longer lasting effects. The latter may allow fewer administrations and better control of IOP. When multiple drugs are used, compliance may be adversely affected because of the need for multiple drug instillations.

Other Antiglaucoma Agents

A number of other drugs or chemicals have been tried and found effective as glaucoma medications. Some of these agents are still in the experimental stages or used clinically only outside the United States.

Alpha Adrenergic Blockers

Thymoxamine is a drug that blocks postsynaptic alpha receptors. This blockade prevents norepinephrine released from the sympathetic nerve terminals from binding to and stimulating the adrenergic receptors. The result is a decrease in the activity of the sympathetic nervous system. Thus, the radial muscle of the iris relaxes causing miosis. The ciliary body is not affected since it has no significant alpha receptor for muscular activity. No significant changes in IOP are seen nificant. Once the decision to treat is made, a management strategy is necessary with the careful monitoring of the optic nerve and visual fields to watch for progression of the disease.

The current approach to the treatment of glaucoma is mainly palliative. Most clinicians have seen the rare case of glaucomatous defects reversed with treatment but these are the exception. At present, there are no drugs available for reversal of the basic histopathological abnormality in the outflow pathways that cause POAG. Epstein raises the basic question of "why not a cure?"[5] He suggests that instead of concentrating our efforts to lower IOP pharmacologically, research should be directed at producing a drug that prevents or stops the glaucomatous damage in the trabecular tissue.[5] For the present, the medications used either decrease aqueous production or improve outflow, all through poorly understood mechanisms that may be harmful to the eye. New pharmaceutical agents have been developed in the past decade for lowering IOP. These agents provide the clinician with a number of options for initiating treatment in glaucoma patients. The medications used exert an ocular hypotensive effect, but may also cause ocular and/or systemic side effects. Therefore, it becomes the clinician's responsibility to choose the medication(s) for maximum efficacy and safety with minimal side effects.

PHARMACEUTICAL AGENTS USED FOR TREATMENT

Adrenergic Antagonists

The topical adrenergic antagonists consist of timolol maleate (Timoptic), levobunolol (Betagan), metipranolol (Optipranolol), and betaxolol (Betoptic). These are commonly referred to as *beta blockers* for their specific action of beta adrenergic receptor blockade, which result in decreased aqueous production. Beta blockers are usually the first medication prescribed for individuals with open-angle glaucoma because of their effectiveness in lowering IOP with few ocular side effects. However, not every person will show a sustained reduction in IOP with beta blockers. A uniocular trial should be used whenever any medication is prescribed, looking for the ocular hypotensive response (using the contralateral eye as a control) and side effects incurred.

Beta blockers cause a decrease in aqueous production in the eye. They also slow the heart rate and decrease pulmonary function capacity. Patients using topical beta blockers must be alerted to their potential systemic side effects since some of the topical medica-

tion is absorbed into the circulatory system, effecting beta-receptors located throughout the body.[6]

Timolol (Timoptic), **metipranolol** (Optipranolol), and **levobunolol** (Betagan) are the available nonselective beta blockers. These drugs work at both the beta 1 and beta 2 receptors. All are administered every 12 hours. In selected individuals, one time per day use may be implemented. When once-a-day dosage is instituted, the IOP must be measured 20 to 24 hours after installation. The contraindications for nonselective beta blockers include cardiovascular disease, second- and third-degree heart block, congestive heart failure, hypotension, asthma, chronic obstructive pulmonary disease (COPD), and emphysema.[7] Every patient considered for a topical beta blocker needs base-line blood pressure and pulse measurements in addition to a review of their medical history. The ocular side effects of nonselective beta blockers include burning, stinging,[11,12] hyperemia, punctate keratitis,[13] and corneal hypoaesthesia,[14] but are not usually a problem of sufficient magnitude to necessitate a change in medications.

Betaxolol (Betoptic) is a cardioselective beta blocker that is not as potent in reducing IOP as either timolol or levobunolol. This selective beta 1 blocker has minimal affinity for the beta 2 receptors of the pulmonary and gastrointestinal tissues, permitting its use with caution in situations where nonselective beta blockers are contraindicated (i.e., past history of asthma, COPD).[17] In addition, while betaxolol is specific for the beta 1 receptors, its affinity to those receptors is also less than timolol. This makes betaxolol a safer drug to use than nonselective beta blockers when concerned about the systemic implications on the cardiovascular, pulmonary, or central nervous system. Betaxolol does not usually exert a significant effect on the cardiovascular system[22] and studies have shown betaxolol to be used safely in patients with pulmonary dysfunction.[17,24,25] Still, betaxolol (Betoptic) is not the initial drug of choice for these individuals. It can be used in patients with relative contraindications when other medications have not performed as required if approved by the patient's internist. Rare cases of exacerbation of asthma and decreased forced expiratory volume have been reported with betaxolol when used in individuals without a history of pulmonary problems.[26,27] Insomnia and depressive neurosis have also rarely been reported.[28]

While not as potent as timolol or levobunolol in reducing IOP,[18] betaxolol may show a greater additive effect with the adrenergic agonist dipivalyl epinephrine (Propine).[19–21] Still dipivalyl epinephrine in combination with any beta blocker will not dramatically reduce IOP. Betaxolol comes in a 0.25% suspension (Betoptic S) and a 0.5% solution. Comparative studies between the 0.25% suspension and 0.5% solution have shown an equal clinical effectiveness in reducing IOP. Each is used every 12 hours. Ocular side effects of betaxolol 0.5% (Betoptic) include stinging and burning that is more intense than that of betaxolol 0.25% suspension or timolol.[22,23] Corneal anesthesia has not been reported with betaxolol.

A dissipation phenomenon, seen with all beta blockers, though particularly with timolol, is known as "short-term escape" and "long-term drift."[8,9] After an initial decrease in IOP from several days to a few weeks of use, short-term escape can occur, resulting in a rise in IOP. After 2 to 4 weeks IOP will stabilize, usually below pretreatment level. Long-term drift is seen as a slow steady rise in IOP after months to years of treatment. Many studies have attempted to identify the mechanism responsible for this decreased efficacy. One study suggests there may be a change in the number of beta adrenergic receptors with continued exposure to adrenergic blockage.[10] Another explanation is that open-angle glaucoma, being a slowly progressive disorder, may be getting worse and becoming more difficult to control.

Cardiac and pulmonary side effects are usually the problems that leads to the modification or discontinuation of topical beta blockers. Other less common but still serious side effects include diarrhea, nausea and cramps, depression, anxiety, and confusion.[15,16]

Cholinergic Agonists

The topical cholinergic and anticholinesterase medications are classified as miotics. These agents are responsible for stimulating the longitudinal fibers of the ciliary muscle resulting in the mechanical opening of the trabecular meshwork and increased aqueous outflow. The cholinergic agonists are direct acting agents that mimic acetylcholine and stimulate the cholinergic receptors in the ciliary muscles. The sphincter muscle of the iris is also stimulated leading to reduced pupil size (miosis). The change in size of the pupil plays no part in pilocarpine's ability to reduce IOP in an open-angle individual. The cholinergic agents available for topical use are pilocarpine and carbachol. They rarely elicit systemic side effects in the concentrations used topically to treat POAG. However, ocular side effects are common. The most frequently reported include globe and orbital pain, browache, blurred vision, secondary accommodative spasm, miosis, hyperemia, visual field constriction, and dimness of vision.[6]

Pilocarpine is the miotic of choice. It is produced in a number of forms and concentration. The solution form is manufactured in 0.5 to 10%, administered four times per day, with 2% and 4% the most commonly prescribed. Concentrations greater than the 4% strength in white or 6% in blacks do little to reduce IOP, but increase the risk of systemic side effects.

Pilocarpine is also available in a gel form (Pilopine Gel HS) in 4% concentration administered at bedtime. One advantage of the gel form is the side effects usually occur while the patient is asleep. Pilopine Gel is especially beneficial for those patients suspected of poor compliance, elderly patients with difficulty with eyedrop insertion, or individuals necessitating miotic use but intolerant to the ocular side effects. Care must be taken so only a small amount (about 1/8″) is applied into the inferior cul-de-sac. The gel is best applied by placing a small measured amount on the tip of the finger and using the tip of the finger to place the gel into the inferior cul-de-sac (Fig. 14–1). Often an excessive amount is applied if the gel is placed directly from the tube into the eye. As with any medication being used one time per day, the IOP must be measured at 20 to 24 hours after installation (before the next dosage cycle) to ensure that no spikes are occurring in the diurnal curve.

Pilocarpine is also available in wafer form for sustained release. Known as Ocuserts, the wafers come in 20 μg/hour release rate (roughly equal to 1% drops) and 40 μg/hour release rate (roughly equal to 2% drops). These are inserted into the inferior or superior cul-de-sac weekly. Ocuserts may be useful in the elderly with poor dexterity in instilling eyedrops or in young patients requiring miotic therapy. The myopic shift associated with miotics, most pronounced in young individuals, is constant and can be corrected with spectacles. Foreign body sensation is one side effect of Ocuserts that may limit their usefulness.

The ocular side effects associated with miotics are usually the reason for poor patient compliance. The side effects are related to both dosage and concentration. A patient may better adapt to the side

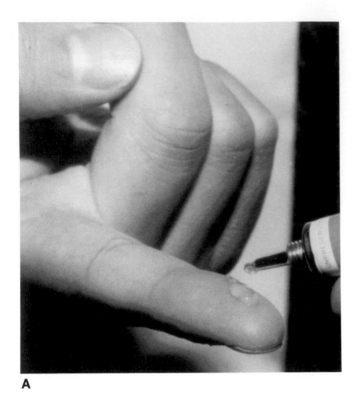

A

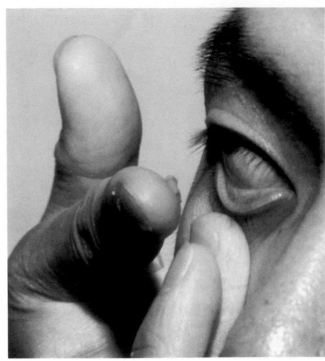

B

Figure 14–1. A. One method for patients to instill ointment into their eyes is by first placing it onto the fingertip. **B.** The ointment is then placed from the fingertip directly into the inferior cul-de-sac.

effects when starting treatment by slowly building up to the full strength and dosage over a few weeks time. For example, miotic therapy is begun with the 1% concentration once a day for 3 days, then increased to twice a day for 3 days, three times a day for 3 days, and finally, four times per day. The IOP and side effects are evaluated at this time and the concentration may be increased to the 2% strength if further IOP reduction is required, provided the side effects are tolerable. During this build-up phase, the IOP may not be properly controlled throughout the day and cannot be used for patients with markedly elevated IOP or advanced glaucoma. The advantage of a slow pilocarpine build-up is improved long-term patient compliance.

Whites with mild glaucoma may be adequately controlled with pilocarpine 1% whereas many blacks require at least the 2% strength for proper control. If greater IOP reduction is needed, the medication is increased to a 4% strength. Compliance tends to be worse for pilocarpine than any other topical glaucoma medication because of the increased dosage schedule and frequent reports of ocular side effects.

Carbachol solution is available in 0.75, 1.50, 2.25, and 3.0% concentrations. The most common concentration prescribed is 3% administered three times a day. Carbachol 3% is a close equivalent to pilocarpine 4% and used when pilocarpine 4% is not effective or tolerated. Carbachol penetrates the cornea poorly such that the IOP can be higher on carbachol 3% than pilocarpine 4%.

Anticholinesterases

The anticholinesterase agents are especially strong miotics because the endogenous acetylcholine action is enhanced by inhibiting cholinesterase enzymes. Because of their severe side effects, these agents are held in reserve for those patients not responding to the direct acting cholinergic agents and showing progression of the glaucoma while on all other glaucoma medications. Candidates for the use of anticholinesterases include pseudophakic/aphakic patients and poorly controlled postsurgical patients.

Echothiophate (Phospholine Iodide) 0.125% administered twice a day is the most commonly used agent. Concentrations of 0.03, 0.06, and 0.25% are less commonly used. Anticholinesterase solutions cannot be used with dipivifrin (Propine) because dipivifrin requires esterase to convert it to epinephrine.

Ocular side effects of echothiophate include miosis, anterior subcapsular cataracts, miotic pupillary cysts, irritation, conjunctival injection, lacrimation, and retinal detachment.[29] Systemic side effects deserve particular attention. Repeated administration can cause depressed serum and erythrocyte cholinesterase levels resulting in urinary incontinence, diarrhea, perfuse sweating, muscle weakness, rhinorrhea, abdominal cramps, apnea, and bradycardia.[29] Individuals receiving anticholinesterase who are exposed to carbamate or organophosphate-based pesticides or insecticides should be warned of the additive effects from absorption of the insecticides via the respiratory tract or skin.[30] The most serious of possible drug interactions with echothiophate involves succinylcholine, a muscle relaxant given before or during general anesthesia. It is vital that physicians attending to patient on echothiophate be aware of its use prior to scheduling the patient for a surgical procedure to avoid the risk of prolonged respiratory paralysis.[30,31]

Other anticholinesterase agents available but rarely used for glaucoma treatment include *demecarium bromide* (Humorsol) in 0.125% solution and *isoflurophate* (Floropryl) in 0.025% ointment.

Adrenergic Agonists
The topical adrenergic agonists used for glaucoma treatment include epinephrine and dipivalyl epinephrine (Propine).

Epinephrine is one of the oldest IOP-reducing agents available. Although the mechanism of action is obscure, it is believed alpha and beta receptor stimulation promotes increased outflow facility.[32] Epinephrine is available in three solution forms: epinephrine borate (0.5, 1.0, and 2.0%), epinephrine hydrochloride (0.25, 0.5, 1.0, and 2.0%), and epinephrine bitartrate (1.0 and 2.0%). The most common forms are 1% borate and 2% hydrochloride, both used twice a day. The bitartrate forms contain approximately one half the concentration as that labeled on the bottle. Epinephrine bitartrate is rarely used except in

eyedrops formulated in combination with pilocarpine 1, 2, 3, 4, and 6% solutions.

Ocular side effects that limit epinephrine's long-term use include hyperemia, allergic follicular conjunctivitis, tearing, adrenochrome deposits, and, in aphakia or pseudophakia, cystoid macular edema.[33,34] Discoloration of soft contact lenses has also been observed.[35] Because of its potential mydriatic effect, epinephrine should be avoided in individuals with narrow angles. Systemic side effects include hypertension, arrhythmia, tachycardia, headache, and browache.[36] Caution should be used in patients with arteriosclerosis, cardiovascular disease, hyperthyroidism, and concomitant use of tricyclic antidepressants.[36]

Dipivalyl epinephrine, or dipivefrin (Propine), a prodrug, is an alternative form of epinephrine. It comes in a 0.1% solution that is instilled twice per day. Dipivefrin (Propine) penetrates the cornea extremely well, being converted to epinephrine after entering the eye. Dipivefrin has become the adrenergic medication of choice because the increased corneal penetration allows a smaller concentration to be used, which in turn reduces the systemic side effects while providing similar IOP reduction. Dipivefrin also provides an alternative for the patient demonstrating an allergic response or side effects to epinephrine. Dipivefrin and epinephrine are not as potent as beta blockers or miotics in reducing IOP but do improve in their efficacy over the first months of treatment.

Carbonic Anhydrase Inhibitors
The final class of pharmaceutical agents used for the treatment of primary open-angle glaucoma are the carbonic anhydrase inhibitors (CAI). At present, these agents are available for oral use only, and are the most potent of the ocular hypotensive drugs. Inhibition of carbonic anhydrase results in decreased aqueous humor production. Generally, CAI are added after maximal topical medical therapy has failed to reduce the IOP to a desired level. The most commonly used agents are acetazolamide (Diamox) and methazolamide (Neptazane). The frequent reporting of systemic side effects often limit their long-term use. These side effects, which are in part related to the concentration used, include paresthesias, anorexia, weight loss, diarrhea, nausea and vomiting, fatigue, loss of libido, bone marrow toxicity, malaise, and metallic taste.[37] Easy bruisability or bleeding

gums may be signs of a developing anemia. Allergy to sulfa drugs contraindicates their use. Acetazolamide can also cause an increased propensity for kidney stone formation. A rare blood dyscrasia, aplastic anemia, has been reported secondary to CAI use.[38] This idiosyncratic reaction may occur after only one dose, though usually seen during the first 2 to 3 months of use. This condition is fatal 50% of the time even with treatment. A routine complete blood count (CBC) may allow earlier diagnosis but would not affect the final outcome and is not ordinarily recommended. A CBC may be warranted before treatment in certain elderly patients with the appearance of or past history of anemia. This anemia should be treated and corrected before initiation of CAI.

Methazolamide (Neptazane) is the CAI of choice due to its reduced frequency for kidney stone formation. Methazolamide is available in 25- and 50-mg tablets. The initial therapy usually begins with a 25-mg tablet twice a day. The dosage regimen is increased by 25-mg steps until satisfactory control of IOP is achieved, up to a maximum dose of 50 mg three times a day. At lower body weights, increasing methazolamide from 100 mg per day to 150 mg per day may not have a clinically significant IOP-lowering effect.

Acetazolamide (Diamox) tablets are held in reserve if the maximum dosage of methazolamide is not sufficient to reduce the IOP to the desired level or if the patient cannot tolerate methazolamide. Acetazolamide is available in 250-mg tablets and in 500-mg time-release capsules (Diamox Sequels). The dosage may be increased up to 250 mg four times a day by tablet form or 500 mg twice a day in capsule form. A reduced dosage is often useful, allowing it to be tailored for each patient. Reducing dosage levels may diminish unwanted side effects while still maintaining proper IOP control. The medication may also be given at specific times of the day to flatten a daily spike in IOP. Mild gastrointestinal upset secondary to the medication may be alleviated by taking the tablets or capsules with meals or using a sodium bicarbonate tablet.[37]

WHEN TO BEGIN TREATMENT

Review of Diagnostic Findings

The clinical evaluation of the glaucoma suspect lies in assessing four areas: IOP, optic nerve and nerve fiber layer, visual field, and anterior chamber angle. Other diagnostic tests may be useful as indicated (*see* Chapter 6).

Open-angle glaucoma usually presents either with elevated IOP higher in one eye, possibly preceding optic nerve and visual field damage or with IOP in the "normal range" with optic nerve cupping. The IOP, while easily measured, is evaluated with caution. Intraocular pressure is viewed as a risk factor for the development of open-angle glaucoma and not the parameter used to define the condition. The higher the IOP, the greater the chance for developing open-angle glaucoma, but individuals may develop POAG with IOP measurements in the so-called "normal" range.

Optic nerve and nerve fiber layer evaluation are crucial to the diagnosis of open-angle glaucoma. A dilated, binocular stereoscopic examination of the optic nerve and surrounding tissue is necessary to detecting subtle changes in the nerve appearance that may occur before visual field loss. By using a 60 D, 78 D, 90 D fundus lens, Hruby, or Goldman fundus contact lens, a detailed examination is possible. Serial stereo color photography permits the comparison of the optic nerve color, depth, size of the optic cup and rim tissue integrity from one examination to the next. The optic nerve appearance is most useful in the diagnosis of open-angle glaucoma with automated visual fields emphasized in following up for progression.

Nerve fiber layer evaluations performed with red-free photography may demonstrate defects that can precede optic nerve changes and corresponding visual field loss. In general, the appearance of asymmetrical optic nerve damage with elevated IOP and full visual fields is diagnostic of open-angle glaucoma. The problem in relying on optic nerve evaluation alone for the diagnosis of glaucoma is in differentiating the large physiological cup from glaucomatous cupping. One guide is physiological cupping tends to be symmetrical, accompanied by full visual fields and healthy neuroretinal rim tissue.

The visual field establishes the level of visual function of the patient. The more sensitive the visual field examination, the more readily visual field defects can be detected resulting in earlier diagnosis and treatment. Automated perimetry permits convenient static threshold testing capable of detecting early visual field changes indicative of glaucoma.

Still, perimetry by any present method has its limitations in the diagnosis of glaucoma. The optic nerve and nerve fiber layer are affected by elevated IOP early in glaucoma, usually, but not always, before visual field changes are evident. A great many nerve fibers must be damaged before visual field changes can be demonstrated, even by the most sensitive methods. Because visual field changes often occur after significant damage to the optic nerve, they are not always required to establish a diagnosis of glaucoma and, when seen, document that damage to the nerve has escalated to a moderate level.

Anterior chamber angle evaluation using the goniolens is necessary to differentiate POAG from secondary open-angle and chronic angle closure glaucoma. Gonioscopy must be performed on all narrow and open-angle glaucoma suspects to understand the type of glaucoma being dealt with since the treatment regimen may vary depending on the form present.

Other diagnostic tests and procedures to aid in the diagnosis include color vision, contrast sensitivity, visually evoked potentials, and fluorescein angiography of the optic nerve. For a more detailed discussion of evaluation, refer to Chapter 11.

Unreliable Diagnostic Evaluation

Occasionally, a complete diagnostic evaluation may not be accomplished because of circumstances beyond the patient's or clinician's control. Examples include poor visual field results due to patients with limited ability to execute the test procedure or the noncommunicating (aphasic) patient. Media opacities, such as corneal leukomas, dense cataracts and vitreous hemorrhage, may cause visual field defects "masking" glaucomatous visual field loss and in addition make visualization of the optic nerve difficult. Also, panretinal photocoagulation creates tiny burns in the retina producing visual field defects. When these defects are located in the arcuate bundle area, visual field defects similar to glaucoma may be seen. Central nervous system or optic nerve disorders, such as cerebrovascular accidents, optic nerve drusen, or retrobulbar optic neuritis, may also mimic glaucomatous visual field loss. Difficulty in the assessment of the optic nerve or visual fields may make the decision to treat difficult. The decision may then depend more on IOP, family history, medical history, other risk factors, and past examination findings.

Review of Risk Factors

The risk factors for glaucoma play a critical role in the decision of when to initiate treatment.[39-42] These risk factors include age, race, family history, medical history (diabetes mellitus, untreated or poorly controlled high blood pressure), refractive error, and secondary glaucoma findings.[43-48] For a more detailed discussion of risk factors, see Chapter 2.

Treatment Guidelines

The goal of treatment in open-angle glaucoma is to reduce the IOP to a level below which optic nerve and visual field damage will not occur or, progression of existing damage is prevented. This level of IOP (target IOP) is different for each individual. The objective is to lower the IOP to that level using the least expensive, most benign method, allowing the patient maximum visual function for the remainder of his or her life.

There are general guidelines to follow when initiating treatment. Based on the diagnostic evaluation, weighing the relative risk factors and considering the risk-to-benefit ratio of treatment, the decision to initiate medical therapy is made. Since open-angle glaucoma is often a bilateral asymmetrical condition, unless an etiology is determined that would support glaucoma in one eye (i.e., angle recession) or the pressure elevation is strikingly asymmetrical, both eyes are treated, with the more involved eye possibly requiring additional therapy.

The glaucoma suspect/OHTN patient whose discs and visual fields are normal and have no associated risk factors should be followed. Patients with IOPs between 21 and 29 mm Hg should be examined, at the very least, every 4 months. The higher the IOP, the greater the chance for developing glaucoma but some individuals may develop glaucoma with IOP in the teens. Optic nerve evaluation, including a dilated fundus evaluation, and automated perimetry should be performed yearly to ensure that findings remain stable.

Treatment becomes optional in cases of OHTN/ glaucoma suspects where the risk for developing glaucoma is increased. This includes patients with suspicious optic nerve findings; suspicious, questionable, or unreliable visual fields; and/or several positive risk factors. Each patient has the right to choose to either accept or refuse treatment after being informed about the examination results, the disease, the relative risk, its treatment, and the long-term implications of therapy. It is in this optional category that more and more individuals are being treated at an earlier stage. As seen in studies by Kass and Epstein,[4,5] without treatment a greater number of cases of OHTN will go on to develop glaucoma than previously thought. Early aggressive treatment will often arrest the condition at an earlier and more manageable stage. For these cases, diagnosis is made on the appearance of the optic nerve, nerve fiber evaluation, and other diagnostic tests along with associated risk factors. Visual fields may be full or only mildly affected at this point in time and provide little diagnostic information.

Treatment becomes mandatory when visual field and/or optic nerve head changes are consistent with glaucoma independent of the IOP. If the pressure is always low (below 17 mm Hg) even with diurnal testing, a normotensive glaucoma evaluation is indicated. Also, because of the increased risk of developing glaucoma with increased IOP, treatment is recommended for patients whose IOP is greater than 30 mm Hg. If the IOP measurements are greater than 21 mm Hg with a previous retinal occlusive vascular disorder, treatment is indicated in both eyes, even if optic nerve and visual fields appear healthy, to reduce the IOP and prevent a branch or central retinal vein occlusion from occurring in the contralateral eye.

The monocular ocular hypertensive individual warrants consideration for early aggressive IOP reduction to enhance all possibilities of preserving maximum visual function. The exception to this may be the patient who refuses treatment because of apprehension, especially if the other eye was damaged due to complications and/or failure with previous therapy. In this situation, patient education is crucial for proper care. All findings and patient wishes should be carefully documented in the chart. The patient diagnosed before the age of 40 also needs to be more aggressively managed and closely followed considering they will have the disease for many years.

INITIATING THERAPY

The objective for instituting therapy is to control the glaucomatous disease process and prevent further damage. Associated with any treatment regimen is an inherent risk of complications and undesired side effects due to the medications. Assessing the relative likelihood of achieving the desired benefits in the face of the possible risk of complications is known as "risk-to-benefit ratio." Glaucoma is not exempt from this association. As is evident from the previous chapter on therapeutic pharmacology, the topical and oral antiglaucoma agents all have the potential for ocular and systemic side effects. The risk-to-benefit ratio must be considered for each individual before treatment is begun.

Uniocular Trials

Once the decision to treat is made, all topical medications are begun in one eye only (uniocular trial) for a short period of time. If the IOP is markedly elevated in both eyes and it is determined treatment must be urgently instituted bilaterally, one approach may be to temporarily use a CAI while a uniocular trial is begun. If the trial is positive, the topical medication is used in both eyes and the CAI withdrawn. The uniocular therapeutic trial is a useful tool in the determination of when to treat the glaucoma suspect and

how each individual will react to a given medication. It is designed to determine both the effectiveness of a medication in decreasing IOP and its side effects, and should be considered whenever a medication is added or changed. Uniocular trials are required because not all glaucoma medications are effective in every individual. The trial is performed by instilling medication in one eye only, preferably the eye with higher IOP, and using the fellow eye as an untreated control. Pilocarpine 1% four times a day or a beta blocker every 12 hours may be used. Intraocular pressure is evaluated at 2 to 7 days after instituting treatment with pilocarpine or 14 days after starting a beta blocker, preferably done at the same time of day as the pretrial checks. Assuming diurnal variation is equal in both eyes, the IOP reduction and difference between the two eyes is evaluated. When using topical beta blockers, the contralateral eye's IOP may be lowered with unilateral installation.[49,50] If a 10% decrease in IOP is noted in the treated eye as compared to the untreated eye, the trial is *positive* and the patient should then use the medication in both eyes. In addition, the side effects, both ocular and systemic, are evaluated to determine if they can be safely tolerated by the patient.

Choosing a Medication

Ocular Considerations. Certain ocular conditions may co-exist with glaucoma prohibiting the use of specific antiglaucoma medications. As more research is performed on new IOP-reducing agents, greater flexibility will be afforded the clinician to institute alternative selections for the initial drug of choice.

Uveal. A history of or an active inflammatory process of the uvea, particularly an anterior uveitis, precludes the use of topical cholinergic agonists. Miotics may enhance the formation of posterior synechia, increase ciliary spasm, and exacerbate a quiescent inflammation. Care must be used to confirm open anterior chamber angles so that pupillary block glaucoma does not occur if pilocarpine treatment is instituted.

Lenticular. Patients under 40 years of age with active accommodation will not tolerate the severe accommodative spasm induced by the cholinergic stimulation of the ciliary muscle. If a miotic is the only medication of choice for a young individual, then the pilocarpine Ocusert should be considered. Miotics should also be avoided in patients with cataracts located centrally along the visual axis to prevent decreased visual acuity. Use of adrenergic agonists should be avoided in aphakic and pseudophakic patients due to the increased risk of cystoid macular edema. Phospholine iodide is not used in phakic patients because of the risk for developing cataracts.

Retinal. Miotics should be used with caution on patients with a history of peripheral retinal holes or tears because of the risk of retinal detachment. A retinal detachment may be pharmacologically induced by the strong contraction of the ciliary body on the peripheral retina. This is a special consideration in highly myopic patients who are more likely to have peripheral retinal changes.

Systemic Considerations

Although glaucoma is a disease confined to the eye, its treatment, especially with topical beta blockers, warrants systemic health considerations. Patients must be educated about the potential systemic side effects secondary to topical medications. Most individuals will recognize a side effect due to a tablet taken orally but do not realize similar side effects may be due to eyedrops. It is important to review an individual's medical history, both past and present, and, when necessary, consult with the patient's primary care physician regarding the use of topical medications. Also, teach all patients to either occlude their punctum or close their eyes for 3 minutes after eyedrop instillation. This will minimize the medication getting into the systemic circulation.

Pulmonary. Topical beta blockers may have specific effects on the pulmonary system. The beta 2 receptors found in the pulmonary smooth muscle if blocked by a beta 2 antagonist cause bronchoconstriction. This can be detrimental if a patient suffers from COPD, asthma, or emphysema. Timolol, a nonselective beta blocker, has been shown to decrease forced expiratory volume in 1 minute in patients with documented asthma or COPD.[17,51] Little published data are available for the other nonselective beta blockers. The cardioselectivity of betaxolol does not completely exclude it from pulmonary side effects. Pilocarpine or dipivefrin is recommended as the first drug for these patients. Betaxolol is used with extreme caution if these medications are not tolerated or are not effective. In addition, instruct patients on punctal occlusion, and obtain base-line pulmonary function tests just prior to and after initiating betaxolol therapy.

Cardiovascular. Systemic beta blockers have been used for many years in the treatment of cardiovascular disease so it stands to reason that systemic absorption of the topical beta blockers may have a secondary effect on the cardiovascular system. Also, the eye can absorb a systemic dosage. One reason that a topical beta blocker may not be effective is because a person is taking an oral beta blocker and their IOP is maximally reduced from beta blockers.

Beta blockers have been reported to cause heart block in susceptible individuals, bradycardia, arrhythmia, hypotension, and exacerbation of congestive heart failure.[51] Although resting pulse rate may not be affected, reduction of exercise-induced tachycardia has been shown with timolol and levobunolol.[52–54] Because of its reduced affinity for beta 1 receptor binding compared to timolol, betaxolol has demonstrated less cardiac blockade than timolol.[55,56] If a patient on a topical beta blocker is to be discontinued after using the medication for a period of time, tapered withdrawal is recommended since one report has documented reflex tachycardia after abrupt withdrawal of timolol.[57]

The adrenergic agonists also warrant consideration with regard to cardiovascular response.[36] Patients with coronary insufficiency and increased arterial blood pressure as well as those on myocardial sensitizing drugs should avoid the use of epinephrine or other adrenergic agonists. Any patient with significant cardiovascular disease or increased propensity for arrhythmia should avoid the use of adrenergic agonists and antagonists. If any of these medications is to be used, the patient should be followed under close supervision of an internist or cardiologist. Also, medications used for the treatment of hypertension or cardiac disease may interact with ocular medications. Carbonic anhydrase inhibitors and other diuretics may upset the potassium balance, affect the required digitalis dosage, or induce cardiac arrhythmia.

Renal. Carbonic anhydrase inhibitors can have significant effects on electrolyte balance and kidney function. Metabolic acidosis, potassium depletion (hypokalemia), and increased propensity for kidney stone formation are side effects that can be significant, especially in the individual with a history of renal disease.[37] Carbonic anhydrase inhibitors should be avoided in these individuals.

Endocrine. At high dosages, CAI may induce a metabolic acidosis that may exaggerate hypokalemia in patients using long-term corticosteroids.[59] In addition, diabetics undergoing an acute angle closure glaucoma attack should avoid all oral hyperosmotic agents if possible.[58] Oral hyperosmotic agents, except isosorbide (Ismotic), require metabolism by the liver. Isosorbide is non-metabolized and if required, may be used with caution in the diabetic patient.[60]

Document baseline exam
Establish diagnosis
Rule out secondary forms
Start with lowest dosage and strength
Uniocular trial
Counsel patient on potential side effects
Teach instillation technique of drops/ointment
Eyelid closure/punctal occlusion for 3 minutes
Always inquire about compliance at each examination

Figure 14–2. Steps in the initiation of therapy in open-angle glaucoma.

The First Drug

Before starting therapy, make sure all findings are carefully documented in detail, establishing a baseline diagnostic record and ruling out secondary forms of glaucoma (Fig. 14–2). Start with the lowest dosage and strength of a medication, doing so with a uniocular trial. A nonselective beta blocker, used twice daily, is generally the drug of first choice in patients without contraindications to their use. The 0.25 or 0.3% strength is used initially and is often effective in whites with a mild form of glaucoma; the 0.5% strength is usually required in blacks. If compliance is a factor, levobunolol 0.25 or 0.5% once a day in the morning may be used.[63,64]

For patients in which beta blockers are contraindicated, pilocarpine or dipivefrin may be the initial drug. Generally, pilocarpine is reserved for older patients and dipivefrin used with younger individuals to avoid accommodative spasm. The pilocarpine Ocusert may be an alternative for the young individual requiring a miotic who has few alternatives. Visual fields should be repeated before miotic therapy is started to eliminate the confusion in interpreting visual field depression secondary to the induced small pupil. Rarely is a CAI the first drug chosen in treating open-angle glaucoma.

OPEN-ANGLE GLAUCOMA MEDICAL MANAGEMENT STARTING THERAPY

Patient Education

Patient education plays an integral role in the management of the glaucomatous individual. The patient must be fully aware that open-angle glaucoma is an asymptomatic, chronic, and progressive disease that is controlled by a lifelong medication and/or surgical

regimen. Up to the time of diagnosis, the patient usually has not experienced any symptoms. This will change since most medications cause some problem that will test the patient's resolve and make him or her question why he or she should continue with therapy. The patient must understand that failure to adhere to the treatment regimen can result in loss of vision. In addition, the use of the medications bears a certain financial cost to the patient, both from medications and the cost of the frequent follow-up examinations.[65] These financial constraints may impact on medication and appointment compliance.

Compliance is a factor that affects many glaucomatous individuals adversely. One measure to improve compliance is in patient education. Reassure the patients that they will not have to change or restrict their lifestyle. Calm their fears and let them know they can use their eyes, read all they want, exercise as before, and continue to drink in moderation. Few systemic medications are a cause for concern in open-angle glaucoma though some may need to be modified in narrow-angle varieties. Communicate with the patient's general physician. Let him or her know what medications are being used and that any change in the treatment regimen will be relayed to him or her. Also, ask for the patient to contact you if there is a change in the patient's health status or medication profile.

The medications' side effects should be discussed with the patient prior to their use with verbal and written dosage schedules provided (Fig. 14–3). Explain to the patient that any systemic side effect may be due to the eyedrops. Have the patient keep a log when side effects occur and to contact you as soon as they happen. In-office education and training on proper eyedrop instillation will aid most individuals. Many elderly have problems putting drops into their eyes and training will be necessary (Fig. 14–4). Teach the patient to squeeze the bottle from the bottom, not the side of the container. Document all forms of patient education in the chart (Fig. 14–5). Remind them to occlude the punctum with a finger or close their eyelids for 3 minutes after eyedrop instillation to reduce systemic absorption and increase the therapeutic index (Fig. 14–6).[66] Try to incorporate the dosage schedule into the patient's daily routine. If possible, patients should refrigerate all medications and feel for the cold sting when a drop hits the eye. Timoptic, with its cost-effective Ocumeter bottle, controls the output of a drop from the container better than other bottles. Individuals with diminished control may still be able to squeeze the Ocumeter bottle at the bottom and instill only one drop at a time into the eye. If multiple medications are used, a separation of 3 to 5

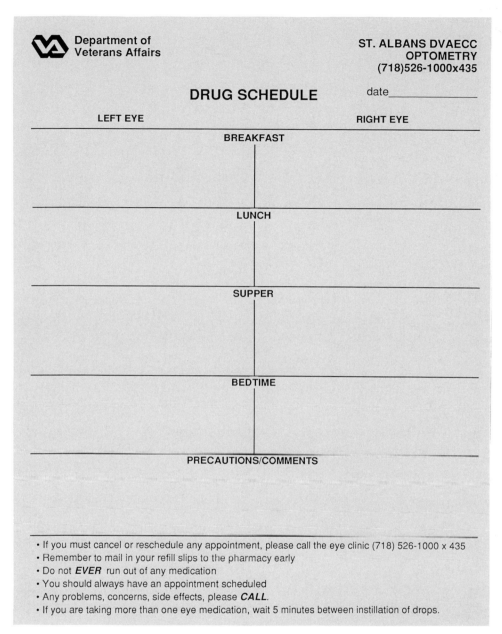

Figure 14–3. Patient information dosage schedule.

minutes between drops increases the therapeutic index by preventing dilution of the first eyedrop. A record is kept when prescriptions are written, the number of refills, and size of the bottle. Patients requiring too frequent refills may be improperly instilling the medications. Patients rarely requiring refills may indicate poor compliance. Be careful with the number of refills and bottle size given to patients of questionable compliance who may not return for their examinations. Compliant patients are given multiple prescriptions for each medication so a separate bottle may be left in the office, at home, or wherever it will be accessible when the time for drop installation occurs. Larger size bottles (10 or 15 mL) are more cost effective than the 5-mL size, so for compliant individuals, prescribe the larger bottle whenever available.

Frequently, patients have difficulty in pronunciation of the names of the medication. Also, several of them sound the same so when medical regimens are reviewed during follow-up visits, some confusion occurs. To avoid confusion for both the patient and clinician, the topical medications may also be identified by the bottle color or bottle cap color (Fig. 14–7). For instance, timolol (Timoptic) 0.5% may be identified as ''the yellow bottle'' or pilocarpine as ''the

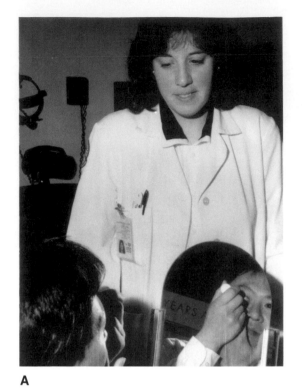

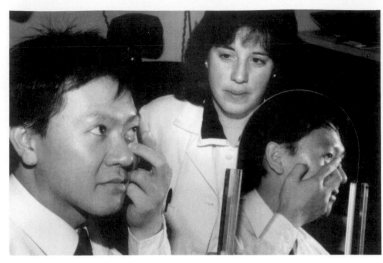

B

A

Figure 14–4. On initiating therapy, instruction is required in the proper technique for eyedrop **(A.)** and ointment installation **(B.).**

Figure 14–5. A stamp placed on the patient's record documents that patient education has been performed.

PROCEDURE FOR PROPER EYE DROP ADMINISTRATION
1) BASIC INSTRUCTIONS FOR EYE DROP INSTILLATION GIVEN
2) ADVISED PT TO:
   1. EYELID CLOSURE FOR 3 MINUTES
   2. WAIT 5 MINUTES BETWEEN DIFFERENT DROPS
3) REVIEWED TIME SCHEDULE OF MEDICATIONS/GIVEN DOSAGE SCHEDULE
4) RETURN DEMONSTRATION DONE:
   GOOD UNDERSTANDING OF TECHNIQUE
   NEEDS REINFORCEMENT
5) STRESSED NECESSITY:
   1. TO KEEP APPOINTMENTS
   2. DO NOT RUN OUT OF MEDICATIONS
   3. TO TAKE DROPS AS ORDERED

SIGN: _____

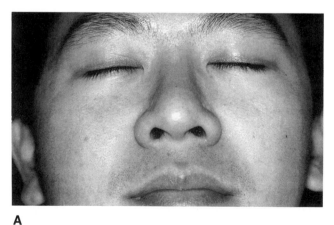

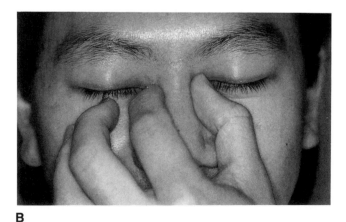

A

B

Figure 14–6. On installation of topical medications, eyelid closure **(A.)** or punctal occlusion **(B.)** will reduce systemic absorption of the medication.

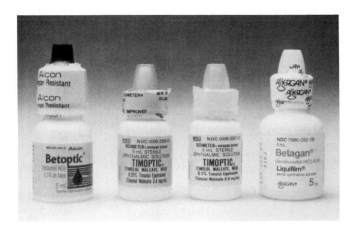

Figure 14–7. Ophthalmic medications may be identified by the color of the bottle or bottle cap.

green-capped drop." A summary of the most common bottle and cap colors is found in Table 14–1. Pilopine Gel may simply be identified as "the gel" and the CAI as "the pill" or "capsule." Still, all patients should have a list of their medications that they carry with them.

Treatment Schemes

Goals for Therapy. The more advanced the glaucoma, the lower the IOP must be maintained in order to stabilize the optic nerve and visual field. The goal is to provide an IOP low enough throughout the day so that optic nerve damage and visual field loss is arrested, using the least expensive, safest drug possible. With this in mind, an individualized therapeutic plan is designed taking into account the patient's medical history, prior damage to the optic nerve and visual field, IOP level, and ocular history along with other factors. The visual field and to a lesser extent the optic nerve are parameters evaluated over time to determine if the glaucoma is controlled.

TABLE 14–1. COMMON BOTTLE AND CAP COLORS OF GLAUCOMA MEDICATIONS

Timoptic, Betagan, Betoptic 0.25%	Light blue cap
Timoptic or Betagan 0.50%	Yellow cap
Betoptic 0.5%	Dark blue cap
Optipranolol 0.3%	White cap
Pilocarpine (all concentrations)	Green cap
Carbachol (all concentrations)	Green cap
Phospholine Iodide (all concentrations)	Clear glass bottle
Propine	Purple cap
Epinephrine (all concentrations)	Brown bottle or white cap/red label

Functional Groups/Target IOP. A functional group scheme, proposed by Richardson,[67] provides general guidelines toward establishing a target IOP. The target or goal IOP is the intended initial level of IOP when treatment is initiated. In theory, when the IOP is consistently at the target level, further damage should be prevented. By using the initial range of IOP measurements, optic nerve, and visual field results along with the risk factors, functional groups are created that depend on the severity of findings. The IOP in the lesser involved eye is another parameter useful in determining the target IOP. Functional groups paint a simplistic picture of the case that is useful in initiating treatment and establishing a target IOP.

For example, an individual with pretreatment IOPs in the mid-20s, a small cup-disc ratio and mild visual field loss may be initially started with medication trying to obtain a target pressure around 18 mm Hg. Another individual with the same IOP level in the mid-20s, mild field loss but a larger cup-disc ratio may need a lower initial target IOP, probably around 16 mm Hg. Pretreatment IOP levels in the low 30s with early disc and field loss may have an initial target pressure in the high teens or low 20s but if pretreatment IOP measurements were never measured higher than the low 20s, with similar early disc and field damage, a more aggressive approach may be required to prevent further deterioration. The initial target IOP is an arbitrary level based on experience and examination findings. Only careful management over time will tell if the target IOP is appropriate for that individual.

At the follow-up visit, the side effects and proximity of the IOP to the target IOP goal is assessed. Compare the pretreatment level of IOP to the present level of IOP after treatment. Is the IOP low enough? If the difference between the post-treatment and target IOP is small, increasing the concentration or dosage (if available) or the addition of dipivefrin to a beta blocker may be appropriate while a large difference may require a change in the beta blocker (if a cardioselective agent is being used), increase in concentration or the addition of a miotic. A miotic along with a beta blocker is the most powerful combination of topical medications.

The tendency is to add medications until the IOP is as low as possible. This approach is not advisable because it may unnecessarily increase patient morbidity and expense. Rather, establish a target IOP level and modify the therapeutic regimen as needed to meet this goal. The target IOP may not be obtainable because of excessive side effects or poor patient response. A decision is made regarding how aggressive therapy must be to meet the target IOP. Care must be taken not to overtreat but, at the same time, if signs of progression occur, consider increasing the strength of the medications, the addition of medication(s), or a surgical evaluation and reset the target IOP to a lower level. A functional grouping only gives an initial target IOP. The ultimate IOP is the one needed to stabilize the optic nerve and visual field over time.

Dosage and Follow-Up Schedule. The first follow-up visit after initiation of treatment is scheduled in 1 to 2 weeks. The return examination should include history (time of last medication instillation, symptoms, side effects, or changes in systemic health), visual acuity, pulse (if on beta blocker), slit-lamp evaluation, IOP measurement, and an abbreviated optic nerve assessment. Most important is the assessment of the patient's acceptance of the treatment regimen and reinforcement of education about the chronic condition.

Reports of side effects must be evaluated. Must the medication be eliminated or is there concomitant management for these side effects? For example, the sting of an eyedrop can be better tolerated if the medication is placed in the refrigerator. Also, miotic side effects may diminish after the adaptation period.

Decreased visual acuity, confirmed with a pinhole, necessitates visual field and dilated fundus examination to rule out new pathology. A dilated fundus exam is also indicated at least yearly in all glaucomatous individuals and in patients with new complaints of photopsia after miotic therapy has been initiated to rule out an acute retinal tear or detachment.

Evaluate the IOP relative to the pretreatment level and desired treatment levels (target IOP). Alterations in the medication regimen are made if the target IOP is not met (Fig. 14–8).

Early in the course of therapy, repeat visits with frequent modifications in the treatment regimen may

be required until the target IOP goal is met. Evaluating the IOP at the end of the dosage schedule is a better indicator of control than an IOP measurement taken just after instillation of the medication. Whenever a medication is added, deleted, or changed, a new dosage schedule is given to the patient and a follow-up examination is scheduled in approximately 2 weeks. Occasionally, a new medication does little to lower IOP. This is usually obvious when the medication is added as part of a uniocular trial. Discontinue the new medication if compliance is not the problem and try a stronger dosage if available, switch to another in its class if available, or a medication from another class. Because medications are not always effective, rarely are two medications started at the same time.

Biomicroscopy should be performed every visit to check for allergic reactions, toxicity, verification of compliance with miotics (small fixed pupil), and subtle ocular side effects such as palpebral conjunctival adrenochrome deposits.

Visual fields may be done with a dilated pupil at the same time as the yearly dilated fundus examination. Dilation will reduce the peripheral field constriction due to a small pupil. It is not imperative that all pupils be dilated before doing visual fields but it is important that the pupil size be consistent from field to field. Dilation is not required if the lens is clear or the pupil size in a dark room is 4 mm or larger. When on a miotic, patients should discontinue them 2 days prior to their visit if dilation is planned. Dilation with a mydriatic and cycloplegic solution is then necessary, especially with darkly pigmented eyes, to provide maximum mydriasis and to prevent posterior synechiae formation. After examination, the patient is instructed to resume miotic therapy and may need to return shortly for additional IOP assessment if the IOP is especially elevated.

Continual evaluation the IOP, disc, and visual fields is required since all can change with time. Patients should be re-examined at 2 weeks, 6 weeks, and 3 months after treatment is initiated. Poorly controlled individuals may need to be seen more often to get the condition under control. Once the IOP and condition are stable, a visit every 3 months is appropriate. The time of each visit is recorded with an attempt made to vary the times of the examination so the IOP is measured at different times of the day. The use of a flowsheet, in addition to the patient record, allows the recording of all findings related to the glaucoma examination (Figs. 14–9 and 14–10). It simplifies follow-up, provides maximum management efficiency, and allows one to see trends in the IOP, optic nerve, or visual field.[68]

Select target pressure based on prior damage, IOP level, history
Maintain IOP below that level with intervention as needed
Monitor visual fields, optic nerve for progression
Reset target pressure (lower) with increasing damage
Minimize side effects of medications
Recognize failure on medications early
Move to advanced therapy as needed (laser, surgery)

Figure 14–8. Open-angle glaucoma management.

Name										

Glaucoma Flowsheet

V

When? Where? What?

Name_____

Address_____

SS#_____

DOB_____

TEL #_____

Type_____

C/D   R
        L

Previous DX_____

Previous TX_____

MH_____

Date	IOP	VF	DFE	GON	PIX	Comments/Exam Results	Meds/Start/Δ	Referral

Figure 14–9. Example of flowsheet open-angle glaucoma.

Modifying the Therapeutic Regimen

Once a drug is started, its effect must be evaluated. If the medication is effective but the IOP is still higher than desired, the medication must either be increased in strength or dosage if possible or a second medication added. This is the "step-method" of management (Fig. 14–11). A medication is modified or another class of medication added (step), always done by a uniocular trial. Each time the IOP is too high (above the target IOP) or progression is seen, another "step" is taken until all medical alternatives are used. The patient is now on maximum tolerated medical therapy. At that time, surgery becomes the next option (step). Side effects due to medications may be a reason to discontinue one medication (step) and go on to the next step.

When the original medication is a beta blocker, dipivyl epinephrine is generally the next drug added if the needed IOP reduction is small (few mm Hg drop required) and pilocarpine is added if the required IOP drop is large. Pilocarpine is increased up to the 4% concentration if further IOP reduction is required. A miotic is usually the last topical medication added prior to the use of adjunctive therapy, either CAI or laser surgery.

Argon laser trabeculoplasty (ALT) has become an effective alternative to oral CAI if maximal topical therapy is inadequate. By applying focal laser burns to the trabecular meshwork in open-angle glaucoma, ALT may lower IOP, though topical ocular hypotensive agents are usually necessary afterwards to maintain control. The use of ALT delays the time interval

Glaucoma Flowsheet

Name _Jack Straw_   s/p Cat. extraction ĉ FILTER OD 1984
Address _Wichita_
SS# _---_   Type _COAG_
DOB _2-22-20_   C/D   R .55/.60   L .5/.5
TEL # _---_

V $\overline{cc}$ 20/20⁻ / 20/20⁻

When? Where? What?
Previous DX _HIP. MANHATTAN VA_
Previous TX _T½ x 20D x 6yrs_
MH ⊕ HTN

Date	IOP	VF	DFE	GON	PIX	Comments/Exam Results	Meds/Start/Δ	Referral
1-11-90	13/23 11³⁰ AM							
1-30-90	13/20 1⁵⁰ PM		✓		✓		START T½ x 2 OU	
2-22-90		✓				pt called to say VF done @ HIP – pt told to bring copy (DR. KRIM)		
2-14-90	12/14 8⁴⁵							
3-14-90	12/13 8³⁰ AM					– pt had D/C T½ for last 2 weeks		
3-19-90		✓	@ HIP - HUMPHREY			VF < sup arc / early sup arc		
4-16-90	10/14 12 NOON							
5-22-90	11/14 9³⁰					D/C T½ due to palpitations	START B½ x 2 OS only	

Figure 14–10. Example of a sample completed flowsheet.

before beginning oral CAI or filtering surgery becomes necessary. On some rare occasions, ALT may be the treatment of choice if poor compliance is likely to hinder adequate medical management.

If CAI are to be added to the topical medications, the patient must be educated on the proper dosage and frequency of administration. Starting with methazolamide (Neptazane) 25 mg two times a day, the dosage is increased in 25-mg steps should the IOP lowering effect not be adequate. The dosage should not exceed 50 mg three times a day. Occasionally, though not recommended, increasing methazolamide to a maximum dose of 100 mg three times a day may demonstrate increased ocular hypotensive effect. These patients must be monitored carefully for side effects. In sensitive individuals, acetazolamide (Diamox) 250-mg tablets may be substituted for methazolamide, starting at 125 mg (one-half tablet) four times a day and building to 250 mg four times a day as needed. If still unsuccessful, Diamox Sequels (500 mg) may lower IOP further. At this point, the patient is considered on "maximum medical therapy" and further IOP control requires referral to a glaucoma specialist for either an ALT, if not already performed, or surgical filtering procedure.

Maximum medical therapy is different for each individual depending on their medical history, ocular history, and response to medications. Maximum medical therapy does not always mean the individual is on every class of glaucoma medication. If some are contraindicated or ineffective, only one or two types of drugs may be usable. An example of this is the elderly gentleman with COPD, history of heart block, sensitivity to propine, and allergy to sulfa drugs. In

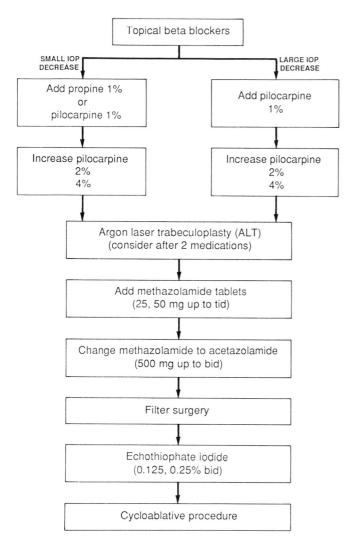

Figure 14–11. Flowchart in the management of open-angle glaucoma.

this case, miotics are the only available class of drugs that are not contraindicated, and therefore would represent maximal medical therapy.

LONG-TERM MANAGEMENT

Primary open-angle glaucoma requires monitoring and follow-up for the lifetime of the patient. Tolerance may develop to any medication over time leading to inadequate control and progression. When glaucoma appears stable, examinations are scheduled for every 3 months. The basic return visit should consist of a history, IOP evaluation, visual acuity, pulse (for beta blockers), slit-lamp examination, and undilated optic nerve examination. The history includes time of last medication, symptoms, any changes in health, and noted side effects. Always ask the patient

exactly how, what, and when the medications are taken, stressing the need for compliance. An extended visit is scheduled at least yearly for gonioscopy, a dilated fundus exam, photography, and visual field testing. The visual fields and optic nerve should be compared with previous slides and fields, looking for change. Depending on the stage of the disease, follow-up examinations may need to be scheduled more frequently than on a quarterly basis.

It may take several visits to determine if progression has occurred by observing changes in the diagnostic data. For example, automated visual field testing needs to be repeated to differentiate long-term fluctuation or ptosis-induced superior field depression from true glaucomatous visual field loss. Do not change the management regimen based on a solitary diagnostic finding. If progression of the visual fields or optic nerves is noted, the treatment regimen needs to be adjusted. Also, the fields or optic nerves may be stable but if the IOP rises to unacceptable levels (above the target IOP), the treatment regimen also needs to be modified. Once extensive damage has occurred to the optic nerve leaving it completely cupped with visual fields constricted to a few degrees, the central 10° field is used for followup. If central vision is lost, then IOP becomes the only parameter to monitor.

The ocular and systemic side effects of medications must be continually assessed. The history from a well-educated patient helps determine if problems are developing. Subtle side effects may occur that are not always appreciated by the patient. If side effects are a problem, can the medication(s) be reduced in any way or does it need to be discontinued (Table 14–2)?

FAILURE OF THERAPY

One of the most disconcerting aspects in the treatment of glaucoma is the failure of medications to adequately control the disease. Maintaining the IOP at a level to prevent optic nerve and visual field deterioration is a goal that is not always achieved with medications, either because of the progressive nature of the disease, its severity, poor response to medications, or noncompliance on the part of the patient.

If advancing visual field loss continues in the presence of an acceptable IOP and compliance is not a factor, progressive optic nerve damage may not be due to glaucoma. Optic nerve or other disorders that mimic glaucomatous field loss or cupping need to be ruled out. Differential diagnosis of optic nerve disease other than glaucoma includes optic nerve dru-

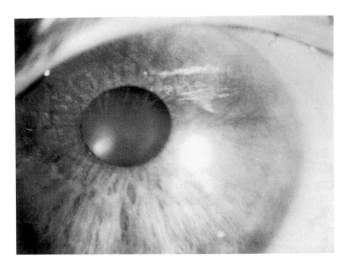

Figure 14–18. Rubeosis irides associated with diabetic retinopathy.

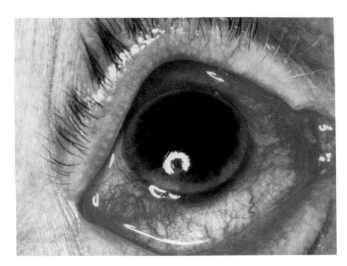

Figure 14–19. Angle closure glaucoma as seen with a red eye and a dilated, fixed pupil.

(Fig. 14–18). Topical steroids and cycloplegic agents may quiet the inflammatory component and relieve ciliary muscle spasm, providing increased comfort. Pilocarpine should be avoided. Surgical intervention for intractable elevated IOP includes filtering procedures, cycloblative procedures, or a Molteno implant (*see* Chapters 15 and 17).

Steroid-induced Glaucoma. Treatment for steroid-induced glaucoma includes discontinuing the steroid, if possible, and using antiglaucoma topical medications to reduce the IOP (*see* Chapter 17). For an external condition, a steroid may be topically applied so it does not penetrate into the eye. For uveitis, if continued steroid use is necessary, switching to a milder steroid (fluoromethylone) may minimize the ocular hypertensive effect. When a potent steroid is required, a topical beta blocker and/or CAI may be used concomitantly.

Acute Angle Closure Glaucoma. The goal of treatment in acute angle closure glaucoma is to move the iris out of the anterior chamber angle, preventing peripheral anterior synechiae and allowing unrestricted outflow of aqueous (Fig. 14–19). Typically, this is accomplished with miotics. However, an IOP greater than 45 to 50 mm Hg causes ischemia of the iris sphincter muscle rendering miotic agents ineffective (*see* Chapter 19). The IOP must first be lowered, either by temporarily opening the angle using indentation gonioscopy or by installation of a topical beta blocker, oral hyperosmotic agents, or CAI followed by a miotic once the IOP drops below 40 mm Hg. Indentation gonioscopy with a Zeiss or Posner 4-mirror lens may be effective in breaking an acute angle

closure attack by mechanically opening the angle when oral agents are not available or warranted.[74] Indentation of the cornea followed by release, done in 15-second intervals is continued for 5 minutes. This push-release method is employed to prevent the risk of a central retinal artery occlusion.[74] If indentation gonioscopy is unsuccessful, an oral hyperosmotic agent may be used.

Osmotics must be used with care in the elderly. Patient nausea from the attack may be aggravated by the agent leading to vomiting. When oral agents are precluded due to nausea, a faster acting dose of intravenous acetazolamide 500 mg or mannitol may be of benefit. A prochlorperazine (Compazine) suppository may be used to reduce the nausea prior to administering glycerin or isosorbide but care is required since prochlorperazine may induce some pupillary dilation.

The treatment regimen for oral glycerin is for the patient to drink a 50% solution in a dose of 1.5 grams per kilogram of body weight (about 4 to 6 fluid ounces). In the case of diabetics, metabolically inactive isosorbide in 45% solution (Ismotic) is used. Pouring the solution over ice will diminish the pungent taste and thin the solution for easier consumption and faster absorption (Fig. 14–20).

After drinking isosorbide or glycerin, one drop of timolol 0.5% and apraclonidine should be administered. The IOP is checked every 30 minutes and on reaching 40 mm Hg or less, one drop of pilocarpine 2% is administered at 15-minute intervals for 1 hour. Increasing systemic symptoms attributed to an ongoing angle closure attack may be due to pilocarpine overdosage and their secondary parasympathomimetic side effects if used in excessive amounts. On

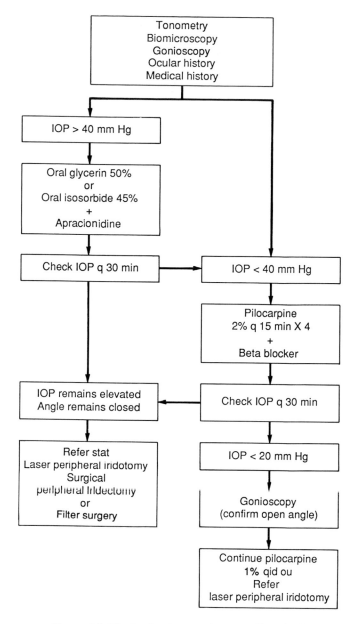

Figure 14–20. Angle closure glaucoma flowchart.

CONCLUSION

Treatment of glaucoma is a challenging endeavor that taxes a clinician's diagnostic and therapeutic skills. The doctor must establish the diagnosis, review the patient's medical and ocular history, and select a medication and target pressure. For all of these decisions, there are numerous choices that can be difficult to make. In addition, the patient must be educated regarding glaucoma: what it is, how it is managed, and potential side effects from the medications used. Periodic monitoring is required to look for medication intolerance, IOP stability, and signs of glaucomatous progression. Finally, the doctor must establish a relationship with the patient built on trust and confidence so that if problems do arise, the doctor will be alerted. For all of this, the best that one can usually hope for is to "break even" and preserve the patient's vision. Glaucoma treatment is a difficult task with few thanks and the preservation of the patient's vision may be the doctor's only reward.

REFERENCES

1. Armaly MF. On the distribution of applanation pressure. I. Statistical features and the effect of age, sex and family history of glaucoma. *Arch Ophthalmol.* 1965;73:11–18.
2. Kass MA. When to treat ocular hypertension. *Surv Ophthalmol.* 1983;28(suppl):229–232.
3. Epstein DL, Krug JH, Hertzman E, et al. A long term clinical trial of timolol therapy versus no treatment in the management of glaucoma suspects. *Ophthalmology.* 1989;96:1460–1467.
4. Kass MA, Gordon MO, Hoff MR, et al. Topical timolol administration reduces the incidence of glaucomatous damage in ocular hypertensive individuals. *Arch Ophthalmol.* 1989;107:1590–1598.
5. Epstein DL. Why not a cure? (editorial) *Arch Ophthalmol.* 1987;105:1187–1188.
6. Jaanus SD, Pagano VT, Bartlett JD. Drugs affecting the autonomic nervous system. In: Bartlett JD, Jaanus SD, eds. *Clinical Ocular Pharmacology.* 2nd ed. Boston: Butterworths; 1989;3:69–148.
7. Burggraf GW, Munt PW. Topical timolol therapy and cardiopulmonary function. *Can J Ophthalmol.* 1980; 15:159–160.
8. Steinert RF, Thomas JV, Boger WP. Long term drift and continued efficacy after multi-year timolol therapy. *Arch Ophthalmol.* 1981;99:100–103.
9. Boger WP III. Short term "escape" and long term "drift." *Surv Ophthalmol.* 1983;28(suppl):235–240.
10. Neufeld AH, Zawistowski KA, Page ED, Bromberg BB. Influences on the density of beta adrenergic receptors in the cornea and iris-ciliary body of the rabbit. *Invest Ophthalmol Vis Sci.* 1978;17:1069–1075.

obtaining an adequate pressure reduction, gonioscopy is repeated to confirm the reopening of the angle. Referral for laser peripheral iridotomy is made as soon as possible once the attack is broken. The patient should be maintained on a mild miotic such as pilocarpine 1% in each eye to prevent repeated angle closure. If the IOP and/or angle configuration does not return to normal, iridotomy or surgical iridectomy should be performed within several hours of the onset of the attack. Treatment of chronic angle closure glaucoma includes laser peripheral iridotomy followed by medical control of any residual pressure elevation. Filtering surgery may be required for adequate control.

11. McMahon CD, Shaffer RN, Hoskins HD Jr. Adverse effects experienced by patients taking timolol. *Am J Ophthalmol.* 1979;88:736–738.

12. Cinotti A, Cinotti D, Grant W, et al. Levobunolol vs. timolol for open angle glaucoma and ocular hypertension. *Am J Ophthalmol.* 1985;99:11–17.

13. Nielsen-Angelo K. Timolol topically and diabetes mellitus. *JAMA* 1980;244:1567.

14. Van Buskirk EM. Corneal anesthesia after timolol maleate therapy. *Am J Ophthalmol.* 1979;88:739–743.

15. Forte EJ, Weber PA. Psychologic effects of topical timolol maleate. *Contemp Ophthalmol Forum.* 1987;5:11–18.

16. Lynch MA, Whitson JT, Brown RH, et al. Topical beta blocker therapy and central nervous system side effects. *Arch Ophthalmol.* 1988;106:908–911.

17. Schoene RB, Abuan T, Ward RL, Beasley CH. Effects of topical betaxolol, timolol and placebo on pulmonary function in asthmatic bronchitis. *Am J Ophthalmol.* 1984;97:86–92.

18. Allen RC, Hertzmark E, Walker AM, Epstein DL. A double masked comparison of betaxolol vs. timolol in the treatment of open angle glaucoma. *Am J Ophthalmol.* 1986;101:535–541.

19. Cyrlin MN, Thomas JV, Epstein DL. Additive effect of epinephrine to timolol therapy in primary open angle glaucoma. *Arch Ophthalmol.* 1982;100:414–418.

20. Allen RC, Epstein DL. Additive effect of betaxolol and epinephrine in primary open angle glaucoma. *Arch Ophthalmol.* 1986;104:1178–1184.

21. Allen RC, Robin AL, Long D, et al. A combination of levobunolol and dipivefrin for the treatment of glaucoma. *Arch Ophthalmol.* 1988;106:904–907.

22. Berry DP, Van Buskirk EM, Shields MB. Betaxolol and timolol: A comparison of safety and side effects. *Arch Ophthalmol.* 1984;102:42–45.

23. Vogel R, Tipping R, Kulaga S, et al. Changing therapy from timolol to betaxolol: Effect on intraocular pressure in selected patients with glaucoma. *Arch Ophthalmol.* 1989;107:1303–1307.

24. Ofner S, Smith TJ. Betaxolol in chronic obstructive pulmonary disease. *J Ocul Pharmacol.* 1987;3:171–173.

25. Van Buskirk EM, Weinreb RN, Berry DP, et al. Betaxolol in patients with glaucoma and asthma. *Am J Ophthalmol.* 1986;101:531–534.

26. Dunn TL, Gerber MJ, Shen AS, et al. The effect of topical ophthalmic instillation of timolol and betaxolol on lung function in asthmatic subjects. *Ann Rev Respir Dis.* 1986;133:264–268.

27. Harris LS, Greenstein SH, Bloom RF. Respiratory difficulties with betaxolol. *Am J Ophthalmol.* 1986;102:274.

28. Topical preparations. In: Kastrup EK, Olin BR, Connell SI, eds. *Drug Facts and Comparisons.* St. Louis, MO: J.B. Lippincott; 1988;10:1717–1961.

29. Schwartz B. Primary open angle glaucoma. In: Duane TD, ed. *Clinical Ophthalmology.* Hagerstown, MD: Harper & Row; 1981;3:1–45.

30. Zimmerman TJ, Wheeler TM. Miotics. Side effects and ways to avoid them. *Ophthalmology.* 1982;89:76–80.

31. Topical preparations. In: Kastrup EK, Olin BR, Connell SI, eds. *Drug Facts and Comparisons.* St. Louis, MO: J.B. Lippincott; 1988;10:1717–1961.

32. Townsend DJ, Brubaker RF. Immediate effect of epinephrine on aqueous in the normal human eye as measured by fluorophotometry. *Invest Ophthalmol Vis Sci.* 1980;19:256–266.

33. Durkee D, Bryant BG. Drug therapy in glaucoma. *Am J Hosp Pharmacol.* 1979;35:682–690.

34. Kolker AE, Becker B. Epinephrine maculopathy. *Arch Ophthalmol.* 1968;79:552–562.

35. Sugar J. Adrenochrome deposits in hydrophilic lenses. *Arch Ophthalmol.* 1974;91:11–12.

36. Ballin N, Becker B, Goldman ML. Systemic effects of epinephrine applied topically to the eye. *Invest Ophthalmol.* 1966;5:125–129.

37. Epstein DL, Grant WM. Carbonic anhydrase inhibitor side effects: Serum chemical analysis. *Arch Ophthalmol.* 1977;95:1378–1382.

38. Mogk LG, Cyrlin MN. Blood dyscrasias and carbonic anhydrase inhibitors. *Ophthalmology.* 1988;95:768–771.

39. Viggosson G, Bjornsson G, Ingvason JG. The prevalence of open angle glaucoma in Iceland. *Acta Ophthalmol (Copenh).* 1986;64:138–141.

40. Quigley HA. The challenge of when to treat in glaucoma. In: Klein EA. ed. *Symposium on the Laser in Ophthalmology and Glaucoma Update.* St. Louis, MO: C.V. Mosby; 1985;1:1–9.

41. Sommer A, Tielsch JM, Katz J, et al. Relationship between intraocular pressure and primary open angle glaucoma among white and black Americans. The Baltimore Eye Survey. *Arch Ophthalmol.* 1991;109:1090–1095.

42. Wilensky JT, Gandhi N, Pan T. Racial influences in open angle glaucoma. *Ann Ophthalmol.* 1978;10:1398–1402.

43. Martin MJ, Sommer A, Gold EB, et al. Race and primary open angle glaucoma. *Am J Ophthalmol.* 1985;99:383–387.

44. Wilson MR, Hertzmark E, Walker AM, et al. A case control study of risk factors in open angle glaucoma. *Arch Ophthalmol.* 1987;105:1066–1071.

45. Schwartz B, McCarty G, Rosner B. Increased plasma free cortisol in ocular hypertension and open angle glaucoma. *Arch Ophthalmol.* 1987;105:1060–1065.

46. Wilensky JT, Kolker AE. Peripapillary changes in glaucoma. *Am J Ophthalmol.* 1976;81:341–345.

47. Buus DR, Anderson DR. Peripapillary crescents and halos in normal tension glaucoma and ocular hypertension. *Ophthalmology.* 1989;96:16–19.

48. Lindenmuth KA, Skuta GL, Musch DC, Buech M. Significance of cilioretinal arteries in primary open angle glaucoma. *Arch Ophthalmol.* 1988;106:1691–1693.

49. Martin XD, Rabineau PA. Intraocular pressure effects of timolol after unilateral instillation. *Ophthalmology.* 1988;95:1620–1623.

50. Kwitko GM, Shin DH, Ahn BH, Hong YJ. Bilateral ef-

fects of long term monocular timolol therapy. *Am J Ophthalmol.* 1987;104:591–594.

51. Zimmerman TJ, Baumann JD, Hetherington J. Side effects of timolol. *Surv Ophthalmol.* 1983;28(suppl):243–249.

52. Affrime MB, Lowenthal DT, Tobert MB, et al. Dynamics and kinetics of ophthalmic timolol. *Clin Pharmacol Ther.* 1980;27:471–477.

53. Shell JW. Pharmacokinetics of topically applied ophthalmic drugs. *Surv Ophthalmol.* 1982;26:207–218.

54. Davidson J, Ribak J, Eckstein D, Barishak R. Timolol maleate: Side effects on healthy nonglaucomatous volunteers. *Aviat Space Environ Med.* 1983;54:360–362.

55. Hernandez HHY, Frati A, Hurtado R, et al. Cardiovascular effects of topical glaucoma therapies in normal subjects. *J Toxicol Cut Ocul Toxicol.* 1983;2:99–106.

56. Atkins JM, Pugh BR Jr, Timewell RM. Cardiovascular effects of topical beta blockers during exercise. *Am J Ophthalmol.* 1985;99:173–175.

57. Ros FE, Dake CL. Timolol eye drops: Bradycardia or tachycardia? *Doc Ophthalmol.* 1979;48:283–289.

58. Becker B, Kolker AE, Krupin T. Hyperosmotics agents. In: Leopold IH, ed. *Symposium on Ocular Therapy.* St. Louis, MO: C.V. Mosby; 1968;3:42–53.

59. Diuretics and cardiovasculars. In: Kastrup EK, Olin BR, Connell SI, eds. *Drug Facts and Comparisons.* St. Louis, MO: J.B. Lippincott; 1988;4:421–684.

60. Becker B, Kolker AE, Krupin T. Isosorbide: An oral hyperosmotic agent. *Arch Ophthalmol.* 1966;62:629–634.

61. Sugar SH. Pitfalls in the medical treatment of simple glaucoma. *Ann Ophthalmol.* 1979;11:1041–1050.

62. Fraunfelder FT, Meyer SM, Bagley CC, Dreis MW. Hematologic reactions to carbonic anhydrase inhibitors. *Am J Ophthalmol.* 1985;100:79–81.

63. Wandel T, Charap AD, Lewis RA, et al. Glaucoma treatment with once daily levobunolol. *Am J Ophthalmol.* 1986;101:298–304.

64. Starita RJ, Fellman RL. Glaucoma treatment with once daily levobunolol. *Am J Ophthalmol.* 1986;102:544–545.

65. Kooner JS, Zimmerman TJ. The cost of antiglaucoma medications. *Ann Ophthalmol.* 1987;19:327–328.

66. Zimmerman TJ, Kooner KS, Kandarakis AS, Ziegler LP. Improving the therapeutic index of topically applied ocular drugs. *Arch Ophthalmol.* 1984;102:551–553.

67. Richardson KT. Medical control of the glaucomas. *Br J Ophthalmol.* 1972;56:272–277.

68. Kowal DJ, Fingeret M. A glaucoma control chart. *J Am Optom Assoc.* 1987;58:734–737.

69. Zimmerman TJ, Zalta AH. Facilitating patient compliance in glaucoma therapy. *Surv Ophthalmol.* 1983;28(suppl):252–257.

70. Van Buskirk EM. The compliance factor (editorial). *Am J Ophthalmol.* 1986;101:609–610.

71. Kass MA, Gordon M, Morley RE, et al. Compliance with topical timolol treatment. *Am J Ophthalmol.* 1987;103:188–193.

72. Airaksinen PJ, Valkonen R, Stenborg T, et al. A double masked study of timolol and pilocarpine combined. *Am J Ophthalmol.* 1987;104:587–590.

73. Kass MA, Meltzer DW, Gordon M, et al. Compliance with topical pilocarpine treatment. *Am J Ophthalmol.* 1986;101:515–523.

74. Anderson DR. Corneal indentation to relieve acute angle closure glaucoma. *Am J Ophthalmol.* 1979;88:1091–1093.

Chapter 15

SURGICAL MANAGEMENT
OF GLAUCOMAS

Elliot B. Werner

THE ROLE OF SURGERY IN THE MANAGEMENT OF THE GLAUCOMAS

The surgical managment of glaucoma is a complex subject because glaucoma is a complex subject. Glaucoma is not a single disease but a family of diseases that share an abnormality of the intraocular pressure and a unique type of optic atrophy called cupping. The various glaucomas, however, have very different underlying mechanisms. The treatment of any particular glaucoma depends on our best current understanding of its pathogenesis and pathophysiology.

Some glaucomas are best treated medically while in others, such as pupil block glaucomas or congenital glaucoma, surgery is the treatment of choice. Even in primary open-angle glaucoma, a disease in which surgery is traditionally employed only if medical therapy fails, evidence is accumulating that early surgery may actually be more beneficial to patients.[1–3]

The goal of any treatment for glaucoma is to reduce the intraocular pressure (IOP) to a level that will prevent progressive optic nerve damage and loss of vision. This must be accomplished without an unacceptably high risk to the patient. Before undertaking any treatment, the clinician must be able to answer the following questions:

1. Does the patient in fact have glaucoma?
2. If so, exactly what type of glaucoma and what is the mechanism?
3. What is the evidence that treatment is beneficial, and how likely is it that this particular patient will benefit from treatment?
4. What is the risk of the treatment and does the potential benefit outweigh the risk?
5. What is the risk of not treating the patient and is it greater or less than the risk of treatment?
6. What treatments are available and which is most likely to achieve the desired result with the least risk?

Once these questions have been answered, the clinician is in a position to recommend treatment. Medical and surgical procedures for glaucoma form a spectrum of treatments that cannot be separated from each other. A clinician managing glaucoma patients must be aware of the full spectrum of treatments available and must feel comfortable with all of them. The goals and role of surgery in glaucoma are no different from those of medical treatment. The procedures chosen to treat a patient must be based on what offers the most benefit and least risk to that patient.

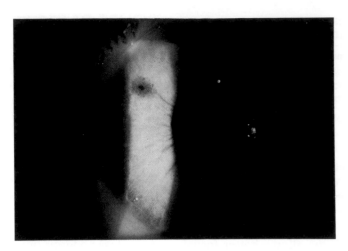

Figure 15–4. Postoperative photograph of a patent laser peripheral iridectomy. To be certain that the iridectomy is patent, the lens capsule should be seen through the iridectomy opening. (*See also* Color Plate 15–4.)

tency is determined by visualizing the vitreous face or intraocular lens surface through the iridectomy.

Complications. Intraoperative complications include failure to penetrate the iris, corneal burns, hemorrhage, and inadvertent retinal damage.[9] Failure to penetrate the iris may result from corneal edema or a corneal opacity that prevents delivery of adequate laser energy to the iris. Some irides are very thick or vascular and are extremely difficult to penetrate. If the iris begins to bleed, or if large amounts of pigment are released into the aqueous, the surgeon may be unable to visualize the iris well enough to complete the procedure. If an iridectomy cannot be created during the initial attempt with the laser, the patient may be brought back in 24 or 48 hours for another attempt. Sometimes, it may be necessary to resort to an incisional iridectomy in very difficult cases.

Corneal burns sometimes result if the laser beam is not aimed and focused properly, or if the iris is very close to the cornea. These burns rarely cause permanent scarring or difficulty, but they may obscure the iris and prevent the surgeon from completing the procedure.

Hemorrhage from the iris is a common occurrence with the Nd : YAG laser. The amount of hemorrhage is usually small and rarely causes permanent sequelae. Blood in the anterior chamber may, however, prevent completion of the procedure and may be associated with a marked increase in IOP postoperatively.

Inadvertent retinal damage from a misdirected laser beam is fortunately rare. If the iridectomy is made in the nasal portion of the iris and the delivery system is directed nasally, damage to the macula will be avoided even if the retina is accidentally coagulated.

Postoperative complications include increased IOP, iritis, posterior synechiae, corneal abrasion, and late closure of the iridectomy.[9] A significant number of patients undergoing laser iridectomy will suffer a marked increase in IOP within the first 2 hours of the procedure. The frequency and severity of this complication can be reduced by the preoperative and postoperative use of apraclonidine drops.[10] All patients should be monitored during the immediate postoperative period. If the IOP increases, the patient may be treated with beta adrenergic blocking agents, carbonic anhydrase inhibitors, and hyperosmotic agents as needed until the pressure returns to normal. This complication rarely causes permanent sequelae, but acutely increased intraocular pressure may be associated with optic nerve infarction or retinal vessel occlusions. In patients with very advanced glaucoma, progressive visual field loss may occur even when the IOP is elevated for only a short time.

Most patients will have some degree of iritis following laser iridectomy.[11] Routine treatment with topical corticosteroids for 3 to 5 days postoperatively will usually prevent any major problems. Some patients will, however, have a prolonged inflammatory response or develop an iritis when the corticosteroid drops are stopped. Even in the presence of a mild anterior chamber reaction, some patients will form posterior synechiae following laser iridectomy.

Corneal abrasions may result in some patients from the contact lens used during the treatment. This is treated like any other corneal abrasion, but may contraindicate the use of topical corticosteroids for several days postoperatively.

Late closure of the iridectomy is a common complication with the argon laser, occurring in anywhere from 10 to 35% of patients. It is much less common with the Nd : YAG laser.[12] If an iridectomy is going to close, it usually will occur within the first 6 weeks. When late closure occurs, it is necessary to repeat the procedure. Sometimes, the previously made iridectomy can be reopened. Alternatively, a new site on the iris may be chosen.

Postoperative Follow-Up. As is true of any surgical procedure, the extent of the postoperative follow-up depends on the occurrence of complications and the patient's course. In an uncomplicated iridectomy in which there has been no postoperative IOP increase, the patient should be treated with topical corticosteroids for 3 to 5 days and seen within a week. If there are no problems, the patient should be seen again 6 to 8 weeks postoperatively. At this point the patient should be gonioscoped to see if the configuration of the anterior chamber angle has changed as a result of the iridectomy. The pupil should also be dilated in order to examine the retina. In patients with pupil block, this may in fact never have been done because of the risk of angle closure. Naturally, postoperative management will need to be modified if the patient has complications or a severe pre-existing glaucoma.

Incisional Peripheral Iridectomy

Indications and Contraindications. Surgical peripheral iridectomy is rarely performed any more due to the safety and high rate of success of laser iridectomy.[13] The indications for surgical peripheral iridectomy are exactly the same as for laser iridectomy (*see* Tables 15–1 and 15–2) in patients where laser iridectomy either fails or cannot be performed. The most common indication for surgical peripheral iridectomy is physical limitation or psychiatric illness, which prevents the performance of a laser iridectomy because the patient cannot sit at a slit-lamp. Examples might include quadriplegia, severe arthritis, deformities of the cervical spine, severe psychosis, mental retardation, and so forth. Patients in whom a patent laser iridectomy cannot be created or maintained despite repeated attempts are also candidates for surgical peripheral iridectomy.

Contraindications for peripheral iridectomy include nanophthalmos, permanent synechial angle closure, and lens-induced angle closure. The uveal effusion syndrome commonly follows intraocular surgery on nanophthalmic eyes and should be avoided if at all possible. Patients with permanent synechial angle closure in whom intraocular surgery is contemplated should probably have filtering surgery rather than iridectomy. Similarly, patients with lens-induced glaucoma should have lens extraction rather than simple iridectomy.

Technique. Surgical iridectomy is usually performed with local anesthesia unless there is a contraindication or a compelling reason for general anesthesia. A small incision is made in the cornea, either under a small conjunctival flap or directly in clear cornea. A peripheral knuckle of iris is drawn out through the incision and excised with scissors. The iris is replaced into the anterior chamber and the corneal incision sutured (Fig. 15–5).

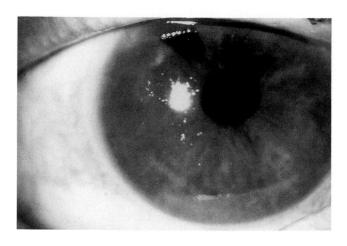

Figure 15–5. Photograph of a patent surgical iridectomy. (*See also* Color Plate 15–5.)

Complications. Since surgical iridectomies are rarely performed, complications are rarely seen. There are complications that can occur following any intraocular surgery, such as infection, hemorrhage, inflammation, retinal detachment, macular edema, choroidal effusions, corneal edema, and optic nerve infarction. Complications of surgical peripheral iridectomy include posterior synechiae, peripheral anterior synechiae, flat anterior chamber, malignant (ciliary block) glaucoma, incomplete iridectomy, and accelerated cataract formation.

Postoperative Follow-Up. Following peripheral iridectomy and any intraocular surgery, the patient must be seen the next day. Visual acuity, IOP, and the results of slit-lamp biomicroscopy must be recorded at each visit. Patients are usually treated with topical corticosteroid drops and a mild cycloplegic until all signs of inflammation have disappeared. Persistent glaucoma if present will also require treatment as necessary, but the possibility of steroid-induced glaucoma must always be considered in a postoperative patient. As with laser iridectomy, the patient should be gonioscoped about 6 to 8 weeks postoperatively, and the pupil dilated in order to examine the fundus.

PROCEDURES TO INCREASE AQUEOUS OUTFLOW

In any patient with uncontrolled glaucoma where the IOP is sufficiently high to pose a major risk of future vision loss, surgery to increase aqueous outflow, if successful, will usually result in better control of IOP. Laser trabeculoplasty can only be performed in patients with an open anterior chamber angle and achieves its best results in primary open-angle glaucoma and a few secondary open-angle glaucomas, such as pseudoexfoliation and pigmentary glaucoma.

Filtering surgery can be performed in the presence of either closed- or open-angle glaucomas. Goniotomy and trabeculotomy are now reserved for treating congenital and juvenile glaucomas. The potential benefit of lowering the IOP must be balanced against the risks of the surgery, the likelihood of progressive visual loss, and the probability that the procedure will succeed.

Laser Trabeculoplasty

Indications and Contraindications. Laser trabeculoplasty is indicated in any patient with an open anterior chamber angle in whom IOP is not low enough to prevent progressive optic nerve cupping and visual field loss. Determining when laser trabeculoplasty is indicated requires careful follow-up of glaucoma patients. Stereoscopic optic disc photographs and visual field examinations should be obtained at frequent and regular intervals.

In general, younger patients and patients with normal or minimally elevated IOP are less likely to respond to laser trabeculoplasty. Certain types of glaucomas are more likely to respond to laser trabeculoplasty than others as shown in Table 15–3.

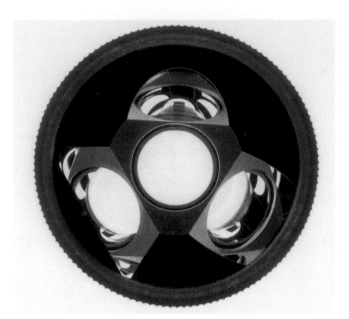

Figure 15–6. Photograph of a Goldmann 3-mirrored lens. The round mirror is designed for gonioscopy and is used for laser trabeculoplasty.

TABLE 15–3. EXPECTED RESPONSE TO LASER TRABECULOPLASTY IN VARIOUS TYPES OF GLAUCOMA

Good (>67% initial success)
Primary open-angle glaucoma
Pseudoexfoliation glaucoma
Pigmentary glaucoma

Fair (33–67% initial success)
Aphakic or pseudophakic patient
Angle recession glaucoma
Following failed filtering surgery
Inactive uveitis
Postiridectomy secondary open-angle glaucoma

Poor (<33% initial success)
Active uveitis
Neovascular glaucoma
Congenital, juvenile glaucoma
Mesodermal dysgenesis
Elevated episcleral venous pressure
Irido-corneal-endothelial syndrome
Steroid glaucoma
Rheumatoid scleritis

Contraindications include corneal edema or opacities that prevent clear visualization of the anterior chamber angle, angle closure glaucoma, and a physical or psychiatric illness that prevents adequate patient cooperation. Relative contraindications include diseases in which laser trabeculoplasty is unlikely to be effective such as those listed in Table 15–3, as well as patients under the age of 35.[14]

Techniques. Although several different types of lasers have been used experimentally, the vast majority of surgeons perform trabeculoplasty with an argon laser. A variety of contact lenses have been devised for use when performing trabeculoplasty. All, however, use a gonioscopic mirror to visualize the anterior chamber angle and are similar to the Goldman 3-mirrored lens (Fig. 15–6). The laser beam is aimed at the anterior half of the pigmented trabecular meshwork (Fig. 15–7).

The number of laser applications and the extent of the angle treated vary from surgeon to surgeon. Some prefer to treat only 180° of the angle initially while others treat 360°. There is no evidence that one technique is safer or more effective than the other. Treatments of less than 50 applications are unlikely to be successful. The ideal number seems to be between 80 and 100 applications. The number of applications and their location on the trabecular meshwork seem

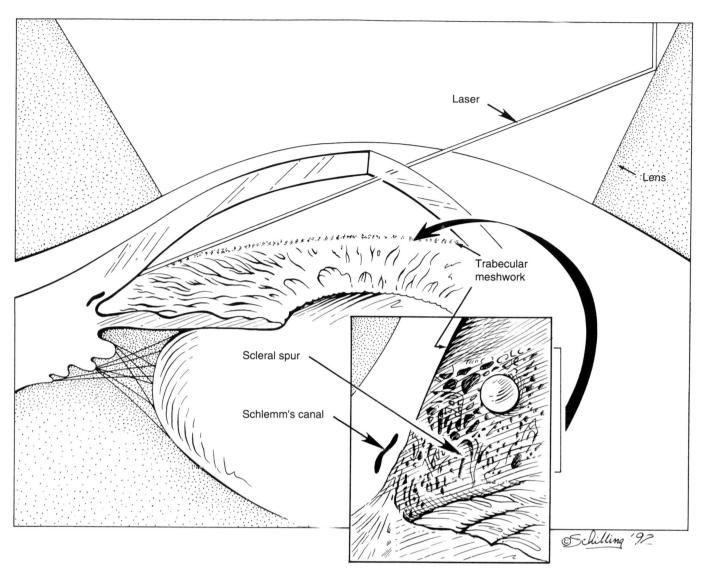

Figure 15–7. In argon laser trabeculoplasty, the laser beam strikes the Goldmann 3-mirrored lens. The beam is reflected onto the anterior portion of the pigmented trabecular meshwork. A small bubble of blanching of the trabecular meshwork after each application indicates the proper power setting has been used.

to be more important in obtaining a good result than the extent of the angle treated.[14]

Laser trabeculoplasty lowers intraocular pressure by increasing facility of aqueous outflow. The mechanism by which this occurs is unknown, but there is evidence suggesting that laser energy increases the metabolic activity of the trabecular endothelial cells and causes them to proliferate. This may result in more efficient movement of aqueous through the trabecular meshwork.

Complications. Serious complications following laser trabeculoplasty are unusual. The reported complications include corneal abrasion, corneal burns, hemorrhage, peripheral anterior synechiae, iritis, a transient or permanent increase in IOP, syncope, allergic or toxic reactions to the eye drops, and failure to lower IOP.

The most common complication is a transient increase in IOP during the immediate postoperative period, sometimes to very high levels. The frequency and severity of this complication can be reduced by using apraclonidine drops preoperatively. Treatment is the same as outlined under complications of laser iridectomy.

The other common complication is failure to

lower the IOP. The response to trabeculoplasty is not usually apparent for 6 to 8 weeks postoperatively. Some patients will show a very marked response in the first week or two only to have no significant change in pressure 8 weeks later. Other patients may show very little effect in the first 2 weeks and still have a successful result later on. Some patients show no effect at all.

In primary open-angle glaucoma, one can expect a satisfactory decrease in IOP in about 70 to 80% of patients. In many patients, however, the effect is not permanent. Late term failures occur in about 10% of patients each year so that by 5 years after trabeculoplasty, less than 50% of patients will still have adequate IOP control.[15]

The other complications of laser trabeculoplasty are similar to those following laser iridectomy and are managed in a similar manner.

Postoperative Follow-Up. Patients should be checked 1 and 2 hours following trabeculoplasty to be sure that there is no postoperative increase in IOP. Topical corticosteroids are used for 5 days after the treatment to minimize the iritis. The patient's glaucoma therapy is usually continued without change.

Barring any complications, patients are usually seen about 2 and 8 weeks postoperatively. If the IOP response is satisfactory, the patient is then followed like any other patient with chronic glaucoma. Stereo disc photographs and visual fields should be obtained at regular intervals. If progression of the disease continues, additional therapy will be needed. In some patients the glaucoma may be controlled with less medication after laser trabeculoplasty, but this is unusual.

In the event of late failure, the options are to increase the medical therapy, repeat the trabeculoplasty, or perform filtering surgery. There is evidence that good results can be obtained following a repeat trabeculoplasty in patients who have had a good result for at least a year following the initial treatment. If the initial effect was not satisfactory, or if the duration of the lowered IOP was less than 1 year, repeat trabeculoplasty is not indicated. In any case, the results following repeat trabeculoplasty are not nearly as good as those following the initial treatment.

Filtering Surgery

Glaucoma filtering surgery aims to create a fistula between the anterior chamber and the subconjunctival space so that the aqueous will drain out of the eye lowering the IOP. When successful, filtering surgery completely bypasses the normal aqueous outflow pathway. In the normal eye, or in the glaucomatous eye that has not had filtering surgery, the IOP is determined by the rate of aqueous production and the resistance to outflow in the trabecular meshwork, Schlemm's canal, and scleral collector channels. Following successful filtering surgery, resistance to outflow is provided by the sclerostomy opening and the subconjunctival tissues. Since there is resistance to outflow in these areas, IOP following filtering surgery is not zero and, in fact, may still be higher than normal despite successful filtration.

Indications and Contraindications. Glaucoma-filtering surgery is indicated in any eye where the IOP cannot be maintained low enough to prevent future vision loss by any other means.[16] In pupil block angle closure glaucoma, filtering surgery is indicated when the pressure cannot be controlled with medication following iridectomy. In non-pupil block angle closure, filtering surgery is indicated when the pressure cannot be controlled by medical therapy. In primary open-angle glaucoma, filtering surgery is indicated when the pressure cannot be controlled by maximally tolerated medical therapy following laser trabeculoplasty. The same indication prevails in secondary open-angle glaucomas unless the patient has a type of secondary glaucoma known to have a poor response to laser trabeculoplasty (*see* Table 15–3).

Contraindications for filtering surgery include blindness, absence of glaucomatous damage, and severe systemic medical problems. The purpose of filtering surgery is to preserve vision. Since there is a small but significant risk of sympathetic uveitis, a life-threatening infection, anesthetic injury, or death from filtering surgery, the operation should not be performed on blind eyes.

In patients with ocular hypertension, that is elevated IOP without evidence of optic nerve cupping or visual field loss, the risk of filtering surgery is probably not warranted, since most patients do not suffer loss of vision. Naturally, any patient with such severe systemic medical illness that anesthesia and surgery pose a major risk of death should not have surgery.

Techniques. There are three types of filtering operations currently in common use: full thickness filtration, partial thickness filtration, and tube or valve implantation. In full-thickness procedures, an opening is made by either cutting (posterior lip sclerectomy) or burning (thermal sclerostomy) through the entire thickness of the sclera (Fig. 15–8). The opening is covered only by conjunctiva and Tenon's capsule.

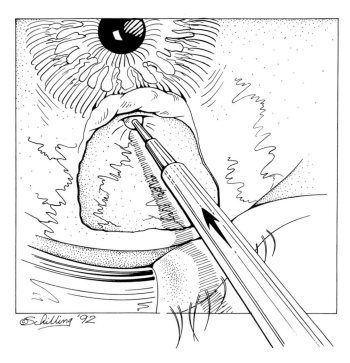

Figure 15–8. Diagram of a posterior lip sclerotomy. A full thickness opening is made through the corneoscleral junction into the anterior chamber using a punch. The opening is then covered with a flap of conjunctiva.

In partial thickness procedures such as trabeculectomy, the scleral opening is covered with a partial thickness flap of the overlying sclera (Fig. 15–9). In tube or valve implantations, a plastic tube is inserted through the sclerostomy into the peripheral anterior chamber to facilitate drainage (Fig. 15–10).

Most filtering surgery can be performed under local anesthesia on an outpatient basis. In certain cases such as one-eyed patients or repeat operations, general anesthesia and hospitalization after surgery may be required.

Full thickness filtering procedures are indicated in younger patients or black patients where trabeculectomy has a high failure rate. Full thickness procedures are also indicated in patients with low-tension glaucoma where very low intraocular pressures are desired postoperatively.[17,18] The partial thickness trabeculectomy is indicated in older, white patients, or in patients with corneal guttata or cataracts where postoperative flat chamber and hypotony should be avoided.[19,20] Tube and valve implantations are usually reserved for patients where a previous standard filtering operation has failed or who have a disease such as neovascular glaucoma where primary standard filtering operations often fail.[21,22]

Drugs such as 5-fluorouracil (5-FU) or mitomycin are used postoperatively in patients undergoing filtering surgery where the risk of failure is very high because of scarring and subsequent closure of the newly created fistula. A fibroblast inhibitor, 5-FU prevents healing of the sclerostomy during the postoperative period. It is given by subconjunctival injection daily for the first 2 weeks following surgery and weekly for the third and fourth week. The major indications for the use of 5-FU are previous cataract surgery or previous failed filtering surgery.[23–25]

Recently, some surgeons have been performing partial thickness procedures with releasable sutures. These sutures may be released with a forceps at the slit-lamp or lysed with a laser during the first postoperative week. This may help avoid hypotony and a flat anterior chamber during the early postoperative period and still provide the patient with the advantages of better IOP control later on by converting the partial thickness procedure to a full thickness procedure without additional surgery.[26,27]

Complications. Table 15–4 lists the more common complications of filtering surgery.[16,28]

Recognition and management of the complications of glaucoma-filtering surgery is often difficult and can be very frustrating for both patient and surgeon. Patients undergoing filtering surgery need to be aware that frequent visits will be required during the postoperative period. Clinicians who manage patients following filtering surgery need to have extensive training and experience in this field.

Full thickness procedures have a somewhat higher success rate and often result in a lower IOP than partial thickness procedures. The complication rate is, however, much higher following full thickness procedures. There is a longer postoperative recovery period and considerably more discomfort following full thickness procedures.

The use of 5-FU increases the risk of wound leaks and corneal epithelial erosions or ulcers. Following tube procedures, the risk of hypotony, choroidal effusions, or intraocular inflammation is increased.

Postoperative Follow-Up. The success rates of glaucoma-filtering surgery depend on several factors.[29,30] First is the definition of success. Success may be defined as creation of a functioning filtering bleb, control of IOP below some predetermined level, or prevention of further visual loss. In evaluating reports of success rates following various types of filtering surgery, it is important to find out how success was defined.

Other factors affecting success rates after filtering

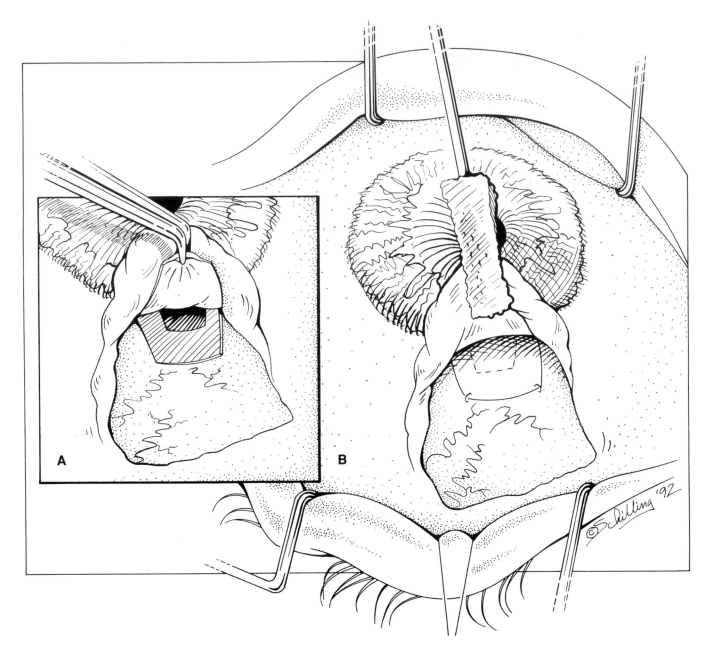

Figure 15–9. Diagram of a trabeculectomy. **A.** The opening into the anterior chamber is first covered by a partial thickness scleral flap. **B.** A conjunctival flap is then sutured over the scleral flap.

surgery are age, race, the nature of the patient's glaucoma, and the type of operation performed. Filtering surgery is generally more successful in older patients. Filtering surgery usually fails in patients under the age of 35, while in patients over 65 success rates of 80 to 90% are often achieved. Filtering surgery is less likely to succeed in black patients than in whites.

Filtering surgery is most successful in primary open-angle glaucoma, chronic primary closed-angle glaucoma, and certain secondary glaucomas such as traumatic, pigmentary, and pseudoexfoliation glaucomas. Filtering surgery is much less likely to succeed in inflammatory glaucomas, neovascular glaucoma, following previous intraocular surgery, or in certain degenerative conditions such as the irido-corneal-endothelial syndrome.

There is evidence that full thickness filtering procedures such as posterior lip sclerectomy have a higher long-term success rate than partial thickness procedures such as trabeculectomy. This seems to be especially true in black patients.

Clinical evaluation of the filtering bleb is impor-

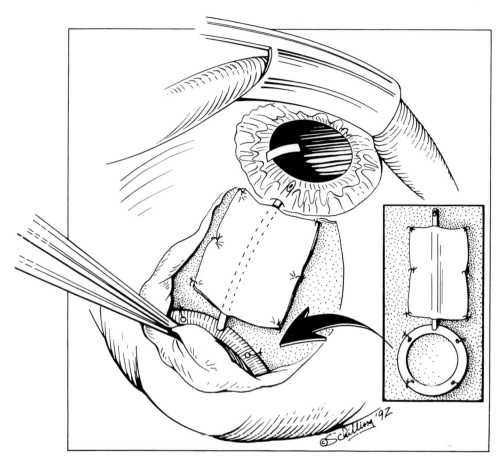

Figure 15–10. Diagram of a tube implantation. The proximal end of the tube is inserted into the anterior chamber. The distal end is connected to a filtration plate that is sutured to the scleral surface 10 mm behind the limbus. The tube is covered with a piece of donor banked sclera to prevent it from eroding through the overlying conjunctiva.

tant in determining if the surgery has been successful. There are certain signs that characterize the functioning filtering bleb. First, the intraocular pressure should be significantly reduced. If not, the bleb is probably nonfunctional.

The functioning bleb may be wide and diffuse with a shallow elevation or it may be localized, markedly elevated, and thin walled. In either case, the normal bleb has an elevated, pale or translucent, avascular appearance and should be white or pale

TABLE 15–4. COMPLICATIONS OF GLAUCOMA-FILTERING SURGERY

Intraoperative complications	Early postoperative complications
Retrobulbar hemorrhage from local anesthesia	Hypotony
Toxic or allergic reactions to anesthetic agents	Flat anterior chamber
Conjunctival buttonhole	Choroidal detachment
Scleral flap disinsertion	Conjunctival wound leak
Intraocular hemorrhage	Suprachoroidal hemorrhage
Choroidal effusion	Malignant (ciliary block) glaucoma
Expulsive suprachoroidal hemorrhage	Iritis
Inadvertent injury to lens or ciliary body	Endophthalmitis
Vitreous loss	**Late postoperative complications**
Descemet's membrane detachment	Encapsulated bleb
Inadequate iridectomy	Bleb failure, increased IOP
Intraocular lens cornea touch	Cataract
	Thin-walled bleb leading to dissection onto cornea, late leakage, rupture, or late endophthalmitis
	Late hypotony, choroidal effusion
	Staphyloma
	Corneal edema
	Sympathetic uveitis

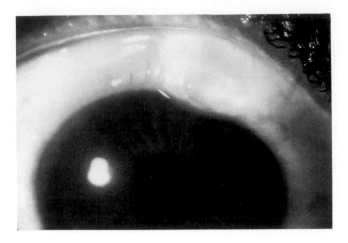

Figure 15–11. Photograph of a functioning filtering bleb. The bleb is translucent, avascular, and demonstrates microcysts at the anterior edge. (*See also* Color Plate 15–11.)

gray in color (Fig. 15–11). A red, vascularized bleb usually fails. When the bleb is functioning well, small, bubble-like cysts are often seen at the very anterior edge of the conjunctiva where it joins the cornea. On gonioscopy, the internal opening of the sclerostomy should be visible and be unobstructed by iris, pigment, or fibrous tissue.

The encapsulated bleb is a common complication usually seen between 2 and 6 weeks postoperatively.[31] The encapsulated bleb has a high-domed appearance. It is often vascularized and a dense, white tissue is seen just below the conjunctiva overlying the bleb (Fig. 15–12). The IOP is usually quite elevated. Treatment consists of topical or systemic medication to lower the IOP, frequent ocular massage, and topi-

cal corticosteroids. The condition often resolves within 6 to 12 weeks, but sometimes additional surgery is required.

Leakage of aqueous through the bleb or the wound may occur at any time following the surgery. Small, asymptomatic leaks can be observed and will often resolve spontaneously. If the leak persists, pressure patching may be tried, but additional surgery to close the leak is often required. Bleb or wound leaks are diagnosed by performing the Seidel test, which involves painting fluorescein over the bleb and looking for a clear stream of aqueous in the midst of the fluorescein.

Endophthalmitis is an uncommon but dreaded complication of filtering surgery.[32] Patients with thin-walled blebs are especially at risk for intraocular infections if they develop conjunctivitis. Any patient with a filtering bleb should be advised to seek medical attention immediately if symptoms of conjunctivitis occur. Intensive antibiotic treatment should be given for any conjunctivitis in the presence of a filtering bleb (Fig. 15–13).

Goniotomy, Trabeculotomy: Surgery for Congenital Glaucoma

Indications and Contraindications. Surgery is the preferred initial treatment for congenital glaucoma or juvenile glaucoma in a young child.[33–35] Filtering surgery is rarely successful in such patients and is used only if goniotomy or trabeculotomy have failed. The purpose of goniotomy or trabeculotomy is not to create a fistula and filtering bleb, but to remove abnor-

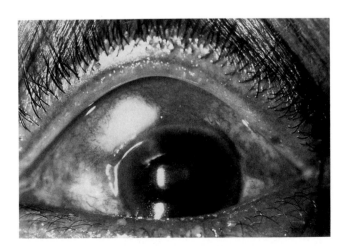

Figure 15–12. Photograph of an encapsulated bleb. The bleb is tense, opaque, elevated, and vascularized. (*See also* Color Plate 15–12.)

Figure 15–13. Photograph of an infected bleb. The eye is markedly hyperemic. The bleb is filled with pus and appears white. (*See also* Color Plate 15–13.)

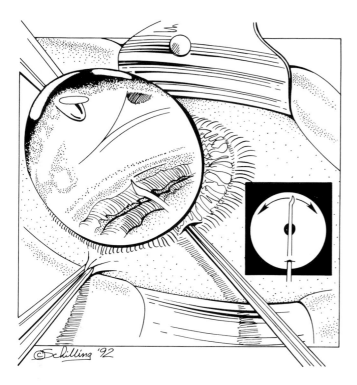

Figure 15–14. Diagram of a goniotomy. A knife is passed through the cornea, across the anterior chamber, and engages the trabecular meshwork. A partial thickness incision is made in the trabecular meshwork over approximately 120°.

mal trabecular meshwork and allow the aqueous freer access to Schlemm's canal.

In goniotomy, a knife is passed through the cornea, across the anterior chamber, and the abnormal trabecular tissue is cut away from the inside (Fig. 15–14). In trabeculotomy, Schlemm's canal is identified by cutting into it from the scleral side. A small probe is placed into the lumen of Schlemm's canal and rotated into the anterior chamber, thus rupturing the inner wall of Schlemm's canal and the trabecular meshwork (Fig. 15–15). Both procedures work equally well. Trabeculotomy is somewhat technically easier to perform, but is associated with a slightly higher complication rate.

Without surgery, children with congenital glaucoma will become blind. Thus, the only contraindication to surgery is severe systemic illness, which would pose an unacceptable surgical risk to the life of the patient.

Postoperative Follow-Up. Once the IOP has been controlled and the glaucoma appears stable, the most important aspect of care is the management of refractive errors and amblyopia. Patients with congenital glaucoma often develop high degrees of myopia, anisometropia, strabismus, and amblyopia. Careful at-

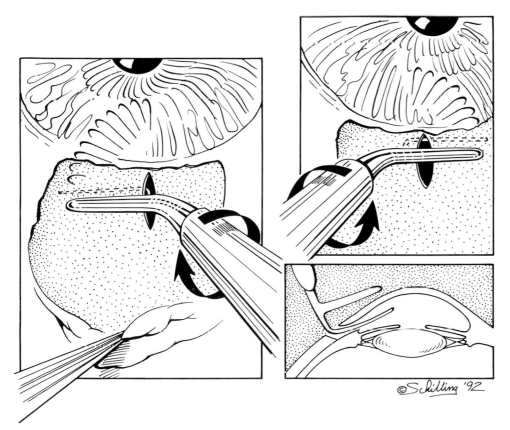

Figure 15–15. Diagram of a trabeculotomy. A small probe is paled into the lumen of Schlemm's canal and rotated into the anterior chamber, rupturing the overlying trabecular meshwork.

tention to these problems is required in order to visually rehabilitate the child.

PROCEDURES TO DECREASE AQUEOUS PRODUCTION

Over the years, several procedures have been developed to destroy the ciliary body epithelium and reduce the IOP by decreasing the production of aqueous humor. The two that are most commonly used at present are cyclocryotherapy and transscleral YAG laser cyclophotocoagulation (TSYLC).

Cyclocryotherapy

Indications and Contraindications. In cyclocryotherapy, extreme cold is used to injure the ciliary epithelium.[36,37] Since the procedure has a high rate of complications and is associated with significant visual loss in many patients, it is reserved for patients with severe glaucoma who have poor vision and in whom other medical and surgical treatments have failed.

The major contraindications to cyclocryotherapy are the presence of a clear lens and good visual acuity.

Technique. A probe with a tip 3 to 4 mm in diameter is attached to a container of a liquid gas such as carbon dioxide or nitrogen. The tip of the probe achieves a temperature of at least −80°C. The probe is applied to the sclera overlying the ciliary body, 2 or 2.5 mm behind the limbus (Fig. 15–16). An ice ball forms whose radius is sufficient to freeze the entire thickness of the ciliary body including the epithelium. Initially six to eight applications are made over 180°. The treatment may be repeated 6 to 8 weeks later if adequate lowering of IOP is not achieved. Treatment over the full circumference of the ciliary body is usually avoided because of the high risk of subsequent phthisis bulbi.

Complications. Complications are common and often severe and permanent after cyclocryotherapy. A severe iritis, which is often quite painful, invariably follows the procedure. The inflammatory response

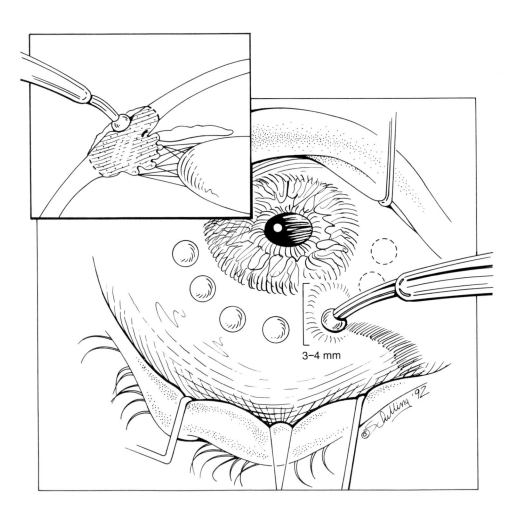

Figure 15–16. Diagram of a cyclocryotherapy. A probe is applied to the outside surface of the eye freezing the ciliary processes. Treatment is usually applied over 90 to 180° and may be repeated if necessary.

3–4 mm

often lasts for months and sometimes long-term treatment with topical corticosteroid is required. Loss of vision due to macular edema is another common complication.

Other complications include cataract, subluxation of the lens, intraocular hemorrhage, corneal edema, pain, hypotony, and phthisis bulbi. A marked degree of lid and conjunctival swelling usually follows the procedure and lasts for several weeks. Most of these complications are the result of the extensive destruction of uveal tissue following cyclocryotherapy.

Postoperative Follow-Up. Cyclocryotherapy is usually done in endstage eyes in an effort to save what is already very poor vision. If cyclocryotherapy fails, the next step is usually enucleation if the eye becomes totally blind or painful.

Postoperative follow-up is similar to other glaucoma procedures. Patients are treated with anti-inflammatory and antiglaucoma medications as needed to control inflammation and IOP. Initially, the pressure after cyclocryotherapy will usually be quite low. Within a few months, however, the pressure sometimes rises and the addition of medication or repeating the procedure may become necessary.

Transscleral YAG Laser Cyclophotocoagulatlon

Indications and Contraindications. In TSYLC, the ciliary epithelium is destroyed with laser energy instead of cold (Fig. 15–17).[38,39] Indications and contraindications are similar to those listed for cyclocryotherapy. This procedure, while quite new, appears

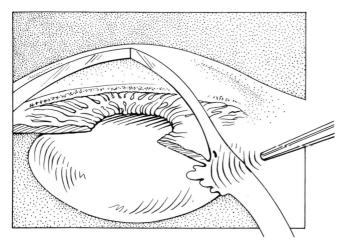

Figure 15–17. Diagram of a transscleral YAG cyclophotocoagulation (TSYLC). Laser energy is delivered through the intact sclera to the ciliary processes.

to be somewhat safer than cyclocryotherapy. Because the laser energy can be focused onto a much smaller area of the ciliary body, much less tissue is destroyed than in cyclocryotherapy. The result seems to be that TSYLC has fewer complications than cyclocryotherapy.

Technique. Using very high levels of laser energy, the beam is directed through the sclera toward the ciliary epithelium. Special optics in the delivery system allow the beam to be focused below the surface of the sclera. In the noncontact mode, delivery is through the optics of a slit-lamp similar to argon laser trabeculoplasty. Recently, contact delivery systems have been developed. Using fiberoptics, the laser beam is directed through a hand piece that is placed directly on the scleral surface of the eye. With either method, between 20 and 40 applications are made around the circumference of the posterior limbus 2.5 to 3.0 mm behind the conjunctival reflection.

Complications. Complications of TSYLC are similar to those of cyclocryotherapy. Postoperative pain and inflammation are often a problem. There seems to be less visual loss following TSYLC than after cyclocryotherapy. The procedure is still fairly new and long-term experience is not yet available. While most surgeons also reserve TSYLC for patients with very poor vision, some are beginning to use it in patients with better central vision, especially in aphakic and pseudophakic patients. More traditional types of glaucoma surgery should, however, be tried before resorting to any cyclodestructive procedure.

Postoperative Follow-Up. Postoperative follow-up is similar to that for cyclocryotherapy. Phakic patients should be carefully followed for the development of cataract.

MANAGEMENT OF COINCIDENT CATARACT AND GLAUCOMA

The patient with poorly controlled glaucoma and a visually significant cataract is a common clinical problem. There are three approaches to such patients. One is to perform filtering surgery and wait 6 to 12 months before removing the cataract. This has the advantage of a high success rate for the filtering surgery but delays visual rehabilitation for the patient.

A second approach is to remove the cataract and try to manage the glaucoma without surgery postoperatively. This is often a successful approach but can be quite dangerous in the patient with advanced glaucoma because of the increase in IOP that often occurs in the immediate postoperative period after cataract surgery. It also reduces the chance for successful filtering surgery if required later because of conjunctival scarring from the cataract surgery.

A third approach is to combine cataract extraction and glaucoma filtering surgery into one operation, the combined procedure.[40–42] If successful, this has the advantage of restoring vision and controlling the glaucoma with a single procedure. The success rate of the filtering portion of combined procedures, however, is much less than that of straightforward filtering surgery.

Combined procedures are technically more difficult, have a much prolonged postoperative recovery time, and have a higher complication rate. Modern techniques of small incision cataract surgery and phacoemulsification seem to give better results when combined with filtering surgery than large incision extracapsular cataract surgery.

Combined Cataract Extraction-Filtering Procedure

Indications and Contraindications. The usual indication for a combined procedure is a visually disabling cataract and inadequately controlled glaucoma in the same patient. Traditional teaching has been that each procedure should be indicated independently of the other procedure before recommending a combined procedure. Many glaucoma surgeons, however, also recommend a combined procedure in the presence of a visually disabling cataract and glaucoma that requires more than one medi-

cation to control. This is thought to decrease the chance of the patient suffering a severe increase in IOP following cataract surgery, a common complication in glaucoma patients.

Another situation in which a combined procedure is often recommended is the patient with uncontrolled glaucoma and an early or moderate cataract. While the cataract itself is not visually disabling, it is likely to become so within a year or two after filtering surgery. In this case, the patient can be spared a second procedure if the cataract is removed at the time of filtering surgery.

Technique. A cataract extraction is performed in the usual manner, either with a large incision extracapsular or small incision phacoemulsification technique (Fig. 15–18). A part of the cataract wound is modified by performing either a posterior lip sclerectomy or a trabeculectomy. This portion of the cataract wound is not sutured in an effort to create a filtering bleb. Posterior chamber intraocular lenses are routinely used. Anterior chamber angle fixated intraocular lenses should be avoided.

Complications. Complications are similar to those listed for filtering surgery. In addition, the clinician must be prepared for all the complications of cataract surgery as well. The most dreaded complication is a flat anterior chamber that allows the intraocular lens to come into contact with the corneal endothelium. This often results in endothelial failure and permanent corneal edema. Careful follow-up is required during the first 2 or 3 weeks after surgery. If a flat

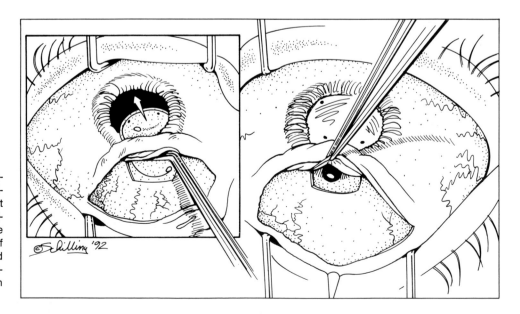

Figure 15–18. Diagram of a combined cataract extraction and filtering procedure. The cataract incision is modified to create a trabeculectomy flap. A portion of the sclera from the posterior edge of the cataract incision is excised and covered with the scleral flap. An intraocular lens is routinely placed in the posterior chamber.

chamber develops, prompt and emergency surgery is indicated to reform the anterior chamber.

Postoperative Follow-Up. Postoperative follow-up is similar to that of a routine filtering procedure. The recovery time will be considerably longer than is usual for either cataract or filtering surgery. The success rate for the filtering portion of the surgery will be lower than expected for routine filtering surgery, and larger degrees of postoperative astigmatism may be encountered than is usual in routine cataract surgery.

REFERENCES

1. Glaucoma Laser Trial Research Group. The glaucoma laser trial (GLT). *Ophthalmology.* 1991;98:317–321.
2. Lavin MJ, Wormald RPL, Migdal CS, Hitchings RA. The influence of prior therapy on the success of trabeculectomy. *Arch Ophthalmol.* 1990;108:1543–1548.
3. Jay JL, Murray SB. Early trabeculectomy versus conventional management in primary open-angle glaucoma. *Br J Ophthalmol.* 1988;72:881–889.
4. Abraham RK, Miller GL. Outpatient argon laser iridectomy for angle closure glaucoma: A two-year study. *Trans Am Acad Ophthalmol Otol.* 1975;79:529–538.
5. Lee DA, Brubaker RF, Ilstrup DM. Anterior chamber dimensions in patients with narrow angles and angle-closure glaucoma. *Arch Ophthalmol.* 1984;102:46–50.
6. Panek WC, Christenson RE, Lee DA, et al. Biometric variables in patients with occludable anterior chamber angles. *Am J Ophthalmol.* 1990;110:185–188.
7. Tomey KF, Traverso CE, Shammas IV. Nd:YAG laser iridotomy in the treatment and prevention of angle closure glaucoma. *Arch Ophthalmol.* 1987;105:476–481.
8. Abraham RK. Protocol for single session argon laser iridectomy for angle-closure glaucoma. *Int Ophthalmol Clin.* 1981;21:145–159.
9. Ritch R, Liebmann J, Solomon IS. Laser iridectomy and iridoplasty. In: Ritch R, Shields MB, Krupin T, eds. *The Glaucomas* St. Louis: C.V. Mosby; 1989:581–603.
10. Zimmerman TJ, Price RE. Apraclonidine for intraocular pressure control. *Ocul Therapeut Man.* 1990;1(2):1–12.
11. Hoskins HD, Kass M. *Becker-Shaffer's Diagnosis and Therapy of the Glaucomas.* 6th ed. St. Louis: C.V. Mosby; 1989:504–505.
12. Schwartz LW, Moster MR, Spaeth GL, Wilson RP, Poryzees E. Neodymium-YAG laser iridectomies in glaucoma associated with closed or occludable angles. *Am J Ophthalmol.* 1986;102:41–44.
13. Morales J, Ritch R. Conventional surgical iridectomy. In: Ritch R, Shields MB, Krupin T, eds. *The Glaucomas.* St. Louis: C.V. Mosby; 1989:645–651.
14. Reiss GR, Wilensky JT, Higginbotham EJ. Laser trabeculoplasty. *Surv Ophthalmol.* 1991;35:407–428.
15. Shingleton BJ, Richter CU, Bellows AR, Hutchinson T, Glynn RJ. Long-term efficacy of argon laser trabeculoplasty. *Ophthalmology.* 1987;94:1513–1517.
16. Katz LJ, Spaeth GL. Filtration surgery. In: Ritch R, Shields MB, Krupin T, eds. *The Glaucomas.* St. Louis: C.V. Mosby; 1989:653–696.
17. Lamping KA, Bellows R, Hutchinson BT, Afran SI. Long-term evaluation of initial filtration surgery. *Ophthalmology.* 1986;93:91–100.
18. Wilson MR. Posterior lip sclerectomy vs. trabeculectomy in West Indian blacks. *Arch Ophthalmol.* 1989;107:1604–1608.
19. Wax MB, Adelson A. Indications for early glaucoma surgery. *Ophthalmol Clin North Am.* 1988;1:175–179.
20. Hutchinson BT, Bellows AR. Glaucoma filtration surgery. *Ophthalmol Clin North Am.* 1988;1:181–186.
21. Minckler DS, Heuer DK, Hasty B, et al. Clinical experience with the single-plate Molteno implant in complicated glaucomas. *Ophthalmology.* 1988;95:1181–1188.
22. Akira C, de Almieda GV, Cohen R, Mandia C, Kwitko S. Modified Schocket implant for refractory glaucoma, experience of 55 cases. *Ophthalmology.* 1991;98:211–214.
23. Liebmann JM, Ritch R. 5-fluorouracil in glaucoma filtering surgery. *Ophthalmol Clin North Am.* 1988;1:125–131.
24. Palmer SS. Mitomycin as adjunct chemotherapy with trabeculectomy. *Ophthalmology.* 1991;98:317–321.
25. Wilson RP, Steinmann WC. Use of trabeculectomy with postoperative 5-fluorouracil in patients requiring extremely low intraocular pressure levels to limit further glaucoma progression. *Ophthalmology.* 1991;98:1047–1052.
26. Savage JA, Condon GP, Lytle RA, Simmons RJ. Laser suture lysis after trabeculectomy. *Ophthalmology.* 1988;95:1631–1637.
27. Cohen JS, Osher RH. Releasable scleral flap suture. *Ophthalmol Clin North Am.* 1988;1:187–197.
28. Liebmann JM, Ritch R. Management of the failing filtering bleb. *Semin Ophthalmol.* 1991;6(2):81–86.
29. Hoskins HD, Kass M. *Becker-Shaffer's Diagnosis and Therapy of the Glaucomas.* 6th ed. St. Louis: C.V. Mosby; 1989:572–582.
30. Stewart WC, Shields MB, Miller KN, Blasini M, Sutherland SE. Early postoperative prognostic indicators following trabeculectomy. *Ophthal Surg.* 1991;22:23–26.
31. Shingleton BJ, Richter CU, Bellows AR, Hutchinson BT. Management of encapsulated filtration blebs. *Ophthalmology.* 1990;97:63–68.
32. Katz LJ, Cantor LB, Spaeth GL. Complications of surgery in glaucoma, early and late bacterial endophthalmitis following glaucoma filtering surgery. *Ophthalmology.* 1985;92:959–963.
33. Luntz MH, Harrison R. Surgery for congenital glaucoma. In: Ritch R, Shields MB, Krupin T, eds. *The Glaucomas.* St. Louis: C.V. Mosby; 1989:707–727.
34. Dickens CJ, Hoskins HD. Diagnosis and treatment of congenital glaucoma. In: Ritch R, Shields MB, Krupin T, eds. *The Glaucomas.* St. Louis: C.V. Mosby; 1989:773–785.
35. Hill RA, Heuer DK, Baerveldt G, Minckler DS, Martone JF. Molteno implantation for glaucoma in young patients. *Ophthalmology.* 1991;98:1042–1046.

36. Bellows AR, Krug Jr JH. Cyclodestructive surgery. In: Ritch R, Shields MB, Krupin T, eds. *The Glaucomas*. St. Louis: C.V. Mosby; 1989:729–740.

37. Rosenberg LF, Holmwood PC. Ciliodestructive surgery. *Semin Ophthalmol*. 1991;6(2):95–104.

38. Wilensky JT. Transscleral laser cyclotherapy. *Ophthalmol Clin North Am*. 1988;1:163–166.

39. Wright MM, Grajewski AL, Feuer WJ. Nd:YAG cyclophotocoagulation: Outcome of treatment for uncontrolled glaucoma. *Ophthal Surg*. 1991;22:279–283.

40. McCartney DL, Stark WJ, Memmen JE, et al. Current management of cataracts in patients with glaucoma. In: Caldwell DR, ed. *Cataracts, Transactions of the New Orleans Academy of Ophthalmology*. New York: Raven Press; 1988:111–126.

41. Lyle WA, Jin JC. Comparison of a 3- and 6-mm incision in combined phacoemulsification and trabeculectomy. *Am J Ophthalmol*. 1991;111:189–196.

42. Crandall AS. Combined trabeculectomy and phacoemulsification. *Semin Ophthalmol*. 1991;6(2):76–80.

Chapter 16

CO-MANAGEMENT OF GLAUCOMA IN THE PRIMARY CARE OFFICE

Susan P. Schuettenberg

With the changing scope of optometric practice, today's clinician is held accountable for the management of additional conditions and diseases, including glaucoma. For optometrists practicing in states without therapeutic privileges, the independent treatment of glaucoma is not yet an option, but a viable alternative is to actively co-manage glaucoma patients with an ophthalmologist. For optometrists who practice in states that allow for the treatment of glaucoma, co-management is likely to resemble a referral-type relationship.

The purpose of this chapter is to provide guidelines for the effective co-management of glaucoma: namely, when to refer, who examines the patient and when, who is responsible for gathering what data, and how to coordinate the care necessary for the proper management of glaucoma. In attempting to define this framework, one must keep in mind that the patient's well-being is of the utmost importance.

GLAUCOMA CO-MANAGEMENT: WHAT IS IT AND WHY DO IT?

There will come a time for every optometrist, even one with therapeutic privileges, when a patient needs care or treatment beyond his or her capabilities. For example, a surgical procedure may be necessary, a stronger medication may be needed but which might be contraindicated due to health concerns, or the patient presents with severe glaucomatous damage. All are valid reasons for referring a patient to a physician. However, with co-management, the patient's care should be coordinated by their *primary eyecare doctor*. They should receive treatment from the appropriate specialist and return to their optometrist for follow-up care. This relationship is similar to that of a general internist who refers a patient to a specialist for a specific problem (i.e., cardiologist, gastroenterologist, or neurologist). After treatment for the specific disorder, the internist will continue to follow the patient on a routine basis until the next time a secondary or tertiary care specialist is needed.

Co-management of glaucoma by an optometrist and ophthalmologist can work in a similar manner. Depending on the particular state, an optometrist

Special thanks to L. Kenneth Bumgarner, OD for his help in the preparation of this manuscript.

295

may have the ability, by law, to treat glaucoma. For those, co-management will entail referring the more difficult glaucoma cases to a glaucoma specialist for advanced medical and/or surgical treatment. Follow-up care may be handled by the optometrist. In a nontherapeutic state or a state that does not allow optometrists to treat glaucoma, a referral is made to the glaucoma specialist for the initiation of glaucoma therapy. Once the patient is stable, he or she should return to the optometrist for follow-up care with periodic consultation with the glaucoma specialist.

FINDING THE RIGHT OPHTHALMOLOGIST

One important consideration when initiating co-management is the selection of an appropriate ophthalmologist or, specifically, a glaucoma specialist. When developing this relationship, the optometrist (OD) should seek an ophthalmologist with a similar treatment philosophy. The OD must be comfortable with the treatment protocol before entrusting patients to the glaucoma specialist. The relationship will most likely evolve over time and is nurtured by the understanding and sharing of a common treatment approach. Just what responsibilities are given to whom will depend on the state practice acts, the confidence that each professional has in the other, the experience of each, and the instrumentation available in each doctor's office.

All ODs are familiar with the difficulties in finding a compatible ophthalmologist, be it a retinal specialist, a cataract surgeon, or a corneal specialist. In the case of glaucoma co-management, this task is especially difficult. When a consultation is sought, a particular treatment modality is often anticipated such as initiating treatment, adding a new medication, or considering surgery.[1] If a different treatment regimen is instituted, the rationale should be communicated to the referring OD.

Open discussion between the MD and the OD should be encouraged at all times. In the beginning, the OD/MD team must decide on the guidelines for the initial patient consultation. Are there certain trigger points level of intraocular pressure (IOP), cup-disc size, visual field, or risk factors that the ophthalmologist feels are critical in the consideration of initiation of treatment? The OD should have input into these guidelines. Since changes in medications, protocols, dosages, and other variables related to caring for patients with glaucoma will occur over time, periodic conferences to update both practitioners should take place. In addition to keeping in touch,

these routine meetings help strengthen the bonds between the OD and the MD.

The co-management relationship should be beneficial to the patient, the OD, and the ophthalmologist. For the OD, it provides a stimulating environment while providing the patient with consistent, coordinated, and effective care. For the ophthalmologist, it allows for more time to concentrate on secondary eyecare. For the patients, it provides for continuity of care by "their" eye doctor, with the expertise of a specialist when necessary. In addition, in rural areas, the optometrist may be the only eyecare practitioner in the area. Thus, a quality co-management relationship can reduce the commuting time for the patient.

ESTABLISHING PROTOCOLS

The second step is to develop the treatment protocols to be used by the glaucoma co-management team. What medication is used first, added second, and when is laser trabeculoplasty or filter surgery considered? Is there agreement concerning target pressures? Is the glaucoma specialist willing to give other treatment suggestions consideration as they arise?

Once a patient has been diagnosed as having glaucoma, started treatment, and successfully set up a co-management regimen, the team needs to decide who is responsible for specific clinical tests. How often does the ophthalmologist want to see the patient? When are visual fields done, and by whom? How often is the patient going to be dilated? How are these clinical findings communicated between parties?

In general, a patient who is stable and *well controlled* is followed every 3 months. Each visit should include a history, biomicroscopy, a check of IOP, and an undilated optic nerve head evaluation. An annual dilated fundus examination with stereo photography, visual fields, and gonioscopy should be performed at one of these visits. Every fourth visit should be with the glaucoma specialist, who most likely will want a stereoscopic view of the optic nerve head, which requires dilation (Table 16–1).

This schedule depends on whether or not the patient is well controlled. For those individuals not controlled, more frequent visits will be necessary to both the OD for IOP measurements, optic nerve assessment, and visual fields, and to the ophthalmologist for a trial of different medications until the IOP is stable.

In those cases where a patient requires laser surgery for treatment of the glaucoma (laser peripheral iridotomy, argon laser trabeculoplasty), the team may

TABLE 16–1. SUGGESTED PROTOCOL FOR CO-MANAGEMENT OF WELL-CONTROLLED OPEN-ANGLE GLAUCOMA

Quarterly Office Visit	OD/MD	Test	Referral?
1	OD	History, slit-lamp, tonometry, gonioscopy, undilated optic nerve assessment	If IOP increased, + side effects from medication, optic nerve assessment shows change (flame hemorrhage, vein occlusion), angle narrow
2	OD	History, slit-lamp, tonometry, VF, DFE, (with stereo photos if indicated)	If IOP increased, C/D has progressed, visual field progression, + side effects from medication, other retinal signs (flame hemorrhage, and so forth)
3	OD	History, slit-lamp, tonometry, undilated optic nerve assessment	If IOP increased, + side effects from medication
4	MD	Yearly examination ± dilation	Back to OD if stable

VF = visual fields; DFE = dilated fundus examination; C/D = cup-disk ratio.

choose to have the OD provide follow-up care. This would be subsequent to the surgeon's day 1 postoperative examination. Any variation from the expected normal recovery would be discussed between the doctors and consultation sought when necessary.

WHEN TO CONSULT/REFER

States Without Glaucoma Therapeutic Privileges

In states that do not allow ODs glaucoma therapeutic privileges, the OD has the obligation to refer to an ophthalmologist, on diagnosis, any glaucoma patient for initiation of treatment.[2] Included may be the glaucoma suspect, ocular hypertensive, those showing visual field or optic nerve changes, or patients presenting with an IOP greater than 30 mm Hg. An IOP of 30 mm Hg or greater is used as a cut-off warranting referral since, even without visual field changes, this

IOP is considered excessively high and may in the long-term damage the optic nerve.[3]

The referral to a glaucoma specialist will result in the choice of a medication appropriate for that patient, the initiation of therapy, and the follow-up of that patient in 1 or 2 weeks. Any change in medication requires that the patient be seen again by the ophthalmologist. If the patient responds favorably to the medication, a 3-month follow-up would be scheduled with the OD, with the information from that visit conveyed to the ophthalmologist. As previously stated, in a well-controlled glaucoma patient, the OD will examine the patient every 3 months with a yearly visit to the ophthalmologist. If there is any change in the patient's status—a red flag—the patient should once again be referred to the glaucoma specialist. Some "red flags" include:

- Optic nerve head changes
- Visual field progression
- Elevated IOP (above target pressure)
- Significant side effects to medications
- Other changes: retinal vein occlusions, flame-shaped hemorrhages

States With Glaucoma Therapeutic Privileges

For those ODs who *are* able to treat glaucoma, consultation with a glaucoma specialist occurs under slightly different circumstances (Table 16–2). Since open-angle glaucoma is a chronic, progressive disease, there often comes a time when a referral is necessary, even for a patient that has been followed closely. Consultation with the specialist should occur with *any* case that the OD does not feel comfortable handling, whether it is a patient requiring advanced medical treatment with a strong miotic, or a patient that may benefit from surgical intervention.

Moreover, those patients who present with end-stage glaucoma need consultation with a glaucoma specialist. In these cases, topical medications may ini-

TABLE 16–2. WHEN TO CONSULT/REFER TO A GLAUCOMA SPECIALIST

ODs without glaucoma therapeutic privileges
1. To initiate treatment
2. To change or add medications
3. For surgical treatment

ODs with glaucoma therapeutic privileges
1. When advanced medical treatment is necessary (carbonic anhydrase inhibitors, strong miotics)
2. For surgical treatment

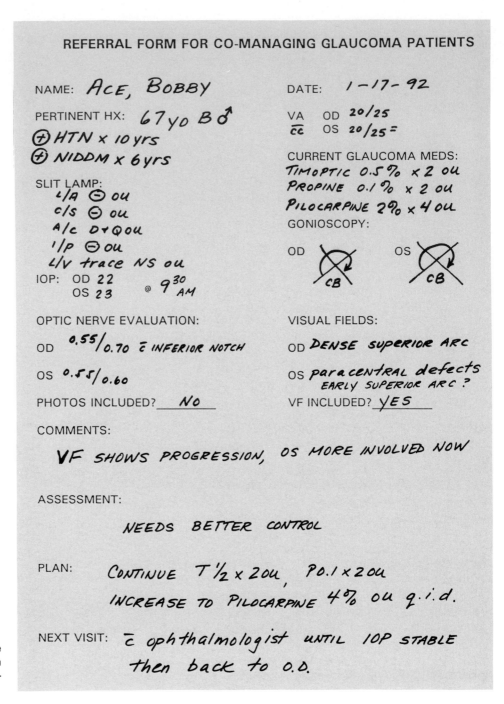

Figure 16–1. This form is to be used for the transfer of information between optometrists and physicians.

tially decrease the IOP, but the disease process will probably continue to injure an already damaged optic nerve. Aggressive therapy is necessary and surgical intervention is often required.

On occasion, a surgical procedure is considered the only effective treatment for certain types of glaucoma. For instance, congenital glaucoma should be referred immediately since surgical intervention is the primary treatment.[4] Medical therapy is used in those cases that have *not* responded to surgical treatment. In addition, long-term medical therapy in children can cause side effects that prove difficult to manage.

Consultation with a glaucoma specialist is also in order if a patient is found to have a narrow angle and is at risk for angle closure. This patient may need to have a peripheral iridotomy performed, after which, the patient is returned to the OD for routine eyecare.

Optometrists with therapeutic privileges will encounter patients that cannot tolerate certain glaucoma medications or may have prevailing medical conditions for which some medications are contraindicated. Consultations with other medical specialties may be indicated to evaluate the appropriate use of certain medications in such situations. An example is the patient with emphysema who requires Betoptic (a cardioselective beta-blocker) to improve control. Here, co-management with a pulmonary specialist is in order to assess the possible respiratory side effects of this glaucoma medication. Does the pulmonary function test support its use?

HOW TO COMMUNICATE

As in all aspects of life, communication is the key to maintaining a successful relationship. This is especially true in a co-management situation. Maximizing the flow of information between the ophthalmologist and OD should be the main objective in order to best serve the patient. This can be accomplished in a number of ways. Consultation by telephone is an often used medium that should be followed by written documentation, both for medical-legal reasons and for completeness of patient records.

In order to facilitate the transfer of pertinent information to the glaucoma specialist, a referral form (Fig. 16–1) is used. The form highlights exactly what the problem is, with space for comments and suggestions as to treatment. Using a form simplifies the transfer process, however, delivering the form to the glaucoma specialist in a timely fashion may be difficult. Many practitioners allow the patient to deliver the information themselves. This may be an easy solution but it carries the risk of the patient losing the form.

One solution would be to mail the information to the MD, but a quicker and more efficient method would be to use fax machines to transmit the data directly to the glaucoma specialist's office. This eliminates delay and allows time for the transmission of additional follow-up data, if necessary.

If both the OD and the ophthalmologist use the same perimeter, the transfer of visual field data and analysis can be facilitated.

In order to insure patient compliance with follow-up, the OD should monitor the appointments scheduled with the glaucoma specialist. Not only will this help guarantee follow-up, but it will serve to remind the patient that the OD is their primary eyecare doctor. In addition, once the OD receives information from the glaucoma specialist, a follow-up letter to the patient may be in order. This note serves to remind the patient of the proper regimen. Moreover, communication between the OD and the MD should occur whenever a patient misses an appointment with either practitioner. In this way, patient recall can be done not only by the glaucoma specialist but also by the OD, reinforcing the importance of follow-up care in glaucoma.

In summary, co-management is an option that gives eyecare professionals the opportunity to provide complete, specialized care for the glaucoma patient. Not only is the patient followed routinely by his or her OD, but access to a glaucoma specialist is available when necessary. By developing a relationship with the ophthalmologist, the OD is able to manage patients more comfortably, knowing that they will be treated following an agreed-on protocol, as well as knowing that the patient will be returning for routine glaucoma care. This dynamic and evolutionary process will not occur overnight; it requires time and effort on the part of both practitioners to make it work.

REFERENCES

1. Fingeret M, Gladstein G. Surgical management of glaucoma. In: Classe JG, ed. *Optometry Clinics: Glaucoma.* Vol. 1. Norwalk: Appleton & Lange; 1991;1:205.
2. Classe JG. *Legal Aspects of Optometry.* Boston: Butterworth; 1989:310.
3. Brumberg J, Ajamian P, Stanfield D. A discussion of primary open-angle glaucoma. *J Am Optom Assoc.* 1987;58:704–706.
4. Dickens CJ, Hoskins HD Jr. Diagnosis and treatment of congenital glaucoma. In: Ritch R, Shields MB, Krupin T, eds. *The Glaucomas.* St. Louis: C.V. Mosby; 1989;42:784.

Chapter 17

SECONDARY GLAUCOMAS

J. James Thimons

Secondary glaucomas result from elevation of intraocular pressure (IOP) leading to damage of the optic nerve caused by factors such as systemic diseases, ocular trauma, intraocular hemorrhaging, degenerative processes, abnormalities of anatomy, and from certain agents. The fundamental etiology of the secondary glaucomas is obstruction of the trabecular meshwork resulting from one of the previously mentioned conditions.

As a group, the secondary glaucomas are complex and present as a broad range of clinical entities that challenge the practitioner's diagnostic and therapeutic acumen. Although primary open-angle glaucoma is the most common of the glaucomas, secondary glaucomas, as a group, have been shown to account for as much as 33% of all glaucomas.[1] The mean age of individuals being treated for secondary glaucomas is considerably less than that for primary open-angle glaucoma. This chapter will deal with those secondary glaucomas that are most commonly seen in clinical practice. These include pigmentary, exfoliative, traumatic, steroid-induced, and neovascular glaucoma.

PIGMENTARY GLAUCOMA

Since the original description of the disease by Sugar and Barbour in 1949,[2] the significance of pigmentary dispersion and its relationship to elevation of intraocular pressure and secondary glaucoma is now better understood.

The release of pigment from the posterior surface of the iris and the subsequent deposition on the corneal endothelium, trabecular meshwork, anterior lens capsule, and the equatorial region of the lens is best classified into two basic presentations. The first is pigment dispersion syndrome, a condition in which the characteristic signs of pigment release are present but intraocular pressure, cup-disc ratio, and visual fields are normal. The second and more important presentation is pigmentary dispersion glaucoma or pigmentary glaucoma. Pigmentary glaucoma is most commonly a bilateral though often asymmetrical disease with onset occurring between age 20 and 40. There is an association with myopia and a greater prevalence in males, where the diagnosis tends to be made at an earlier age.[3,4] Little evidence exists to show an hereditary component to the development of pigmentary glaucoma but there have been recorded cases of the disease occurring in family members.[5] It is seen more commonly in whites than in blacks.

Pathogenesis. The pathophysiology of pigmentary glaucoma is more easily understood if separated into two distinct components. The first is the mechanism by which pigment release is generated and the second is the actual process that disrupts aqueous outflow.

In 1979, Campbell described a theory that brought together several older diverse concepts.[6] He postulated that the mechanism for the release of pigment was secondary to the mechanical contact of the posterior iris surface with the anterior insertion of the zonular fibers into the lens. The constant movement of the pupil produces the necessary abrasive action between the surfaces, which liberates small pigment

particles into the posterior chamber and, subsequently, following the flow of the aqueous, deposits them in the trabecular meshwork (Fig. 17–1). Supporting this theory are anatomical studies that show a correlation between zonular insertion and the area of erosion on the posterior iris surface.[7] The theory is also substantiated by anatomical evidence of the growth pattern of the normal young myopic eye, in which enlargement of the globe produces an expansion of the ciliary body ring with subsequent backward bowing of the mid-peripheral iris causing iridozonular contact.[8] Another finding, which lends credibility to this mechanism, is the decline in incidence of pigmentary glaucoma with age, probably due to the development of a miotic pupil and an increase in the iridolenticular contact area secondary to enlargement of the lens. The aged, enlarged lens causes a mild forward peripheral bowing of the iris surface with relief of the iridozonular contact.

Although the theory developed by Campbell[6]

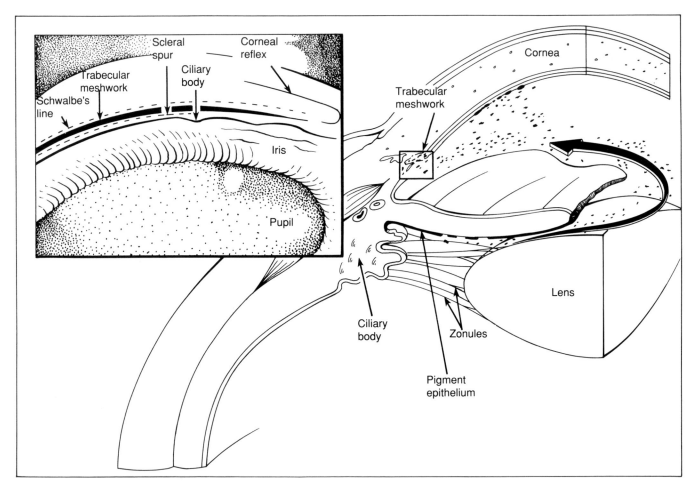

Figure 17–1. Presumed pathogenesis of pigment dispersion syndrome. Pigment is liberated from the posterior iris pigment epithelium due to iris-zonular touch. The pigment circulates in the anterior chamber, being deposited on the lens, iris, cornea, and in the trabecular meshwork.

proposes a logical explanation for the mechanical basis of this disease, there is still the underlying question as to the observed difference in incidence of pigmentary dispersion glaucoma between blacks and whites. In the age group in which pigmentary glaucoma is most prevalent in whites, there is a decreased incidence in non-whites, including both blacks and Orientals.

The pathophysiology for the elevation of IOP is less clear than that of the mechanism for pigment release. Pigment accumulation in the trabecular meshwork can produce acute elevations of IOP.[9,10] Also, dilation of the pupil in susceptible individuals will produce pigment particle release that creates significant elevation of IOP.[11] There is, however, a relatively large group of individuals who demonstrate release of pigment on dilation or exercise and do not demonstrate an acute elevation of IOP. It also does not account for individuals who demonstrate pigmentation of the trabecular meshwork without subsequent rise in IOP. Therefore, it is not strictly an issue of obstruction of aqueous outflow that produces the elevation in IOP.

Rohan and Van Der Zypen demonstrated that the trabecular endothelial cells have a significant role in phagocytosis of particulate matter exiting the anterior chamber.[12] The endothelial cells, when presented with normal amounts of material, phagocytize the particles and return to a normal appearance. When significantly increased levels of pigment are released into the anterior chamber, the endothelial cells may be unable to adequately perform this function leading to their disintegration and migration from the trabecular beams. Histological studies in individuals with advanced pigmentary glaucoma have shown denuding of the trabecular beams and the blockage of the juxtacanalicular spaces with the non-phagocytized debris.[13]

Clinical Presentation. The clinical features of pigmentary glaucoma involve the identification of the deposition of pigment on a variety of surfaces and the presence of iris transillumination defects. There have also been cases in which the peripheral retina has shown pigmentary deposition.[14]

Typically, on slit-lamp examination, the cornea shows bilateral deposition of fine pigment granules on the endothelial surface. This pigment most commonly presents in an elongated vertical pattern called Krukenberg's spindles (Fig. 17–2). The appearance of this pigment is unlike the diffuse pigment seen in some patients with corneal guttata or the scattered pigment deposits occasionally seen in pseudophakic patients. The amount of pigment can vary considera-

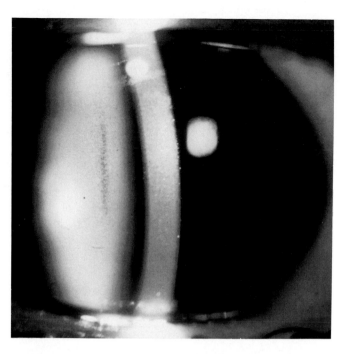

Figure 17–2. Typical pattern of fine pigment deposition on the corneal endothelial surface (Krukenberg's spindle) associated with pigment dispersion syndrome. Note the vertical orientation.

bly between individuals and the level can increase during the active phases of the disease process and decrease in later years.[15] Between 5 and 10% of patients with Krukenberg's spindles eventually develop pigmentary glaucoma.[16,17]

The iris may demonstrate several different appearances in pigmentary glaucoma. The first is a generalized stippling of the iris surface with small pigment granules. This dust-like coating is sometimes difficult to observe in brown-eyed patients. Since the disease can present asymmetrically, heterochromia may be present. The more commonly noted change is the development of transillumination defects,[18] classically located in the mid-periphery of the iris. The defects can vary from being relatively isolated to a circumferential presentation. There may be a relationship between the number of iris transillumination defects and the severity of glaucoma.[19]

The best way to observe iris transillumination defects is by directing a small circular beam of light from a biomicroscope through the pupil in a very dimly lit room and observing the presence of the retroilluminated defects in the iris (Fig. 17–3). Gross observation of retrodefects can be achieved with the use of the Finhoff transilluminator positioned inferior to the globe and in contact with the eyelid. In those individuals in which the disease process is suspected but slit-lamp assessment is unable to identify the

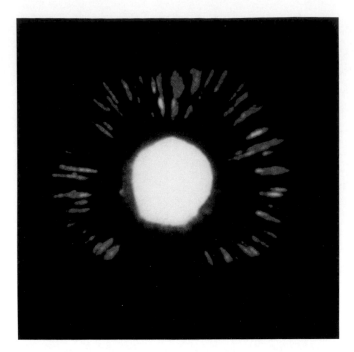

Figure 17–3. Iris transillumination defects, associated with pigment dispersion syndrome, occur in the mid-periphery and are circumferential in appearance. (*See also* Color Plate 17–3.)

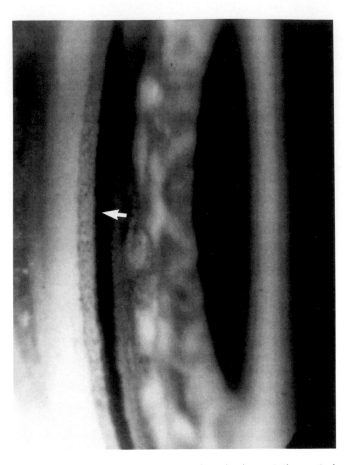

Figure 17–4. Dense trabecular meshwork pigmentation noted in an individual with pigmentary glaucoma. (*See also* Color Plate 17–4.)

presence of iris defects, the use of intra-red videography to detect and record transillumination defects has been successful.[20]

Gonioscopically, pigmentary glaucoma patients generally present with deep anterior chambers and circumferential pigmentation of the trabecular meshwork. The pigment deposition is most commonly located over the filtering portion (posterior) of the trabecular meshwork but is frequently seen diffusely deposited over the entire meshwork surface and Schwalbe's line (Fig. 17–4).[21] The grading of the anterior chamber pigmentary deposition is on a scale of 0 through 4+ with 0 representing no visible pigment in the trabecular meshwork and 4+ representing severe pigmentary deposition that approximates a chocolate-like coloration of the trabecular area.

Other areas of pigment deposition include the surface of the lens and, in some patients, a circumferential ring of pigment at the equator of the lens often detected as a distinct line of pigment visible on gonioscopy through a fully dilated pupil. The retina, although infrequently involved in the process, can show peripheral pigment deposition and, in some cases, peripheral retinal degenerations.

In pigmentary glaucoma IOP can be quite variable and has been shown to reach extremely high levels. Heavy exercise or exertion in certain susceptible individuals is capable of causing acute elevation of

IOP secondary to the release of pigment granules. These patients are frequently symptomatic (blur, eye pain) secondary to the high IOP and will seek consultation. Unfortunately, the large majority of pigmentary glaucoma patients are asymptomatic even when significantly elevated IOPs are observed on routine clinical examination. In a study by Scheie of those patients who presented with pigmentary dispersion syndrome, 37% showed elevation of IOP. Approximately 35% of these individuals developed glaucoma over a 10- to 20-year period.[22] It is not uncommon to have patients show a reduction in IOP over time due to a decrease in the release of pigment that is associated with increasing age.

Differential Diagnosis. The differential diagnosis of pigmentary glaucoma is related to those diseases that mimic the pigment dispersion process. Primary among them is exfoliative glaucoma in which the patient can present with classical signs of Krukenberg's spindles, iris transillumination defects, and pigmentation of the trabecular meshwork.[23] There is usually less pigmentation of the trabecular meshwork in exfoliative glaucoma, and careful slit-lamp examination of the anterior segment will reveal pseudoexfoliative debris on the lens capsule. Other conditions that must be considered in a differential diagnosis of pigmentary glaucoma include uveitis, which can stimulate pigment release secondary to the inflammatory process. Uveitis is easily differentiated from pigmentary dispersion by the presence of inflammatory cells and protein in the anterior chamber. Intraocular lens (IOL) implantation has been shown to produce pigment dispersion-like signs in the immediate postoperative period, but the pigment release is stable long term and rarely produces elevations of IOP.[24] Ciliary body and iris cysts as well as tumors in the eye can produce melanoma cell deposits in the anterior chamber angle.

Prognosis. Many individuals with pigment dispersion syndrome do not develop elevated IOP or glaucoma. Unfortunately, in those individuals who develop glaucoma, management can sometimes be more difficult because of the significant fluctuations in IOP as well as the inability on the part of the practitioner to stop the fundamental cause of the damage to the trabecular meshwork. Management of the disease is very similar to that used in primary open-angle glaucoma in that topical beta blockers, as well as other ocular antiglaucoma drugs are effective in controlling IOP in the majority of patients. Some clinicians recommend the use of miotics, if the patient will tolerate them, to reduce the iridozonular contact and decrease the release of pigmentation. This can be accomplished with the use of Pilogel at night, the weekly Ocusert system, or by using pilocarpine 1% twice daily. Once pigment release is reduced, IOP usually decreases significantly. The use of laser trabeculoplasty and filtering procedures is warranted in individuals with progressive disease.

EXFOLIATIVE GLAUCOMA

Etiology. In 1917, Lindbergh described the ocular appearance of what is today termed pseudoexfoliative syndrome. This condition was subsequently identified by Vogt, Wilson, and eventually Dvorak,[25] who coined the term pseudoexfoliation and identified it as a disease of basement membranes affecting tissues of the anterior segment of the eye. It is differentiated from true exfoliative disease, which is associated with exposure of the eye to intense heat or infra-red radiation, and is usually seen in glass blowers. Termi-

nology used to describe this condition varies considerably in the professional literature. The term "pseudoexfoliation syndrome" is the most common, but exfoliation syndrome is also used, as well as capsular glaucoma when the condition progresses past that of a syndrome to a true glaucomatous state.

The incidence of exfoliative changes in open-angle glaucoma patients varies from 3% in the United States up to 75% in Sweden.[26] Historically, it has been felt that the disease process was limited to certain subpopulations, particularly those of the Scandinavian countries. It has now been shown that the disease is universal in its distribution, and not confined to any ethnic group or geographic area. The one common finding throughout population studies done worldwide is that pseudoexfoliation syndrome and exfoliative glaucoma are directly related to age, with the onset being most common between the sixth and eighth decades. Interestingly, unlike pigmentary dispersion syndrome, which is almost always a bilateral disease, pseudoexfoliation begins most commonly as a monocular condition. But in over 40% of patients with monocular pseudoexfoliation syndrome, the second eye develops similar findings within a 7-year period.[27,28] Much like pigmentary dispersion syndrome, there does not appear to be a pattern of inheritance associated with pseudoexfoliation syndrome. Studies involving both steroid responsiveness testing and human leukocyte antigen (HLA) typing have been inconclusive in establishing an hereditary relationship.[29]

Pathogenesis. Pseudoexfoliation syndrome is a disease in which a fibrilogranular material of a protein nature, similar to amyloid, is deposited in the anterior segment of the eye (Fig. 17–5). Investigators have identified a relationship between the deposited material and glycosaminoglycans[30] as well as similarities in staining patterns to lens zonular material. Others have related the exfoliative debris to be secondary to disturbances in the biosynthesis of basement membranes.[31] The origin of the exfoliative material continues to be somewhat elusive but it is currently thought that the lens epithelium, at least in part, contributes to the exfoliative process of the anterior lens capsule. Exfoliative material is also found in the conjunctiva, the anterior iris surface, trabecular meshwork, zonules, vessel walls, and ciliary body.[32] Pigment released during pseudoexfoliation is rubbed off the back of the iris near the pupil by the roughened surface of the lens.

The pathogenesis of the glaucoma itself is still somewhat unclear,[33] but most likely the dispersion of pigment and the release of the exfoliative material

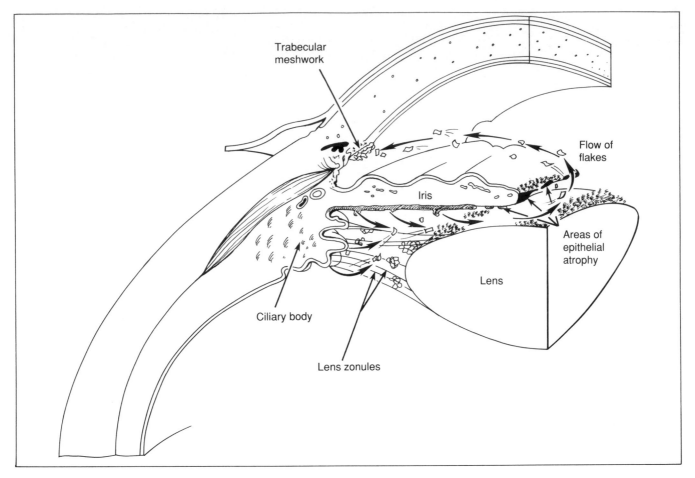

Figure 17–5. Exfoliative material, produced in the anterior segment, is deposited on the lens surface, zonules, iris, and trabecular meshwork. Also seen are areas of iris epithelial atrophy.

produces significant obstruction of the aqueous outflow pathways and, subsequently, an elevation in IOP. There is a decrease in the facility of aqueous outflow in some but not all patients with exfoliative disease.[34] Therefore, significant questions remain unaswered regarding the pathogenic mechanism that produces the underlying elevation of IOP.

Clinical Presentation. Pseudoexfoliation syndrome affects all tissues of the anterior segment but has classically been associated with the anterior lens capsule. Jundall was the first to grade the severity of the disease process. He divided pseudoexfoliation syndrome into three levels. Stage 1 shows the development of small pigmented dots on the lens capsule in radial clusters near the margin of a nondilated pupil.[35] Occasionally, at this location, small areas of local transillumination defects of the iris are noted, but no significant alteration in the pupillary frill is present. In stage 2, the pigmented dots that were originally noted on the lens capsule lose their colora-

tion and increase in size to gray flake-like structures that coalesce. Also noticeable is an alteration of the pupillary frill and an increase in the transillumination zones at the pupillary margin (Fig. 17–6). Stage 3 shows the flecks merging into larger areas of granular membrane-like structures that form geographic patterns. This final stage accounts for the picture most commonly associated with pseudoexfoliation syndrome, a central translucent disc with curling of the margins surrounded by an annular zone of clear lens tissue most likely secondary to the lens-iris contact and, finally, a peripheral granular zone that frequently presents with a slit-like striation pattern (Fig. 17–7).

Changes in the anterior chamber angle represent another important clinical feature of this disease. Although the level of trabecular pigmentation is variable, it is a consistent finding from the earliest stages of the disease process. Pigmentation of the trabecular meshwork is generally less than that seen with pigmentary dispersion syndrome (Fig. 17–8). Pigment

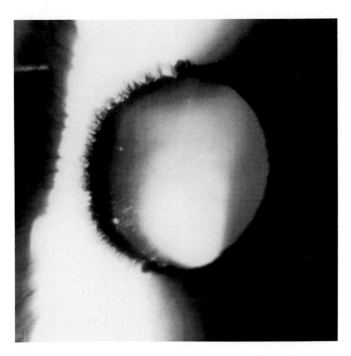

Figure 17–6. Stage 2 pseudoexfoliation of the lens. Note the gray flakes at the pupillary margin.

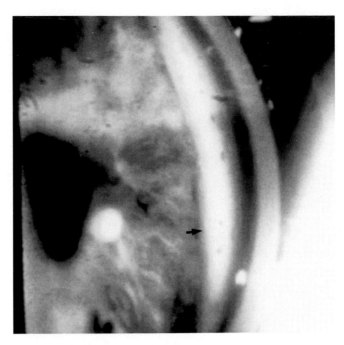

Figure 17–8. Gonioscopic findings in exfoliative disease. Note the pigmentation visible in the trabecular meshwork.

released from the iris surface is the most likely cause of this presentation. The most prominent area of pigmentation is inferiorly and slightly nasal to the 6 o'clock position. Pigment accumulating anterior to Schwalbe's line is known as Sampaolesi's line. In

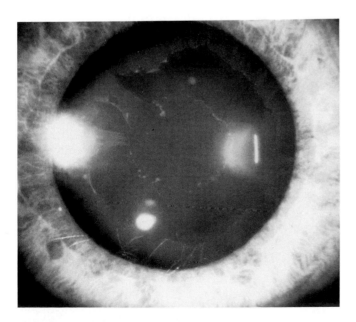

Figure 17–7. Classical pseudoexfoliative "bulls-eye" pattern on the anterior lens surface. (*See also* Color Plate 17–7.) (*Courtesy of Rodney Gutner, OD.*)

some individuals with pseudoexfoliation syndrome, rapid elevations of pressure occur secondary to the release of pigment following dilation with epinephrine.[36] This is not dissimilar to the pigment showers noted in pigmentary dispersion syndrome following exercise. There is also a significant increase in narrow angles in pseudoexfoliation syndrome patients,[37] as well as higher levels of transillumination defects than in normal patients with the same eye color.

Deposits of exfoliation material have been noted in zonular fibers, possibly explaining the high incidence of spontaneous subluxation of the lens in exfoliative disease.[38] An incidence of 8.4% of phakodonesis has been found in patients with exfoliative glaucoma, secondary to marked degenerative changes in the zonular fibers. This may result in the possible displacement of IOLs in extracapsular cataract surgery. In extreme cases, it has been associated with IOL dislocation. Corneal changes similar to those seen in pigmentary dispersion syndrome are also noted in pseudoexfoliation syndrome, but the frequency and intensity of the Krukenberg's spindles is significantly less.[39]

One of the unusual findings in this disease process are fluorescein angiographic abnormalities of the peripupillary iris, such as abnormal permeability as well as frank neovascularization. The significance of this has yet to be defined.[40]

Ocular hypertension occurs in 22 to 81% of individuals with pseudoexfoliation syndrome.[41,42] In newly diagnosed pseudoexfoliation syndrome patients IOP is generally higher compared to primary open-angle glaucoma patients,[43] and the progression of the glaucoma tends to be more rapid.[44] Once exfoliative glaucoma has developed, the IOP tends to be more difficult to control with topical medications, and laser trabeculoplasty and filtration surgery are used earlier compared to those patients with open-angle glaucoma of the same duration.

Differential Diagnosis. The differential diagnosis of exfoliative glaucoma is similar to pigment dispersion since both conditions result in the dissemination of iris pigment throughout the anterior chamber, producing a similar clinical picture. Fuch's heterochromic iridocyclitis as well as melanin-producing iris and ciliary body tumors must also be considered. Iritis is most easily distinguished from pseudoexfoliation syndrome by the presence of flare and cells in the anterior chamber as well as both anterior and posterior synechiae. The clinician may frequently encounter areas of sector iris atrophy that are consistent with the placement of the IOL haptic in the capsular bag of pseudophakes. These individuals also show mild release of pigment that deposits on the anterior IOL surface as well as the posterior cornea.

Prognosis. Not all patients with pseudoexfoliation syndrome develop glaucoma but the incidence rates are significantly greater than those individuals with ocular hypertension unrelated to pseudoexfoliation syndrome.[45] In long-term studies following patients with pseudoexfoliation syndrome and normal IOPs, 5% develop increased IOP over a 5-year period, while 15% develop ocular hypertension in 10 years.[46] In individuals with unilateral exfoliative glaucoma and normal IOP in the fellow eye, 75% develop elevated IOP in the fellow eye within 6 years,[47] with 20% of those eyes going on to develop glaucoma.

The prognosis for long-term success in the treatment of pseudoexfoliative disease does not appear to be as good as in open-angle glaucoma but has been demonstrated to be successful in those patients in which significant reduction in IOP is accomplished. Although the treatment of pseudoexfoliative disease is generally considered more difficult than in primary open-angle glaucoma,[48] argon laser trabeculoplasty is more successful in exfoliative glaucoma. This improved effect is present in the first year only and drops to a success rate of 50% after a 2-year follow-up.[48,49] Filtration surgery is also more effective in exfoliative glaucoma than in open-angle disease.[50,51]

Historically, there was thought to be a relationship between IOP and cataract extraction because of the assumption of the lens capsule as the only source of the pseudoexfoliative materials. Subsequently, it was shown that the basement membrane changes are present throughout the anterior segment and cataract surgery, although frequently showing initial relief for IOP, does not produce long-term resolution of the disease process.[32] Cataract surgery in exfoliative glaucoma patients has an increased risk of lens displacement secondary to zonular abnormalities.[51] Combined procedures of filtration surgery, extracapsular cataract extraction, and IOL implantation have been shown to be successful in managing both the lenticular changes frequently associated with the disease and the IOP.

POST-TRAUMATIC GLAUCOMA

Elevation in IOP following trauma to the globe can arise from a wide variety of etiologies. These include angle recession, hyphema, inflammation, lens dislocation and rupture, and pathological changes resulting from perforating injuries to the globe.

Frequently, the first noted evidence of damage to the anterior chamber angle is the presence of hyphema, sphincter tears of the pupillary margin, and/or lens subluxation, all of which are observable on slit-lamp examination.[52] Gonioscopy is required for the patient presenting with blunt trauma, but the view of the angle may be precluded at initial examination by anterior chamber inflammation or hyphema.

Because of the complexity of the secondary glaucomas resulting from trauma, it is easiest to separate them based on the time in which they arise following the trauma. The first type occurs within hours or days following the trauma and is primarily related to inflammation, hyphema, and early changes in the trabecular meshwork secondary to blunt trauma. The second type can occur weeks or years after the traumatic incident, and is more commonly seen in patients with severe angle recession, peripheral anterior synechiae, or those who suffered significant tissue damage secondary to perforating injuries of the eye.

EARLY ONSET POST-TRAUMATIC GLAUCOMA

Blunt trauma to the globe can produce damage to various tissues of the anterior segment including iris sphincter tears, iridodialysis, cyclodialysis, hyphema, trabeculodialysis, inflammation, zonular rupture, and lens dislocation. The individuals most likely to suffer blunt trauma are males in their second to third decades. There is also a significant relationship between blunt trauma and athletics, industrial settings, and home activities.[53] Over 4% of all emergent care rendered in a major urban hospital was for trauma to the globe.[54]

Hyphema

Hyphema, which is red blood cells in the anterior chamber, is one of the most common clinical presentation following blunt trauma to the globe. In a study of 149 cases of hyphema, 88.59% were due to blunt trauma, with over 80% of that trauma acute in nature.[55] Histopathologically, hyphema is most commonly due to a tear in the ciliary body between the longitudinal and circular muscle fibers, resulting in damage to the major arterial circle (iris) located in this area (Figs. 17–9 and 17–10). The mechanism by which the tear is induced is thought to be shortening of the anterior/posterior length of the eye that forces aqueous fluid, under pressure, toward the anterior chamber angle causing tissue damage. The bleeding can ocur at the time of trauma or anytime within the first 7 days following the event.

Clinical Presentation. On clinical examination hyphema can present as minute levels of circulating red blood cells in the anterior chamber or be grossly observable as either layering of blood or as complete filling of the anterior chamber known as an "eight-ball" hyphema. In those patients with a full eight-ball hyphema, it is postulated that the clot formed in the anterior chamber is primarily responsible for the marked increase in IOP.

Clinical assessment of patients with hyphema includes measuring the level of hyphema and the magnitude of the IOP. It is not uncommon to see IOP vary from normal levels to as high as 75 to 80 mm Hg, depending on the level of obstruction of the trabecular meshwork.

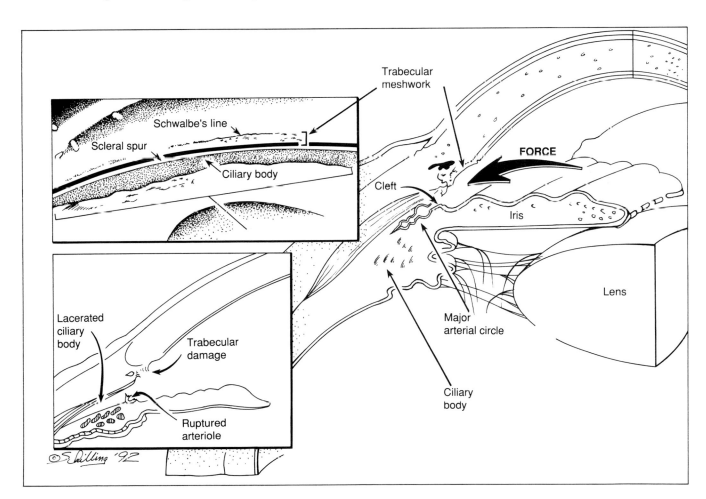

Figure 17–9. Diagram illustrating the structural changes to the anterior segment from ocular trauma. Any part of the angle may be damaged leading to a compromised outflow system. The angle may be recessed or lacerated with either potentially leading to elevated IOP.

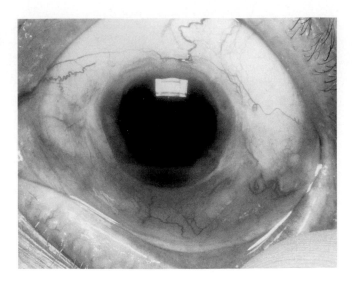

Figure 17–10. Hyphema following blunt trauma to the globe. (*Courtesy of Rodney Gutner, OD.*)

The IOP following an hyphema is most influenced by whether there is a single episode of bleeding followed by resolution of the hemorrhagic material or a secondary bleed or rebleed. Most patients who suffer from a single episode of hemorrhagic activity resolve well with appropriate management. Those who suffer secondary rebleeds are at considerable risk for the development of a secondary glaucoma.[56,57] Rebleeding is one of the most serious complications of hyphema and commonly occurs in the first 5 to 7 days following the initial episode. Incidence rates for secondary hemorrhage following the initial traumatic episode range from 10 to 19%. In patients with sickle hemoglobinopathies, there is a tendency toward elevated IOP following a hyphema.[58,59] This is due to the inability of the sickled cells to pass through the trabecular meshwork because of their lack of pliability.

The relationship between traumatic hyphema and glaucoma is also related to the magnitude of the hemorrhage present at the initial examination. Coles showed that in those individuals whose hemorrhage involved less than half of the anterior chamber, 13.5% developed glaucoma, while in those cases of total hyphema, 57% developed glaucoma.[57] Other factors that assist in determining those most likely to develop increased IOP following hyphema include associated cataract and more than a 2-mm Hg increase in IOP when the patient changes from a sitting to a prone position.

Sequelae following the resolution of the hyphema include angle recession, present in over 50% of hyphema patients; subluxation or dislocation of

the lens; vitreous hemorrhage, which can cause a delayed increase in IOP; and corneal blood staining, which occurs secondary to hemosiderin deposits in the cornea following prolonged elevation of IOP. An increased risk of central retinal artery occlusion occurs in patients presenting with a hyphema due to a prolonged increase in IOP.

The management of the patient with hyphema has undergone a great deal of scrutiny over the last 20 years. Initially, it was felt that bedrest accompanied by bilateral patching and sedation was the appropriate mechanism for limiting the secondary sequelae. Recent studies have demonstrated that this regimen results in no better outcome than permitting limited activities and no patching. In addition, a randomized controlled study of 51 patients showed no significant difference in the rate of rebleeding between those receiving aspirin versus placebos following a hyphema.[60] The use of aminocaproic acid has been shown to significantly lower the incidence rate of rebleed following hyphema.[61,62] The early surgical management of patients who demonstrate prolonged elevation of IOP with the presence of hyphema is not advisable due to the difficulty encountered in persistent hemorrhage following the procedure. The optimal time for the removal of the clot of blood resulting from a hyphema is at 4 days, because the adherence of the clot to the adjacent structures is least at this time. The complete removal of the clot is not necessary in the majority of cases and in many instances will increase the risk of new hemorrhage.

Prognosis. Between 2 and 10% of patients who suffer blunt trauma will develop secondary glaucoma. In individuals who suffer a mild-to-moderate hyphema, the progression to glaucoma is less than 15%. The prognosis for post-traumatic glaucoma is directly related to the severity of the disease and the ability to minimize initial damage secondary to the extreme elevation of IOP. In most instances, topical antiglaucoma therapy is sufficient to manage the short-term rise in IOP. In those instances in which this rise is severe, the necessity for surgical intervention also increases the likelihood for the development of a secondary glaucoma as a sequela to the initial traumatic episode. The only significant success demonstrated in the management of these patients is the use of aminocaproic acid and, more recently, oral steroids to limit the rate of rebleeding and subsequently to decrease the severity of the complications.[63]

Trabecular Injury
Along with hyphema, one of the most common forms of damage to the anterior chamber following blunt

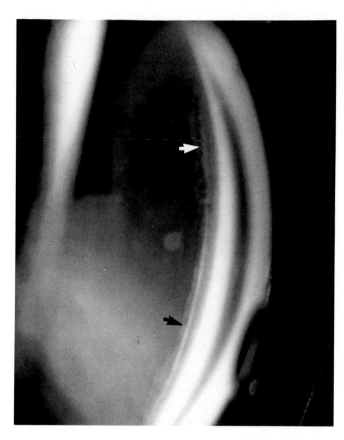

Figure 17–11. Moderate angle recession following blunt trauma. Note the variation in color and depth of the angle at the ciliary recess.

trauma is trabecular injury. The relationship between hyphema and damage to the ciliary body and trabeculum has been well established.[64,65] Angle recession and the associated trabecular injury is a primary cause of both early and late onset glaucoma secondary to blunt trauma, and, as such, represent a significant clinical challenge to the practitioner (Fig. 17–11). Ciliary body injury is the primary clinical sign of the underlying trauma to the trabecular tissue. The healing of the ciliary body results in eventual sclerosis of the trabecular meshwork in that area.[66]

Clinical Presentation. Damage to the ciliary body and the trabecular meshwork can produce a variety of clinical presentations from mild trabecular swelling to complete ciliary body detachment. Examination of the patient with anterior segment trauma must be performed bilaterally in order to adequately assess subtle clinical variations. Signs of angle damage include increased visibility of the scleral spur and ciliary body in one quadrant or, if more extensive, in one eye relative to the other. Also, the trabecular meshwork may be torn with small tags of iris tissue found adherent to the scleral spur and the anterior portion

of the ciliary body. Another subtle finding, immediately following the trauma, is the presence of hemorrhages in the trabecular meshwork accompanied by minor tears in the tissue structure. These clinical signs of angle damage are frequently missed because of their transient nature.

The level of IOP elevation in most instances is related to the amount of damage incurred at the time of trauma. One of the most common causes of short-term elevation of IOP is aqueous blockage secondary to mild iritis or trabecular swelling. Individuals who present with this form of elevated IOP are usually easily managed with short-term topical beta blockers, topical steroids, and carbonic anhydrase inhibitors. They show no long-term secondary effects from the IOP elevation.

More substantial damage to the anterior chamber angle can result in ciliary body recession and tearing of the trabecular meshwork. Elevation of IOP following this type of injury presents in two basic patterns. The first and most common is a temporary rise in IOP, which is managed with topical beta blockers and/or carbonic anhydrase inhibitors and usually produces no immediate damage to the nerve head or visual field. These individuals require chronic observation just like a glaucoma suspect because of the relatively high incidence of late-onset glaucoma.[64] The second type of elevation of IOP was described by Chandler and Grant[5] and occurs within several days to weeks following the original trauma but can occur as late as 2 years later.

In more significant cases of trauma, the disruptions of the anterior chamber angle involves cleavage of the longitudinal muscles of the ciliary body, which produces a widening and deepening of the anterior chamber angle in that area. This is known as angle recession. Angle recession can vary from a few degrees to a circumferential appearance and is generally quite striking when compared to adjacent normal tissue in the same eye or in comparison to the fellow eye.[67] Ciliary body coloration can be a clue to the extent of the recession. The ciliary muscle appears light gray or tan, with the normal ciliary body adjacent to the damaged area substantially darker. In those cases in which the damage is extensive with a full thickness rupture of the muscle, the scleral wall will be exposed as in a cyclodialysis cleft (Fig. 17–12).[67,68] Occasionally, accompanying a full thickness tear of the ciliary body, one can visualize small anterior ciliary arteries on the scleral surface. A rare finding following blunt trauma to the globe is peripheral anterior synechia, which, if significant, can actually obscure the view of the underlying angle recession.

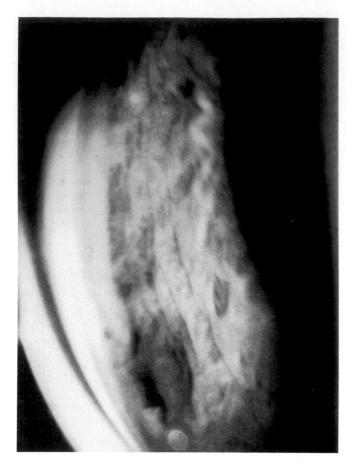

Figure 17–12. Severe angle recession. Note how wide open the angle appears. (*See also* Color Plate 17–12.)

Differential Diagnosis. The differential diagnosis of the individual with acute anterior segment trauma and elevation of IOP is primarily related to the exclusion of those entities, which can also produce an elevation of IOP, and were present but undiagnosed in the patient prior to the trauma. These include pseudoexfoliation syndrome, pigmentary dispersion syndrome, primary open-angle glaucoma, and subacute or intermittent angle closure glaucoma. All of these conditions present with clinical signs and symptoms not typical of those seen in traumatic angle disease and should be readily differentiated with a thorough physical examination.

Prognosis. Armaly found that individuals who suffer an acute rise in IOP after trauma to the globe, show a positive steroid response in their fellow uninjured eye at a rate consistent with patients with primary open-angle glaucoma.[69,79] This leads to speculation that these individuals have a genetic pre-

disposition for development of elevated IOP, which could help explain why many patients suffer blunt trauma to the globe, but only a few eventually develop glaucoma.

Still, the degree of angle recession appears to be the most sensitive indicator for long-term prognosis relative to the development of IOP and early onset glaucoma.[69,70] Chandler and Grant[5] feel that in individuals in which only a small portion of the anterior chamber angle is involved in traumatic recession, the incidence of intractable glaucoma is relatively low. Patients who develop an elevation of IOP soon after trauma are usually managed with standard treatment regimens and followed as glaucoma suspects once IOP has returned to normal.

LATE ONSET POST-TRAUMATIC GLAUCOMA

Unlike those individuals who experience an elevation in IOP shortly following a traumatic episode, some do not develop elevated pressure until years after the original event. The major causes of this late development of glaucoma are angle recession and penetrating injuries.[70]

Angle Recession

Clinical Presentation. As previously mentioned, angle recession is common following blunt trauma to the globe. Late onset glaucoma occurs in a relatively small number of people who suffer blunt trauma. Those individuals who are most likely to develop late onset glaucoma have significant angle damage, which involves approximately two thirds to three quarters of the anterior chamber angle and may include tearing of the longitudinal muscles of the ciliary body, recession or retraction of the anterior chamber, and damage to the trabecular meshwork. They also have a much higher incidence of full thickness tears with evidence of exposure of the scleral wall. Occasionally, damage to the trabecular meshwork will be present as incision-like gaps in the area that overlies Schlemm's canal and may well involve the canal itself. Initially, the IOP is low, which is likely due to the direct access of the aqueous to the outflow channel. Once this access has been blocked secondary to the deposition of fibrotic tissue and subsequent scarring, the IOP usually elevates dramatically.[71]

Sclerosis of the trabecular meshwork is one possible mechanism for the development of late onset glaucoma syndrome. Another is the presence of a hyaline-like membrane that extends from the corneal endothelium following trauma, blocking the outflow of aqueous through the trabecular meshwork.[62,69]

Prognosis. Although IOP is initially normal in late onset glaucoma, occasionally individuals present with relative hypotony secondary to either a decrease in aqueous production or the establishment of a small suprachoroidal cleft that allows for direct shunting of aqueous fluid. Unfortunately, once the IOP elevation starts, it tends to be dramatic and difficult to manage. In some instances, the glaucoma is so severe as to be unresponsive to medical management.

The overall outlook for success in late onset glaucoma is difficult to assess. There is evidence that the damage to the ciliary body is not necessarily the cause of the eventual rise in IOP, but is instead a clinical sign that underscores the level of trauma to the corneoscleral trabecular meshwork and other components of the outflow system. Interestingly, it has been demonstrated that in those individuals who develop late onset angle closure glaucoma, the facility of outflow and the IOP in the fellow eye were both abnormal. This gives rise to the possibility that individuals may well have a predisposition for glaucoma, which is present prior to the traumatic episode, and may help explain the late onset of the disease.

Penetrating Injuries

One of the most devastating insults to the eye is that of a penetrating injury. It may produce a number of significant alterations in tissue structure and physiological function. Penetrating injuries include mechanical disruption of the anterior chamber angle or ciliary body, lens damage with subsequent intraocular inflammation, and retained foreign bodies. The source of these injuries is diverse. In a large study of penetrating injuries, 22% were secondary to blunt force, 37% were the result of lacerations, and 41% were caused by high velocity objects.[72] It is not surprising that the incidence of penetrating injuries to the globe is significantly greater in males and in younger age groups. This is consistent with data on the incidence of other conditions such as hyphema and blunt trauma.

There are several mechanisms that produce elevation of IOP following perforating injury. Most common is the anatomical disturbance secondary to peripheral anterior synechiae (Fig. 17–13).[73] Peripheral anterior synechiae can occur from prolonged presence of a flattened anterior chamber and iridocorneal contact. This is most commonly seen when inadequate wound closure is present. The wound leak causes continued reduction in IOP. Another cause of

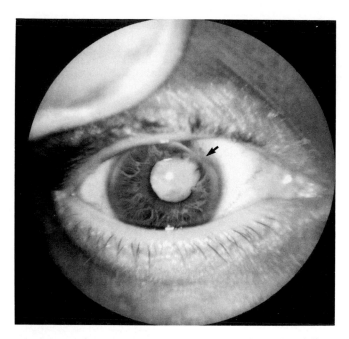

Figure 17–13. Peripheral anterior synechiae formation following anterior segment trauma.

peripheral anterior synechia is the inflammatory response that occurs following the traumatic episode. Topical cycloplegics are required during the immediate post-traumatic period along with anti-inflammatory agents to limit the inflammatory response. Unsuccessful cycloplegia may lead to seclusion of the pupil resulting in pupillary block. In some instances, the inflammatory response is severe enough to produce a cyclitic membrane that can also cause closure of the anterior chamber angle.[74]

Another significant sequela of a penetrating injury that can cause glaucoma is epithelial in-growth. It appears as a grayish membrane on the posterior corneal surface that can cause obstruction of the trabecular meshwork.[75] The mechanism for epithelial in-growth is thought to be related to the introduction of epithelial cells either from the trauma itself or the subsequent wound repair.

Intraocular foreign bodies present a unique challenge to the clinician. The secondary effects of siderosis (iron rust) and chalcosis (copper oxidation) result in significant tissue damage which can result in the development of glaucoma. The mechanism is believed to be related to the impairment of aqueous outflow secondary to iron and copper damage.[76,77]

Clinical Presentation. In individuals with peripheral anterior synechiae secondary to hypotony, the central chamber will be somewhat formed but the periphery shows consistent contact of the iris to the posterior cornea. The IOP is usually quite low, frequently at 1 to 2 mm Hg, and is difficult to measure because of the softness of the globe. The presence of an idiopathic filtration bleb is possible but not necessary to justify the low IOP. The clinician may also see an irregular crocodile shagreen to the corneal surface, due to the gross reduction of IOP.

Present in the early course of the inflammatory response to the injury will be areas of iris adhesion to the anterior lens surface, posterior synechiae. This appears as mounded zones of pigment at the pupillary margin, and, on dilation, as points of adhesion that produce an irregular pupillary border. As the disease progresses, if the clinician is unable to fully dilate the pupil and relieve these iridolenticular adhesions, the initial areas may progress to a full 360° iris-lens touch. This effectively stops the forward flow of aqueous from the posterior chamber, producing iris bombé. Cyclitic membrane development is seen primarily in those individuals who have a severe inflammatory response, which presents a sticky, thick protein component (4+ flare) in the anterior chamber. This is followed by the development of a membrane that can span either the pupil or, using anterior chamber tissue, scaffold the anterior chamber angle producing either iris to corneal adhesion and/or pupillary seclusion.

Approximately 50% of eyes injured by metallic intraocular foreign bodies show lens capsule damage. Other clinical findings are heterochromia, siderotic or chalcotic staining of the anterior segment tissue, unexplained unilateral mydriasis, or the presence of a corneal scar with aligned transillumination defect of the iris. These findings in the presence of unilateral elevated IOP should alert the practitioner to the possibility of glaucoma secondary to a retained intraocular foreign body.

Differential Diagnosis. The differential diagnosis of late onset glaucoma includes conditions that can produce unilateral glaucoma such as asymmetrical primary open-angle glaucoma, exfoliative glaucoma, and pigmentary dispersion. These present with a variety of clinical signs and symptoms that assist the clinician in their differential diagnosis.

The entities that can produce clinical findings similar to those of penetrating injury are few in number. Among the most common are Fuch's heterochromic iridocyclitis, phakoanaphylactic glaucoma secondary to hypermature lens rupture, and blunt trauma without penetration, but with significant sequelae. In Fuch's heterochromic iridocyclitis, there is no history or physical findings indicative of a penetrating foreign body. The asymmetry of iris color, unilateral elevated IOP, and the presence of cataract in many of these individuals is not dissimilar to that noted in retained intraocular foreign body. In phakoanaphylactic glaucoma, it is likely that the patient's age and the examination of the fellow eye, which will show advanced lens changes in most instances, will be sufficient to steer the clinician toward the correct diagnosis.

Blunt trauma without penetrating injury may be the most difficult to differentially diagnose. Because of the many similarities seen in these two conditions, it is initially a clinical challenge to assure oneself that penetration is not the cause of the underlying problems. Radiographic evaluation including the use of computed tomography scans may be needed to effectively establish the diagnosis.

STEROID-INDUCED GLAUCOMA

Etiology. Francois demonstrated that prolonged use of hydrocortisone in certain individuals resulted in an elevation in IOP that was relieved by the discontinuation of the drug.[78] Topical, systemic, periocular injections, facial creams or lotions containing corticosteroids can cause this effect. Steroids are used clinically in the prolonged treatment of ocular conditions such as uveitis and systemically for the treatment of asthma, collagen vascular diseases, and in immunosuppressive therapy. Agents such as prednisolone acetate are most likely to initiate an IOP rise while steroids in the fluoromethalone category produce a minimal response due to low concentration and penetration of the drug. These factors can be used in intelligent drug selection, routes of administration, the selection of patients who should receive steroid treatment, and the frequency of follow-up.

A substantial amount of the research in steroid-induced glaucoma has been directed at identifying those individuals most susceptible to this type of reaction. These studies indicate patients with primary open-angle glaucoma, myopia, and direct relatives of primary open-angle glaucoma patients are more likely to demonstrate a positive response than the general population.[79-81]

TABLE 17–1. POSITIVE CORTICOSTEROID RESPONSE

Low response	<5 mm Hg	60%
Intermediate response	6–15 mm Hg	35%
High response	>15 mm Hg	5%

Armaly in his classical series of studies on steroid responders was able to demonstrate three distinct response levels (Table 17–1). The low response group showed an increase in IOP of less than 5 mm Hg after 4 weeks of steroid use, while the intermediate and high response groups had a pressure rise greater than 15 mm Hg.[82,83] The low response group (one) showed an elevation in pressure for only the first 2 weeks after which the pressure began to decline, whereas the intermediate response group (two) and the high response group (three) showed continued elevation of pressure throughout the 4-week cycle, the only difference being the magnitude of that rise. Armaly also found that increased concentrations and/or dosage of steroids were more likely to elicit a response.

Steroid-induced ocular hypertension in normal eyes is genetically determined. Becker and associates proposed that primary open-angle glaucoma is a genetically determined disease, expressed by a single gene.[81] Using the results of IOP responses to steroids in normal individuals, Armaly contradicted this concept and proposed that glaucoma is determined by multifactorial inheritance. He hypothesized that the three types of IOP responses to topical steroids were phenotypes for an allele pair, P^l, P^h, where P^l determined a low level of response, and P^h a high level of response. Thus, the genotype P^lP^l, P^lP^h, and P^hP^h represented the low, intermediate, and high response groups to topical steroids.[82] Armaly's studies of offspring of glaucoma patients demonstrated the various genotypes in the frequency predicted from their parental genotype classification. Individuals with genotype P^lP^h had an 18 times and those with P^hP^h a 100 times greater probability of developing glaucoma than an individual with P^lP^l.[83]

Steroid-induced effects can result from abnormal levels of endogenously produced steroids such as adrenal corticotropin hormone (ACTH). In individuals who suffer from adrenal syndromes such as Cushing's disease, IOP is reduced and the facility of outflow is improved following adrenal surgery.

Pathophysiology. The mechanism of steroid-induced elevation of IOP is believed to be due to alterations in the outflow of aqueous.[84] Investigators have identified several possible mechanisms. These include the accumulation of glycosaminoglycans in the outflow channels, the potentiation of 5-beta dihydrocortisol, and a decrease of phagocytic activity in the trabecular endothelium.[85,86] Glycosaminoglycans located in the anterior chamber angle become hydrated creating an obstruction secondary to edema, which increases the resistance to aqueous outflow.[87] 5-beta dihydrocortisol has been shown to potentiate the hy-

pertensive effects of dexamethasone in animal studies and has been postulated to have a similar effect in humans.[86] Decreased levels of phagocytic activity in the trabecular endothelium may be responsible for the accumulation of debris noted in electron microscopic studies of the trabecular meshwork in individuals with steroid-induced glaucoma.[88] No single mechanism has been proven as the sole pathophysiological process responsible for steroid-induced glaucoma, and it may well be that a combination of all these effects produces the elevation of IOP.

Clinical Presentation. Clinically, corticosteroid-induced elevation of IOP is asymptomatic, similar to primary open-angle glaucoma. The IOP rise is generally bilateral, unless the patient is being treated for a unilateral problem. In steroid responders IOP can rise to dramatic levels but rarely does the patient achieve symptomatology similar to a closed angle attack.

The physical examination findings are typical of primary open-angle glaucoma, including an open anterior chamber angle without evidence of secondary changes, glaucomatous changes in the optic nerve, and abnormalities of the visual field consistent with glaucomatous damage. The response to corticosteroids is more common with topical treatment than oral regimens but any patient on steroid therapy should receive a base-line IOP evaluation and follow-up should occur at intervals appropriate to the level of steroid treatment. All patients being treated with steroids should have IOP measurements at every office visit.

Differential Diagnosis. The differential diagnosis of steroid-induced glaucoma includes primary open-angle glaucoma. The differentiating factor is the awareness of the relationship between steroid use and an elevation in IOP. Particular attention should be paid to the potential use of over-the-counter medications that may contain corticosteroid-based products.

Prognosis. The first phase of management for individuals with steroid-induced glaucoma is that of discontinuation of the drug. In most instances, the IOP returns to relatively normal levels within 1 to 4 weeks. There appears to be a relationship between the duration of IOP elevation following discontinuation and the length of time that the patient was treated. Espildora showed that in patients treated for less than 2 months, the pressure normalized in all instances, but, in those treated for greater than 4 years, there remained a chronic elevation of IOP.[89] In individuals with a positive corticosteroid response who cannot be taken off the anti-inflammatory agents, treatment with topical antiglaucoma medications can be initiated until the underlying disease resolves and steroids can be discontinued. In those instances in which the glaucoma is refractory to topical control, the use of laser trabeculoplasty or filtering procedures must be considered. Undoubtedly, the worst prognostic indicator for individuals with steroid-induced glaucoma is the lack of recognition on the part of the practitioner of the underlying etiology.

NEOVASCULAR GLAUCOMA

Etiology. Neovascular glaucoma is a condition associated with elevation of IOP due to synechial closure of the anterior chamber angle secondary to the formation of fibrovascular membranes that obstructs the outflow of aqueous.[90] The fibrovascular membranes result from rubeosis irides, a network of fine vessels that arborize on the surface of the iris, and eventually grow into the anterior chamber angle (Fig. 17–14). There has been a great deal of confusion regarding the terminology used to describe this disease. It has been called thrombotic glaucoma, hemorrhagic glaucoma, congestive glaucoma, and, in some instances, confused with hemolytic glaucoma. Hemolytic glaucoma is due to the blockage of aqueous outflow by the accumulation of ghost cells in the trabecular meshwork, following a vitreous hemorrhage. Weiss, in 1962, coined the term neovascular glaucoma, which is the one most commonly used today.[91]

Pathophysiology. There appears to be little controversy that hypoxia is the stimulus for the neovascular response in the eye. A vasoproliferative factor similar to that postulated as the cause of proliferative retinopathy seems to also cause rubeosis irides. This vasoproliferative or angiogenic factor is thought to be elaborated by hypoxic retinal tissue in an attempt to

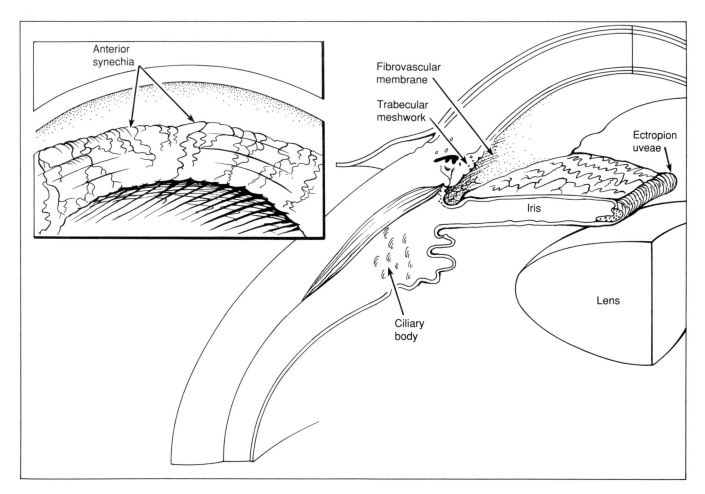

Figure 17–14. New blood vessels occur at the pupil margin, growing over the iris surface towards the angle. The fine vessels grow into the angle, accompanied by a fibrovascular membrane that may contract zippering the angle shut.

revascularize the areas. The factor diffuses through the vitreous and posterior chamber to the iris and induces a similar neovascular response to that occurring in the retina. Agents that have been postulated as potential angiogenic factors include prostaglandins,[92] biogenic amines,[93] and activated macrophages.[94]

Predisposing Factors. Neovascular glaucoma develops following a wide variety of ophthalmic diseases.[95,96] Among the more common are central retinal vein occlusion, branch retinal vein occlusion, central retinal artery occlusion, carotid occlusive disease, diabetic retinopathy, chronic retinal detachment, and heterochromic iridocyclitis. The two most common disease states associated with retinal neovascularization are central retinal vein occlusion and diabetic retinopathy.[96]

Central Retinal Vein Occlusion

Central retinal vein occlusion is a relatively common cause of neovascular glaucoma although the incidence rates are quite variable.[97] The difficulty in managing patients with central retinal vein occlusion has been in predicting those most likely to advance to neovascular glaucoma so that appropriate intervention can occur. Hayreh, in his study on central retinal vein occlusion, was able to demonstrate two distinct categories of patients based on the presence or absence of retinal ischemia.[98] Other investigators have also shown that ischemic central retinal vein occlusion results in a markedly higher incidence of rubeosis irides than the non-ischemic varieties.[99]

Rubeosis irides following central retinal vein occlusion frequently leads to "90-day" glaucoma. This is due to the natural history of the disease in which the majority of patients have the initial onset of rubeosis and an increase in IOP within 3 months following the retinal vascular event.

Some clinical studies have found a relationship between primary open-angle glaucoma and central retinal vein occlusion.[100,101]

The relationship between IOP and central retinal vein occlusion is somewhat complex. Initially following the inciting episode, the IOP may be low. Yet, a significant percentage of patients with central retinal vein occlusion either have ocular hypertension or glaucoma at the time of the retinal vascular accident.

Branch retinal vein occlusion, although more common than central retinal vein occlusion, results in a lower incidence of neovascular glaucoma.[102] Interestingly, even though branch retinal vein occlusion rarely causes anterior segment neovascularization, it

has been implicated in the development of neovascularization of the retina.

Diabetic Retinopathy

Patients with diabetic retinopathy reveal striking differences with respect to the development of neovascular glaucoma depending on the presence of proliferative changes. In patients with background retinopathy, the incidence of neovascular glaucoma is approximately 5%.[103] In those with proliferative retinopathy, the incidence may be as high as 50%.[104]

Other factors that influence the development of neovascular glaucoma in patients with diabetic retinopathy include cataract extraction, vitrectomy/lensectomy procedures, and retinal attachment surgery. The risk of the development of neovascular glaucoma in patients with diabetic retinopathy is considered to be less after extracapsular cataract extraction than intracapsular primarily due to the maintenance of the anterior hyaloid surface and posterior capsule, which are thought to act as a barrier to the movement of the angiogenic factor from the retina to the iris. The time frame for development of neovascular glaucoma following cataract surgery is within the first month postoperative, necessitating careful surgical follow-up. The development of neovascular glaucoma is five times greater in patients with a combined vitrectomy/lensectomy than with only a vitrectomy.

Chronic retinal detachment unrelated to diabetic retinopathy has also been implicated in the development of neovascularization of the anterior segment. These cases are frequently associated with other underlying conditions that may be instrumental in the pathogenesis of neovascular glaucoma, such as malignant melanoma, Coat's disease, retrolental fibroplasia, and sickle cell retinopathy.

Clinical Presentation. The clinical presentation of neovascular glaucoma is relatively consistent regardless of the underlying etiology. Initially, the disease presents with small dilated capillaries at the pupillary margin and, occasionally, vessel arborization on the surface of the iris near the pupil (Fig. 17–15). The anterior chamber angle is usually clear of vessel activity, in this early phase, although some individuals show a very delicate network of fine capillary activity. Fluorescein angiography demonstrates leakage in and around the pupillary margin. Unfortunately, this pattern of peripapillary leakage is also noted in some elderly non-diabetic patients. Therefore, its predictive value is somewhat limited.[105] The IOP in the early phase is usually normal.

The mid-phase in the development of neovascular glaucoma occurs when the anterior chamber angle

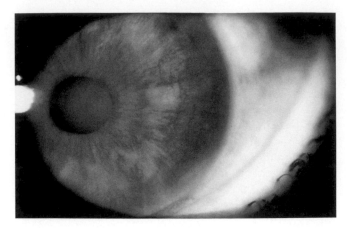

Figure 17–15. Early neovascular changes seen at the pupillary zone and mid-periphery of the iris. (*See also* Color Plate 17–15.)

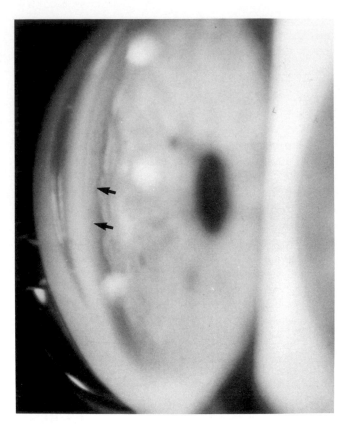

Figure 17–16. Moderate neovascular glaucoma. New blood vessels are seen in the angle. (*Courtesy of Rodney Gutner, OD.*)

becomes involved. The new vessels growth and fibrovascular membrane on the surface of the iris are clearly defined, frequently showing radial progression with areas of arborization that have an irregular pattern. The time frame to achieve this level of neovascularization is variable. Gonioscopy shows these vessels crossing the ciliary body band and scleral spur and occasionally appearing to derive directly from vessels in the ciliary body (Fig. 17–16). Chandler and Grant[5] found that all normal vessels are located posterior to scleral spur. Therefore the vessels that arborize over the trabecular meshwork up to Schwalbe's line are assumed to be abnormal vascularization of the angle. During this mid-phase, some patients may present with a hyphema. The IOP is elevated and subject to spikes, due to the obstruction of aqueous outflow (Fig. 17–17).

In the late phase of neovascular glaucoma, the fibrovascular membrane contracts, producing peripheral anterior synechiae that usually begin in one quadrant. The synechiae can progress to a complete 360° closure of the angle, described as being "zippered shut" (Fig. 17–14). There is also a loss of texture of the iris surface and the appearance of ectropion uvea. Ectropion uvea is secondary to the retraction of the pupillary margin by the fibrovascular membrane exposing the posterior pigmented surface of the iris. A potentially confusing appearance on gonioscopy is the presence of an endothelial sheet contiguous with the endothelium of the cornea. This endothelial change follows synechial closure, creating a pseudoangle. In this phase, the patient usually has a significant reduction in visual acuity, extreme elevation of IOP, corneal edema, gross congestion of the globe, and inflammatory activity in the anterior chamber.

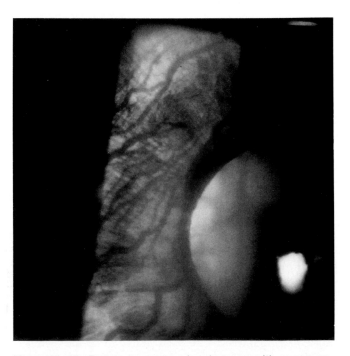

Figure 17–17. Endstage neovascular glaucoma with severe vessel development in the anterior chamber angle.

Differential Diagnosis. The differential diagnosis of neovascular glaucoma involves consideration of conditions that can independently produce rubeosis irides without the underlying retinal vascular disease. Primary among these is Fuch's heterochromic iridocyclitis, which can present with rubeosis irides and an elevation of IOP. Fortunately, these patients usually present with a white quiet eye as opposed to the intense engorgement of the globe seen in the late phase of neovascular glaucoma. The appearance of new vessel growth on the iris in heterochromic iridocyclitis tends to be finer in texture relative to the coarse, somewhat engorged vessels seen in neovascular glaucoma. Intraocular inflammation must also be considered in any differential diagnosis of neovascular glaucoma. Classically, these eyes present with a significant anterior chamber reaction, with the neovascular component usually resolving following treatment with topical anti-inflammatory agents. Intraocular hemorrhage (hyphema) of unknown etiology should always be considered as a prelude to neovascular glaucoma even when presenting with normal IOP. A physical examination of the anterior chamber angle and iris is required to rule out neovascular changes.

Prognosis. It was not long ago that the only expected outcome of neovascular glaucoma was an extremely painful blind eye that required enucleation. The current use of photocoagulation of the retina as the primary step in management of proliferative retinopathy has resulted in a significant reduction in neovascular glaucoma, and an improvement of the management of the glaucoma if it occurs.[106] Recent studies have demonstrated reasonable levels of success along with significant complications in the use of drainage implants to treat neovascular glaucoma.[107]

TABLE 17–2. COMPARISON OF SECONDARY GLAUCOMAS

Type of Glaucoma	Biomicropscopic Findings	Gonioscopy	IOP	Characteristics	Prognosis
Pigmentary	Krukenberg's spindle Iris transillumination Pigment on lens/iris surface	Pigment of trabecular meshwork	Variable increase Diurnal fluctuation	Bilateral Onset 20–40 y/o Myopia	Generally good Diminish with age
Exfoliative	Gray flake-like deposits at pupil frill Anterior lens annular zone Iris transillumination	Pigment in trabecular meshwork (less than PDS) Increased incidence of narrow angle	Variable, can show rapid increase	Onset 60 y/o and greater	IOP difficult to control ALT effective
Steroid induced	No characteristic findings	No abnormalities	Usually noted 4–6 weeks after initiation of topical steroid therapy	Family history of glaucoma Concurrent disease treatment with steroids	IOP usually decreases on cessation of steroid
Traumatic	Hyphema Sphincter tear Inflammation Lens subluxation	PAS[a] Angle recession (variable degree) Iris tags Variation in color of ciliary body	Hypotony to extreme elevation, depending on extent of trauma	No specific factors	Variable depending on degree of trauma
Neovascular	Vessels visible on iris surface Hyphema	Arborized vessels in angle PAS Fibrovascular membrane	Initially low, rises with time to extreme levels	Diabetes CRVO BRVO Intraocular surgery	Poor prognosis
Congenital	Corneal edema Descemet's tears Increased corneal diameter	Anterior insertion of iris root Abnormality of trabecular meshwork	IOP lower than adult to produce same level of damage, 20–40 mm Hg	Can be associated with systemic disease	Related to age of onset and severity of disease

y/o = years old; IOP = intraocular pressure; PAS = peripheral anterior synechiae; PDS = pigment dispersion syndrome; CRVO = central retinal vein occlusion; BRVO = branch retinal vein occlusion.

CONCLUSION

The diagnosis and treatment of secondary glaucomas is an important and challenging aspect of the overall management of glaucomas (Table 17–2). Because of the variation of their presentation and the frequent association with underlying ocular and/or systemic disease processes, the primary care clinician is required to have a firm understanding of the anatomy, pathophysiology, differential diagnosis, and treatments for this category of glaucomas.

REFERENCES

1. Teikari JM, O'Donnell J. Epidemiologic data on adult glaucomas. Data from the Hospital Registry of Right to Free Medication. *Acta Ophthalmol.*1989;67(2):184–191.
2. Sugar HS, Barbour FA. Pigmentary glaucoma: Rare clinical entity. *Am J Ophthalmol.* 1949;32:90.
3. Epstein DL. Pigment dispersion and pigmentary glaucoma. In: Chandler PA, Grant WM eds., *Glaucoma.* Philadelphia: Lea & Febiger; 1979:122.
4. Farrar SM, Shields MB, Miller KN, et al: Risk Factors for the Development and Severity of Glaucoma in the Pigment Dispersion Syndrome. *Am J Ophthalmol.* 1989;108(3):223–229.
5. Chandler PA, Grant WM. *Glaucoma.* Philadelphia: Lea & Febiger; 1986:201.
6. Campbell DG. Pigmentary dispersion and glaucoma. A new theory. *Arch Ophthalmol.* 1979;97:1667–1672.
7. Kampik A, Green WR, Quigley HA, et al. Scanning electron micrograph studies of two cases of pigment dispersion syndrome. *Am J Ophthalmol.* 1981;91:573.
8. Davidson JA, Brubaker RF, Ilstrup DM. Dimensions of the anterior chamber in pigment dispersion syndrome. *Arch Ophthalmol.* 1983;101:81.
9. Peterson HP. Can pigmentary deposits on the trabecular meshwork increase the resistance to aqueous outflow? *Acta Ophthalmol.* 1963;47:743–749.
10. Grant WM. Experimental aqueous perfusion in enucleated human eyes. *Arch Ophthalmol.* 1963;69:783–801.
11. Kristensen P. Mydriasis induced pigment liberation in the anterior chamber associated with acute rise in intraocular pressure in open-angle glaucoma. *Acta Ophthalmol.* 1965;43:714–716.
12. Rohen JW, Van Der Zypen E. The phagocytic activity of the trabecular meshwork endothelium: An electron microscopic study of the vervet. *Graefe's Arch Clin Exp Ophthalmol.* 1988;175:143–146.
13. Richardson TM, Hutchinson BT, Grant WM. The overflow tract in pigmentary glaucoma: A light and electron microscopic study. *Arch Ophthalmol.* 1989;227(4):335–339.
14. Piccolino FC, Calabria G, Polizzi A, et al. Pigmentary retinal dystrophy associated with pigmentary glaucoma. *Graefe's Arch Clin Exp Ophthalmol.* 1989;227(4):335–339.
15. Speakman JS. Pigmentary dispersion. *Br J Ophthalmol.* 1986;65:249–253.
16. Richter CV, Richardson TM, Grant WM. Pigment dispersion syndrome and pigmentary glaucoma. A prospective study of the natural history. *Arch Ophthalmol.* 1986;104:211–215.
17. Wilensky JT, Buerk KM, Podos SM. Krukenberg's spindles. *Am J Ophthalmol.* 1975;79:220–224.
18. Donaldson DD. Transillumination of the iris. *Trans Am Ophthalmol Soc.* 1974;LXXII:89.
19. Scheie HG, Fleischhaver HW. Idiopathic atrophy of the epithelial layers of the iris and ciliary body. A clinical study. *Arch Ophthalmol.* 1958;59:216.
20. Alward Wl, Munden PM, Verdick RE, et al. Use of infrared videography to detect and record iris transillumination defects. *Arch Ophthalmol.* 1990;108(5):748–750.
21. Lichter PR. Pigmentary glaucoma—Current concepts. *Trans Am Acad Ophthalmol Otol.* 1974;78:309–312.
22. Scheie HG, Cameron JD. Pigment dispersion syndrome: A clinical study. *Br J Ophthalmol.* 1981;65:264.
23. Laydon WE, Ritch R, King DG, et al. Combined exfoliation and pigment dispersion syndrome. *Am J Ophthalmol.* 1990;109(5):530–534.
24. Pignalosa B, Toni F, Liguori G. Pigmentary dispersion syndrome subsequent IOL implantation in P.C. *Doc Ophthalmol.* 1989;73(3):231–234.
25. Dvorak TG. Pseudoexfoliation of the lens capsule: Relation to "true" exfoliation of the lens capsule as reported in the literature and role in production of glaucoma capsulocuticucare. *Trans Am Ophthalmol Soc.* 1953;51:653.
26. Layden WE, Shaffer RN. The exfoliation syndrome. *Am J Ophthalmol.* 1974;78:835.
27. Hansen E, Sellevold OJ. Pseudoexfoliation of the lens capsule. II. Development of the exfoliation syndrome. *Acta Ophthalmol.* 1969;47:161.
28. Aasved H. The frequency of fibrillopathia epitheliocapsularis (so called senile exfoliation or pseudoexfoliation) in patients with open angle glaucoma. *Acta Ophthalmol.* 1971;49:194.
29. Slagsvold JE, Nordhagen R. The HLA system in primary open angle glaucoma and in patients with pseudoexfoliation of the lens capsule (exfoliation or fibrillopathia epitheliocapsularis). *Acta Ophthalmol.* 1980;58:188.
30. Ringvold A, Husby G. Pseudoexfoliation material—an amyloid like substance. *Exp Eye Res.* 1973;17:289.
31. Harnisch JP, Barrach HJ, Hassell JR, et al. Identification of a basement membrane proteoglycan in exfoliation material. *Graefe's Arch Ophthalmol.* 1981;215:273.
32. Ritch R, Shields B. *The Secondary Glaucomas.* St. Louis, C.V. Mosby; 1982:108.
33. Toriyama K, Maezawa N. Electron microscopic study

on the trabecular tissues in glaucoma capsulare. *Acta Soc Ophthalmol Jpn*. 1976;80:780.

34. Aasved H. Intraocular pressure in eyes with and without fibrillopathia epitheliocapsulars (so-called senile exfoliation or pseudoexfoliation). *Acta Ophthalmol*. 1971;49:601.

35. Junndal T. In: Cairns JE, ed. Open angle glaucoma and pseudoexfoliation syndrome. Philadelphia: Grune & Stratton; 1986.

36. Prince AM, Ritch R. Clinical signs of the pseudo-exfoliation syndrome. *Ophthalmology*. 1986;93:803–807.

37. Layden WE, Schaffer RN. Exfoliation syndrome. *Am J Ophthalmol*. 1974;78:835.

38. Bartholomew RS. Lens displacement associated with pseudocapsular exfoliation. *Br J Ophthalmol*. 1970;54:744.

39. Sugar HS, Harding C, Barksy D. The exfoliation syndrome. *Ann Ophthalmol*. 1976;10:1165.

40. Ghosh M, Speakman JS. The iris in senile exfoliation of the lens. *Can J Ophthalmol*. 1974;9:289–297.

41. Sugar S. Pigmentary glaucoma associated with the pseudoexfoliation syndrome: Update. *Ophthalmology*. 1984;91:307.

42. Kozart DM, Yanoff M. Intraocular pressure status in 100 consecutive patients with exfoliation syndrome. *Ophthalmology*. 1982;89:214.

43. Valle O. Prevalence of simple and capsular glaucoma in the central hospital district of Kotka. *Acta Ophthalmol*. 1988;814:116.

44. Lindblom B, Thornburn W. Prevalence of visual field defects due to capsular and simple glaucoma in Halsingland, Sweden. *Acta Ophthalmol*. 1982;60:353.

45. Slagsvold JE. The follow-up in patients with pseudoexfoliation of the lens capsule with and without glaucoma. 2. The development of glaucoma in persons with pseudoexfoliation. *Acta Ophthalmol*. 1986;64:241.

46. Henry JC, Krypin T, Schmitt M, et al. Long-term follow-up pseudoexfoliation and the development of elevated intraocular pressure. *Ophthalmology*. 1987;94:545.

47. Brooks AM, Gices WE. The presentation and prognosis of glaucoma in pseudoexfoliation of the lens capsule. *Ophthalmology*. 1988;95:271.

48. Hetherington J Jr. Capsular glaucoma: Management philosophy. *Acta Ophthalmol*. 1988;184:138.

49. Svedbergh B. Argon laser trabeculoplasty in capsular glaucoma. *Acta Ophthalmol (Suppl)* 1988;184:141.

50. Raitta C. Filtering surgery in capsular glaucoma. *Acta Ophthalmol*. 1988;184:148.

51. Jerndal T, Kriisa U. Results of trabeculectomy for pseudoexfoliative glaucoma. *Br J Ophthalmol* 1974;58:927.

52. Petti TH, Keats EV. Traumatic change of the chamber angle. *Arch Ophthalmol*. 1963;69:438.

53. Canavan YM, Archer DB. Anterior segment conse-quences of blunt ocular injury. *Br J Ophthalmol*. 1982;66:549.

54. Yospaiboon Y, Sangveejit J, Suwanwatana C. Traumatic hyphema: Clinical study of 149 cases. *J Med Assoc Thailand*. 1989;72(9):520.

55. Howard GM, et al. Hyphema resulting from blunt trauma. *Trans Am Acad Ophthalmol Otolaryngol*. 1965;69:294–306.

56. Edwards WC, Layden WE. Traumatic hyphema. A report of 184 consecutive cases. *Am J Ophthalmol*. 1973;75:110.

57. Coles WH. Traumatic hyphema: An analysis of 235 cases. *South Med J*. 1968;61:813.

58. Goldberg MF. The diagnosis and treatment of secondary glaucoma after hyphema in sickle cell patients. *Am J Ophthalmol*. 1979;87:43.

59. Goldberg MF, Tso MOM. Sickled erythrocytes, hyphema and secondary glaucoma. VII. The passage of sickled erythrocytes out of the anterior chamber of the human and monkey eye: Light and electron microscope studies. *Ophthalmol Surg*. 1979;10:89.

60. Marcus M, et al. Aspirin and secondary bleeding after traumatic hyphema. *Annal Ophthalmol*. 1988;20(4):157.

61. Wilson TW, Jeffers JB, Nelson LB. Aminocaproic and prophylaxis in traumatic hyphema. *Ophthalmol Surg*. 1990;21(11):807.

62. Kutner B, Fourman S, Brein K, et al. Aminocaproic acid reduces the risk of secondary hemorrhage in patients with traumatic hyphema. *Arch Ophthalmol*. 1987;105:206.

63. Blantan FM. Anterior chamber angle recession and secondary glaucoma. A study of the after effects of traumatic hyphema. *Arch Ophthalmol* 1964;72:39.

64. Tonjun AM. Gonioscopy in traumatic hyphema. *Acta Ophthalmol*. 1966;44:650.

65. Bron A, Aury P, Salagnac J, et al. Pre-equatorial contusion syndrome. Analysis appropos of 59 cases. *J Francais D Ophthalmol*. 1989;12(3):211.

66. Mooney D. Angle recession and secondary glaucoma. *Br J Ophthalmol*. 1973;57:608.

67. Miles DR, Boniuk M. Pathogenesis of unilateral glaucoma. *Am J Ophthalmol*. 1966;62:493.

68. Alper MG. Contusion angle deformity and glaucoma. *Arch Ophthalmol*. 1963;69:455.

69. Lauing L. Anterior chamber glass membranes. *Am J Ophthalmol*. 1969;68:308.

70. Gilles WE. Traumatic glaucoma. *Trans Ophthalmol Soc Aust*. 1967;XXVI:54.

71. deJuan E Jr, Sternberg P Jr, Michaels RG. Penetrating ocular injuries. Types of injuries and visual results. *Ophthalmology*. 1983;90:1318.

72. D'Ombrain AW. Traumatic monocular chronic glaucoma. *Trans Ophthalmol Soc Aust*. 1945;V:116.

73. Richardson K. Acute glaucoma after trauma. In: Freeman HM, ed. *Ocular Trauma*. New York: Appleton-Century-Croft; 1979.

74. Jensn P, Minckler DS, Chandler W. Epithelial ingrowth. *Arch Ophthalmol*. 1977;95:837.

75. Simmers RJ, Kimbrough RL. Late glaucoma after trauma. In: Freeman HM (ed). *Ocular Trauma.* New York: Appleton-Century-Crofts; 1979.

76. Rosenthal AR, Marmor MF, Levenberger P. Chalcosis: A study of natural history. *Ophthalmology.* 1979;86:1956.

77. Rosenthal MJ. Intraocular foreign bodies, prognosis. *Int Ophthalmol Clin.* 1968;8(1):257.

78. Francois J. Cortisone et tension. *Ann Oculist.* 1954;187:805.

79. Armaly MF. Effects of corticosteroids in intraocular pressure and fluid dynamics. II. The effect of dexamethasone in the glaucomatous eye. *Arch Ophthalmol.* 1963;70:492.

80. Becker B, Podos SM. Elevated intraocular pressure following corticosteroid eye drops. *J Am A.* 1963; 185:884.

81. Becker B, Hahn KA. Topical corticosteroids and heredity in primary open angle glaucoma. *Am J Ophthalmol.* 1964;57:543.

82. Armaly MF. Statistical attributes of the steroid hypertensive response in the clinically normal eye. II. The demonstration of three levels of response. *Invest Ophthalmol.* 1965;4:187.

83. Armaly MF. Inheritance of dexamethasone hypertension and glaucoma. *Arch Ophthalmol.* 1967;77:747.

84. Kayes J, Becker B. The human trabecular meshwork in corticosterdoid induced glaucoma. *Trans Am Ophthalmol Soc.* 1969;67:354.

85. Francois J. The importance of the micropolysaccharides in intraocular pressure regulation. *Invest Ophthalmol.* 1975;14:173.

86. Weinstein BI, Gordon GG, Southern AL. Potentiation of glucocorticoid activity by 5B-dihydrocortisone: Its role in glaucoma. *Science.* 1983;222:172.

87. Sherwood M, Richardson TM. Evidence for in vivo phagocytosis by trabecular endothelial cells. *Invest Ophthalmol.* 1958;59:216.

88. Bill A. The drainage of aqueous humor. *Invest Ophthalmol.* 1975;14:1.

89. Espildora J, Vicuna P, Diaz E. Cortisone induced glaucoma: A report on 44 affected eyes. *J Fr Ophthalmol.* 1981;4:503.

90. Smith RJH. Rubeotic glaucoma. *Br J Ophthalmol.* 1981;65:606.

91. Weiss DI, Shafer RN, Nehrenberg TR. Neovascular glaucoma complicating cavernous sinus fistula. *Arch Ophthalmol.* 1963;69:304.

92. Federman JL, Brown GC, Felberg NT, et al. Experimental ocular angiogenesis. *Am J Ophthalmol.* 1980;89:231.

93. Ben Ezr D. Neovasculogenesis: Triggering factors and possible mechanisms. *Surv Ophthalmol.* 1979;24:167.

94. Polverini PJ, Cotran PS, Gimbrone MA Jr, et al. Activated macrophages induced vascular proliferation. *Nature* 1977;269:804.

95. Laatikamen L. Development classification of rubeosis irides in diabetic eye disease. *Br J Ophthalmol.* 1979;63:150.

96. Gutman FA, Zegarra H. The natural course of temporal retinal branch vein occlusion. *Trans Am Acad Ophthalmol Otol.* 1974;78:178.

97. Hoskins HD Jr. Neovascular glaucoma. Current concepts. *Trans Am Acad Ophthalmol Otol.* 1974;78: 330.

98. Hayreh SS. So called "central retinal vein occlusion." I. Pathogenesis, terminology, clinical features. *Ophthalmolgia.* 1976;172:1.

99. Magaral LE, Brown GC, Augsburger JJ, et al. Neovascular glaucoma following central retinal vein occlusion. *Ophthalmology.* 1981;88:1095.

100. Bertelsen TI. The relationship between thrombosis in the retinal vein and primary glaucoma. *Acta Ophthalmol.* 1961;39:603.

101. Dryden RM. Central retinal vein occlusion and chronic simple glaucoma. *Arch Ophthalmol.* 1965; 73:659.

102. Heyreh SS, Podhagsky P. Ocular neovascularization with retinal occlusion. II. Occurrences in central and branch neutral artery occlusion. *Arch Ophthalmol.* 1982;100:1585.

103. Ohrt V. The frequency of rubeosis in diabetic patients. *Arch Ophthalmol.* 1971;49:301.

104. Aiello LM, Ward M, Liang G. Neovascular glaucoma and vitreous hemorrhage following cataract surgery in patients with diabetes mellitus. *Ophthalmology.* 1983;90:814.

105. LaatiKaninen L, Blach RK. Behavior of the iris vasculature in central retinal vein occlusion: A fluorescein angiographics study of the vascular response of the retina and the iris. *Br J Ophthalmol.* 1977;61:272.

106. Cashwell LF, Marks WP. Pan-retinal photocoagulation in the management of neovascular glaucoma. *South Med J.* 1988;81(11):1364.

107. Phillip W, Klima G, Miller K. Clinicopathological findings 11 months after implantation of a functioning aqueous drainage silicone implant. *Graefe's Arch Clin/ Exp Ophthalmol.* 1990;228(5):481–486.

Chapter 18

LOW-TENSION GLAUCOMA

David M. Cockburn
Ian F. Gutteridge

Glaucoma is often described as an enigmatic disease and no form of glaucoma is more of an enigma than that termed low-tension glaucoma (LTG), perhaps more properly referred to as "normal-tension glaucoma." The condition was originally described by von Graefe in 1857.[1] Indeed, there are those who dispute the existence of LTG as a separate entity or believe it to be extremely rare.[2] Their view is that glaucomatous damage occurs during spikes of undetected raised intraocular pressure (IOP), or during more extended episodes at night that also go undetected. Others believe that the clinical signs of LTG, although similar to those of primary open-angle glaucoma (POAG) with raised IOP, differ in some respects and represent a different pathological mechanism from that classical form of glaucoma. It appears that in one school of thought there is an ideological difficulty in dissociating the pathology of glaucoma from a causal role of raised IOP. Accordingly, strategies are devised to explain the signs of LTG in terms consistent with a pressure-induced model by arguing that eyes having LTG have a lower pressure threshold for damage than do normal eyes. On the other hand, the view has been expressed that raised IOP may be no more than a sign of glaucoma, rather than its underlying cause.[3] If accepted, this latter argument would imply

that LTG is simply a form of open-angle glaucoma in which one of the signs, raised IOP, is absent.

DEFINITIONS AND NOMENCLATURE

Open-angle glaucoma associated with raised IOP (POAG) is customarily defined in terms of three clinical entities: raised IOP, characteristic visual field defects, and optic disc damage in the form of tissue loss at the optic disc. The presence of any two of these signs is traditionally accepted as sufficient clinical evidence of the presence, or impending development, of POAG. On the other hand, LTG by its definition is recognized clinically in terms of only two signs, visual field defects and optic disc damage. In LTG, both signs must be present to confirm the diagnosis and raised IOP must, by definition, be absent. If these definitions are accepted then, logically, LTG is simply a variant of POAG because two of the requirements for POAG are present in LTG. These semantics aside, definitions of both POAG and LTG presuppose unobstructed trabeculae, since this differentiates both conditions from angle closure glaucoma. Other ocular disease capable of producing glaucoma must be ab-

assumed to be a whitening of the disc substance as occurs in the stark white appearance of the disc following primary optic atrophy. However, in glaucoma, and especially LTG, the remaining optic disc rim tissue frequently has a distinctly dark gray and moth-eaten appearance. The gray color is probably caused by atrophy of both glial and axonal components of the rim tissue following a reduction in the amount of vascular support.

Clinical assessment of the color of the optic disc is influenced by the spectral nature of the illumination of the ophthalmoscope or biomicroscope, by absorption of light passing through the ocular media, and by objective influences, including bias when other clinical factors are known to the clinician. These limitations make clinical judgments of pallor somewhat hazardous and, although there are techniques for objective determination of pallor, these methods are not as yet clinically applicable.

Optic disc color is certainly a useful measure of the health of this tissue and may provide the first detected sign of glaucoma. Changes in the extent of pallor as measured by computer image analysis are significant during the transition from the ocular hypertension state to that of frank glaucoma. However, once optic disc cupping becomes well established in glaucomatous eyes, disc pallor is not very useful in assessing progress of the damage and does not always correlate with visual field loss.[58] However, it is unlikely that there are differences between the changes that occur in LTG and POAG that allow clinical differentiation.

With these limitations, it appears that the clinically assessed degree of pallor, or grayness of the disc, is not a sensitive sign of glaucoma and provides little or no assistance in further categorizing the disease into LTG or POAG.

Peripapillary Halo and Atrophy. Primrose[59] reported that peripapillary halo might be a useful sign of early glaucomatous damage. He suggested that this sign might be due to ischemia of the choroid and damage to the retinal pigment epithelium overlying this region. Since the lamina and the peripapillary region are both supplied by vessels originating from the short posterior ciliary arteries, this association might lend further weight to the ischemic model of disc damage in LTG. The appearance of peripapillary crescent or halo consists of a more or less regular pale annulus surrounding the optic disc. The suggestion that this sign might be useful in detecting glaucoma did not survive a study[60] in which photographs of normal and glaucomatous eyes were graded by three observers. However, these observers also graded the presence of peripapillary atrophy that was defined as the presence, in addition to the halo or crescent, of a definite red-brown outer edge to the halo that is noticeably darker than the surrounding normal retina. With this added sign, there was a statistically significant greater extent of peripapillary atrophy in glaucomatous eyes than in normal eyes.

Anderson[61] postulated that misalignment of the retinal pigment epithelium and choroid with the optic disc is the underlying cause of the peripapillary halo and may predispose the disc to ischemic damage. He found a correlation between the extent of the crescent, the location of the disc excavation, and the field defect. These were most striking in the cases of glaucoma having lower pressures. He reasoned that the presence of a peripapillary crescent or halo might participate in determining the susceptibility of the disc to damage from elevated IOP and facilitate this damage at low pressures as occurs in LTG.

It should be noted that peripapillary atrophy and crescents or halos are not found solely in LTG but occur commonly in POAG and also in normal eyes. The discovery of a peripapillary halo or crescent should be a trigger to lower the clinician's threshold of suspicion for the glaucomas and perhaps for undertaking of a visual field analysis. Clearly, there is a need for a better understanding of the etiology of the mechanism behind the production of peripapillary atrophy, following which its association with both POAG and LTG might lead to a better understanding of the pathology in the glaucomas. Figure 18–3 illustrates the appearance of peripapillary atrophy.

Greve and Geijssen[43] compared the optic discs of patients having conventional POAG and those having LTG. The LTG eyes were categorized as being either senile sclerotic LTG or focal ischemic LTG on the basis of the presence or absence of other ischemic disease and retinal, choroidal, and peripapillary atrophy. They addressed the question of the existence of recognizable differences in discs and fields between POAG and LTG by looking for differences in the appearance of the optic disc and in optic disc-visual field relationships. They found that the senile sclerotic LTG group had a relatively large visual field defect and a relatively small degree of cupping (high visual field/cup disc ratio) compared to both POAG and the ischemic LTG subjects. The senile sclerotic LTG group discs were characterized by "pale moth-eaten sloping excavation." By contrast, the ischemic LTG disc cupping was found to be predominantly in the vertical direction and steep sided, while POAG cupping was larger overall and less steep. The authors

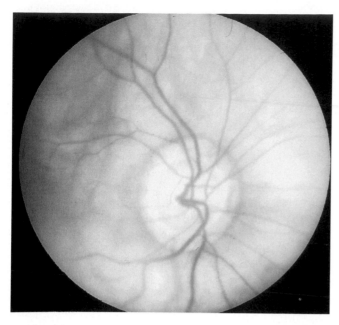

Figure 18–3. The pale atrophic irregular annulus centered on the optic disc and bordered by a brown line is known as peripapillary halo or atrophy. Although common in normal eyes, peripapillary atrophy is over-represented in patients having glaucoma and particularly low-tension glaucoma. (*See also* Color Plate 18–3.)

point out that, at least in the early stages of the disease, the clinician can differentiate between two classes of LTG on the basis of the cup disc-visual field ratio and the appearance of the disc cupping and surrounding fundus.

The cited differences in the optic disc changes of LTG and POAG are summarized in Table 18–2.

Visual Field Defects. The loss of visual field in LTG and the nature of that loss is the subject of controversy centering on reports of similarities and differences between the visual field loss in LTG and POAG. If the diseases have similar etiologies, it would be expected that there would be comparable field defects. Equally, significantly different patterns of visual field loss would suggest that the two diseases arise from different pathological mechanisms. Therefore, studies comparing field losses have been used to impact on arguments relating to the etiology of LTG and POAG.

By definition, the visual field changes in LTG are "typical" of primary open-angle glaucoma. The basic unit of visual field loss in optic nerve disease in general, and in glaucoma in particular, is the nerve fiber bundle defect. In its classical form, this is manifest as the arcuate scotoma. Single or multiple arcuate scotomas are undoubtedly features common to both LTG and POAG. However, they represent relatively advanced field deficits. The lack of sensitivity of perimetry has obscured subtleties of their development. There is a need to consider earlier aspects of visual field loss where differences in LTG and POAG defects might be detected.

There has been much interest in the earliest observed field defects in POAG, particularly since the advent of static perimetric techniques has enabled ex-

TABLE 18–2. COMPARISON OF OPTIC DISC AND VISUAL FIELD CHANGES TYPICAL OF LTG AND COAG[a]

Feature	LTG	POAG
Optic Discs		
Location of rim damage	Focal as inferior temporal notch	At vertical poles and more diffuse
Cup sides	Tend to be steep	More sloping
Hemorrhages	Frequent and recurrent	Uncommon
Baring of circumlinear vessels	Common	Common
Peripapillary halo (atrophy)	Common	Occasional
Visual Fields		
Field loss relative to duration	More severe?	Less severe?
Affected hemisphere	Superior hemifield	Superior = inferior hemifield most common
Proximity to fixation	Commonly within 10°	Commonly 10–15° from fixation
Margin of defect	Steep sided	Steep or sloping margins
Depth of depression	Deep	Less deep relative to duration
Uniformity of defect	Tend to uniformity?	Less uniform over defects?
Unaffected visual field	Thresholds relatively normal	Increase of threshold in remaining field
Mean defect index	Relatively lower than POAG	Relatively higher than LTG
Corrected loss of variance index	Relatively higher than in POAG	Relatively lower than in LTG
Laterality	May be unilateral but mostly bilateral	Unilateral presentation uncommon

[a] Note that the listed features are those most commonly observed but the differences are not totally reliable. Disputed or unlikely differences are shown with a query. See text for full discussion of the significance of these possible differences.

tremely sensitive estimates of visual fields at differential thresholds. The recognized early defects in glaucoma include isolated paracentral scotomas,[62,63] nasal steps,[64,65] and local increases in threshold such as the wedge-shaped defect[66] demonstrable with static profile perimetry. Field defects in LTG have a low probability of being detected early because IOP is not elevated and cupping of the disc probably not advanced at this early stage. Routine field screening of optometric patients may minimize the problem of late detection. However, there is probably no means of ensuring that POAG and LTG can be compared at similar stages of progression, and studies purporting to show particular features of field loss in either form of glaucoma are inherently difficult to analyze.

Patterns of early POAG visual field loss and preferentially involved regions[62,63] are useful in identifying patients with glaucoma. It has been shown, for example, that isolated scotomas in the arcuate area (described as stage 2 defects by Aulhorn[63]) have an interesting frequency distribution. First, the superior and inferior hemifields are involved with equal frequency. Second, when the upper field is involved, there is equal involvement on the nasal and temporal side of the vertical midline. Also, these scotomas are heavily concentrated within 5 to 15° of fixation. Third, when the lower hemisphere is involved, the nasal field is more seriously affected and has a greater likelihood of extension beyond 15°. This extension into the nasal field may be analogous to the nasal step, also considered to be a sign of early glaucomatous damage when it involves the periphery.[65] Aulhorn's widely accepted report provides a basis for comparison with other forms of glaucoma. Reports have subsequently suggested that in LTG there were frequent variations from this pattern, particularly with involvement inside 5° and a higher probability of defects in the superior field.[41] These findings have, in turn, been contested, leading to controversy on the nature and underlying cause of LTG visual field loss and casting further doubt on the differences, if any, between POAG and LTG visual field losses.

The following characteristics have been reported in LTG studies and merit analysis and comment:

1. It is commonly believed that scotomas in LTG, when compared to POAG, occur closer to fixation (and frequently within 5°), are steeper sided and deeper when examined both by kinetic perimetry[41] and static perimetry.[67,68] At first sight, this appears to be an attractive means by which to differentiate the two conditions, but the differences cannot be considered to be diagnostic of LTG since dense sco-

tomas also may lie close to fixation in POAG when visual field loss is advanced.[41,69] Levene[41] reported that a defect was found within 5° of fixation in 20% of patients in his POAG series although he found 94% in this region in his LTG series.

Several studies, however, have failed to confirm these field characteristics in LTG. Greve and Geijssen[69] compared POAG with LTG which was further subdivided into senile sclerotic and focal ischemic LTG. They concluded that there was no significant difference between the three groups with respect to the proximity of visual field loss to fixation. When attempts were made to match the degree of cupping in LTG and POAG series,[70] no significant difference was found between groups, although both groups exhibited defects within 5° in 80% of cases. Maximum luminance defects were also seen in approximately 80% of cases in both groups. Phelps, Hayreh, and Montague[71] compared patients having mild, moderate, and severe LTG, POAG, and AION and failed to show that LTG caused early visual field defects within 5° any more frequently than occurred in POAG. One study,[72] in which static perimetry profiles were generated by the Octopus Program 32, in LTG patients (IOP < 21 mm Hg) and POAG patients (IOP > 25 mm Hg) having similar degrees of cupping, found the opposite trends. When the scotoma closest to fixation was examined, the defects were closer, deeper, and steeper in the POAG group, although the differences shown for depth and steepness were not statistically significant.

It seems from the currently available evidence that, while defects close to fixation are a common feature of LTG, this finding cannot be used alone to specifically differentially diagnose LTG from POAG (Fig. 18–4). There is, however, good evidence that in POAG dense scotomas are found close to fixation when the total field loss is greater, while in LTG, such defects can occur when there is relatively little general field involvement.[68]

2. The superior hemifield is preferentially affected in LTG, with studies showing superior arcuate defects occurring between two and four times more frequently than inferior defects.[21,69–71] Unfortunately, this feature of LTG is also characteristic of POAG and thus does not assist in differentiating the two conditions.[69–71] Conversely, it is well established

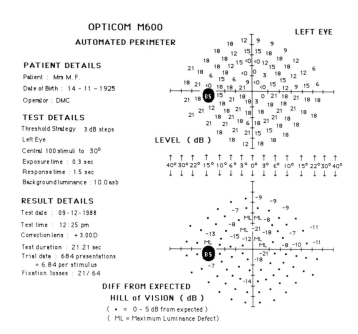

Figure 18–4. Visual field (OS) of a patient diagnosed with low-tension glaucoma. Note the superior arcuate field loss associated with defects close to fixation.

that AION causes an inferior visual field defect more frequently than a superior one,[69–73] lending weight to the argument that acute AION and LTG are different entities.

Since the superior field seems preferentially affected in both LTG and POAG, it follows that the inferior portion of the prelaminar optic nerve appears to be more vulnerable to the glaucomatous process while the superior disc (and inferior visual field) is more at risk from ischemia of acute vascular origin, as in AION. An interesting corollary is the finding that most disc hemorrhages seen in POAG occur in the inferotemporal region of the disc.[48] It is attractive to think of LTG as being a chronic ischemic disease and POAG as causing damage as a result of raised IOP. However, it is possible that damage may also occur in POAG from the same ischemic factors, thus explaining the characteristic finding of superior field loss in both POAG and LTG.

3. A high prevalence of unilateral field loss has been claimed to occur in LTG,[41] but more recently a similar prevalence of unilaterality was found in POAG and LTG.[71] Therefore, it seems that unilateral field loss is not a reliable means of differentiation between LTG and POAG. Of particular interest from the point of view of the etiology of LTG is the early report of Drance[74] in which he describes cases of uni-

lateral LTG and cases of LTG in one eye with POAG in the other. This suggests that a patient can be subject either to visual field loss from two different diseases, one on either side of the body, or to a disease that is essentially the same but lacking one of the signs (raised IOP) in one eye.

4. LTG is said to be associated with an early loss of fixation or central scotoma.[21,41] Chumbley and Brubaker[21] reported that 25% of their LTG patients had papillomacular involvement, implying acute symptoms of visual loss. This suggests papillomacular bundle vulnerability in LTG, not unlike AION, where acute visual loss is a common symptom and correlates with pathological evidence of vascular occlusion.[75] However, it seems that neither POAG nor LTG commonly have central scotomas as an early finding. If a central scotoma is an early finding, there appears to be no significant difference in prevalence between POAG and LTG.[71]

5. Visual field defects in LTG may have a sudden onset.[21] Since there is a possible association between LTG, hemodynamic crises, and disc hemorrhages, it is not surprising that field defects may develop acutely in response to these insults. It is also stated that such defects are less likely to progress, particularly in those patients who have suffered a hemodynamic crisis,[15] unless, of course, a further hemodynamic event occurs.

6. Patients with LTG are more likely to have normal visual field thresholds in uninvolved hemifields than those found in POAG.[76] In a study using static perimetry results of eyes having defects involving only the upper *or* lower field, it was found that POAG patients had significantly higher thresholds in the "normal" hemifield than LTG patients. This is consistent with the theory that high levels of IOP such as may occur in POAG cause diffuse nerve fiber damage in field areas that are without arcuate characteristics.[77]

7. The tendency for field loss to progress clearly depends on whether the patient suffers from a progressive or nonprogressive form of LTG. Drance[74] reported that 99% of LTG cases associated with hemodynamic crises did not progress unless new crises occurred. As described above, optic disc hemorrhage is a commonly reported finding in LTG, is believed to be a sign of microinfarction, and is frequently associated with fresh nerve fiber

bundle field defects.[47] Therefore, it follows that LTG visual loss may be progressive, but perhaps in a step-like fashion related to recurrent microinfarction of the disc. Since it is difficult to determine the depth of a scotoma in LTG, progression may relate more to new scotomas rather than worsening of pre-existing defects. Gramer and colleagues[78] commented that the depth and extent of field loss in LTG tended to increase proportionately, in contrast to POAG where defects tended to increase in size initially and to increase in depth later in the course of the disease.

A retrospective study of progression of field loss in LTG using a single kinetic isopter[79] showed that as many as 60% of cases did not deteriorate in the region of this isopter in a mean follow-up period of 10.5 years. If progression did occur, it could take up to 4 years to manifest and the probability that it would occur in an already damaged hemifield, or a previously undamaged hemifield, was found to be 50 and 25%, respectively. These results, although demonstrated by kinetic perimetry, suggest that the upper and lower fields behave with some independence, that IOP spikes are not associated with field deterioration, and monitoring of LTG cases with perimetry may, with safety, be relatively widely spaced in time.

8. Uniformity of scotomas has been suggested to be a feature of LTG. This implies that defects have consistent depth, a view which is supported by the generally steep-sided nature of defects and the acute involvement of nerve fiber bundles after a disc hemorrhage, rather than the more diffuse cumulative effects of elevated IOP. However, there is little evidence to support this contention. Visual field results are difficult to interpret in this manner because many of the scotomas are defects to maximum luminance available with an automated perimeter both in LTG and POAG.

9. An interesting new dimension of visual field loss in glaucoma has recently emerged as a result of detailed statistical analysis of static perimetric results, particularly those results of Octopus and Humphrey perimeter studies. This form of analysis has led to the development of indices or numbers, which are thought to indicate specific field loss characteristics. It is now possible to differentiate diffuse from focal visual field loss using global indices.

Since these indices are considered to be sensitive to different types of field loss, they have been studied in LTG and the results compared with those found in POAG.[42,80] Caprioli and Sears[42] looked at the visual fields of a small number of eyes having relatively early glaucoma and allocated them to the category of "diffuse" or "localized" field loss on the basis of global indices. They retrospectively studied IOP and optic disc cupping and found that the IOP was consistently higher in eyes with diffuse loss. These eyes also tended to have round optic disc cups with relatively even rims. Eyes with localized defects tended to have lower IOPs in the range typical of LTG and also had more eccentric cupping in which the axis of cupping was shifted inferotemporally. The resultant hypothesis was that higher IOPs were responsible for diffuse field damage, which represented diffused axonal dysfunction and later death, while LTG cases tended to have localized field damage without diffuse loss. Such indices may provide clinical evidence helpful in the differential diagnosis of LTG and POAG and perhaps provide clues to the pathophysiology of the glaucomas.

The cited differences in the visual field changes observed in LTG and POAG are summarized in Table 18–2.

Intraocular Pressures in LTG and POAG. By definition, the IOP of a patient with LTG is always within the "normal" range; yet a normal range of pressures is not easily defined. Furthermore, the level of IOP chosen as the junction between normal and abnormal will impact on the definition, prevalence, and diagnosis of LTG. Whether a group of patients having LTG have IOP measurements at the high end of the normal range (as suggested by Kolker and Hetherington[24]) or undetected spikes of pressure is an exercise in semantics that does not greatly assist in the diagnosis of individual cases. It can be said that the difference between the IOP in LTG and POAG is, in the words of C.S. Calverley, "As to the meaning, it's what you please."

It is commonly held that POAG is mistakenly referred to as LTG, because random or clinical tonometric estimates fail to demonstrate the full range of IOP. There is probably no indisputable time of day when IOP estimates correctly predict the presence of POAG or LTG. Although IOP is normal in LTG, there may be some characteristics of IOP that would assist in identifying LTG patients. First, some definitions of

LTG require that facility of aqueous outflow be normal,[81] which is consistent with normal IOP measurements. However, some studies have shown that a high proportion of LTG cases have low facility of outflow.[16,21] As tonography is not commonly performed in the clinic and there is some controversy on its interpretation in LTG, it is unfortunately an unreliable means of distinguishing between POAG and LTG. Second, the posture of the patient may influence the level of IOP. For instance, there is a reversible increase in IOP when both normal and glaucomatous patients change from seated to supine positions.[82,83] This may have significance in LTG where IOP estimates are found to be normal at all times when measured with the patient seated. The inference is that glaucomatous damage may occur during sleep when the subject is supine and the pressure raised. Indeed, IOP in normal patients has been shown to increase by 3 to 6 mm Hg within 30 minutes of sleep and to remain above the waking level.[84] Diurnal IOP variation in glaucoma patients may fluctuate widely, with one study showing a mean increase in POAG of 15 mm Hg in a 24-hour period.[85] However, POAG and LTG patients suffer similar rises in IOP when supine and thus this form of assessment per se does not help differentiate between the two conditions.

Third, it has been suggested that LTG patients have lower amplitudes of ocular pulse than normal, ocular hypertensive, and POAG patients.[86] Since the ocular pulse is a function of the influx of blood into the eye with systole, lower tonometric fluctuation or ocular pulse in LTG implies that blood flow is in some manner reduced. However, the role of arterial insufficiency in LTG is poorly understood and, since the techniques of ocular pulse recording are complex, the characteristics of the ocular pulse does not appear to be a useful clinical means of differentiating between LTG and POAG.

Clinical Course

The clinical course of LTG, like that of POAG, is variable, between the extremes of apparently nonprogressive cases through to those that relentlessly proceed to blindness in spite of maximum medical and surgical intervention. When nonprogressive cases are excluded, the course of LTG in the remaining cases is usually marked by continuing loss of visual field; increased cupping, especially in the vertical direction; and marked grayness of the remaining neural rim of the disc. Recurrent disc hemorrhages are common and may be followed by notching and worsening of the visual field defect.

Fortunately, LTG is a disease usually found in the later years of life when progression is halted by death from other causes and before the patient becomes seriously affected or blind. It is also fortunate that central vision is usually retained until late in the disease. Progressive LTG in patients having a relatively long life expectancy has a poor prognosis and the most common view is that it should be treated vigorously from the time of diagnosis. Although there is but scant evidence to support the view that maintaining IOP at very low levels retards, or prevents the visual damage, it is the only treatment available at this time. For ethical reasons, it is unlikely that we will be able to compare the progress of eyes by means of masked prospective trials of the treatment versus placebo. This is the unfortunate legacy of an unscientific approach to treatment in the past, complicated by a blind faith that IOP is the cause of glaucoma damage to the exclusion of other possible etiologies or treatments.

SPECIFIC RISK FACTORS FOR LOW-TENSION GLAUCOMA

Migraine. We have already discussed the role of migraine in LTG when considering ischemia of the optic nerve. Migraine is a relatively common vascular disease associated with decreased cerebral blood flow. Attacks of migraine cause ischemia of the brain, optic nerve, and retina. Optic disc ischemia is considered a possible cause of LTG. A sample of 54 patients having LTG, 182 having POAG, and 126 with ocular hypertension, together with 493 normal subjects, were questioned for a history of migraine.[13] The LTG group reported a significantly higher prevalence of migraine and other forms of headache than did the other three groups. These reports suggest there is some association, although possibly not causal, between migraine and LTG. They recommend that patients suffering from progressive LTG and migraine should be given a clinical trial using systemic beta adrenergic blocking drugs.

Myopia. Myopic eyes are significantly more frequently associated with ocular hypertension and open-angle glaucoma than would be expected from their prevalence. This holds equally for both POAG and LTG.[87] It appears that myopic patients are more likely than hypermetropic patients to develop frank glaucoma during the course of ocular hypertension; indeed, 32% of myopic ocular hypertensive subjects developed glaucoma during follow-up, whereas only 3% of the emmetropic and hypermetropic group advanced to glaucoma.[87] It should be noted that it is more difficult to evaluate optic disc appearance and visual field defects in myopic subjects which may result in a later diagnosis and treatment of LTG in myopic eyes.

It has been argued earlier that glaucomatous damage is due to either axoplasmic transport block, mechanical damage, or ischemic changes in the region of the lamina. The association of myopia and glaucoma may be explained by any one, or combinations of the following:

1. Raised IOP in glaucoma may stretch the eye (as seen in juvenile glaucoma) and cause both the glaucoma and the myopia. However, this hypothesis does not explain the association of myopia with LTG, where pressures, by definition, remain normal.
2. Anatomical differences in the myopic eye, other than stretching of its coat, may predispose it to mechanical or vascular insult or to interruption of axoplasmic transport.
3. Both myopia and glaucoma may be genetically determined with the inheritance factors linked, but not necessarily causally associated. Myopic patients are known to be overrepresented in subjects who have IOP increases during topical steroid administration and this feature is known to be genetically determined.
4. As a result of stretching of the globe, myopic eyes may be rendered more susceptible to later damage even at normal IOP or because of slight increases in IOP. This hypothesis could explain the ischemic, axoplasmic, or mechanical mechanism and could apply in cases of LTG.

Although an explanation of the association between myopia and both POAG and LTG remains to be elucidated, the clinician has a valuable clue to the management of patients having discs or fields that are equivocal for glaucoma damage. It is clear that myopia should be considered a risk factor and a lowered threshold for concern for LTG disc and visual field damage adopted for these patients.

Carotid Artery Insufficiency. Since the vascular supply of the ophthalmic artery depends on the carotid system, insufficiency of supply in these arteries can cause ischemic changes in the eye. Acute occlusion of the internal carotid artery causes a reduction in IOP of a few mm Hg, which might be considered to be a protective factor against ischemia because it improves the overall perfusion pressure. However, this effect only occurs in severe insufficiency of carotid supply and probably plays no part in the chronic and less intensive form of carotid artery disease. The most commonly recognized ocular manifestations of carotid insufficiency are amaurosis fugax and venous stasis retinopathy. It is conceivable that selective ischemia of the lamina region of the optic disc could result from this condition and because of the absence of raised IOP, a diagnosis of LTG would be appropriate. In the event of chronic carotid artery insufficiency, the LTG damage would be progressive or follow a pattern of stepwise deterioration in synchrony with deterioration of vascular flow or continuing embolic obstruction of downstream arteries.

A study[88] of five patients having LTG and eight patients having POAG showed that cerebral circulatory deficits were present in both groups but are more pronounced in LTG. The authors concluded that insufficiency in the carotid circulation is a factor in both POAG and LTG but is more prevalent in LTG. The value of this study is limited by the small number of subjects and its dependence on the rather limited reliability of the results of ophthalmodynamometry. Another study[89] failed to identify, during 3 to 12 years of follow-up, any visual field loss or optic disc damage in five patients with raised IOP and severe carotid artery disease. If carotid disease had a causal role in LTG, it would be expected that the combination of ocular hypertension and carotid insufficiency would have led to visual field and disc damage during the course of the study. Levene[41] reviewed the literature reporting the association between carotid artery disease and LTG and concluded that the evidence for a causal relationship was unconvincing and inconsistent.

Regardless of any role in glaucoma, carotid artery disease confers a serious risk of stroke, central retinal artery occlusion, and venous stasis retinopathy and is treatable in many cases. Cervical bruits commonly accompany carotid insufficiency and are readily detected by auscultation over the bifurcation of the common carotid artery in the neck. These bruits are common in patients of optometrists,[90] occurring in 4.4% of all patients over 50 years of age. It is important that this sign be recognized, and the patient referred appropriately. Until the question of a causal association is finally settled, LTG should be considered in the management of patients found to have carotid artery insufficiency and, conversely, cervical auscultation should be carried out on all glaucoma patients.

The Empty Sella Syndrome. The sella turcica is the saddle-shaped depression on the mid-line of the sphenoid bone, which contains the pituitary gland.

Empty sella is the term used to describe the absence, or partial absence, of the pituitary in the presence of a normal-sized or even larger than normal sella. The cause is frequently not found; however, the condition may follow necrosis after childbirth (Sheehan's syndrome) or necrosis following a pituitary tumor. Clinically, the patient may be asymptomatic, or exhibit frank hypopituitarism.[91] A variety of visual field defects is frequently associated with the empty sella syndrome,[92] the most recognizable being bitemporal in nature. However, there is a report of this condition being associated with typical glaucomatous changes in the optic discs and fields of a patient in whom the IOP was normal.[93] The authors are at pains to point out that the two conditions might be present in this patient by chance alone, but they suggest that an examination for intracranial disease should be carried out in all cases of low-tension glaucoma.

Diabetes. Diabetes mellitus is a disease known to cause microvascular occlusions in the retina, in larger vessels elsewhere in the eye, and in other target organs. It would seem likely that similar changes could interfere with the vascular supply to the lamina region of the disc and, thereby, be a primary cause of LTG by causing ischemia of the disc in the presence of normal IOP. This proposition is not borne out by the result of multivariate analysis of predictive risk factors for LTG.[94]

Other Systemic Factors in LTG. Patients with LTG appear to have a greater prevalence of multiple systemic abnormalities than are present in a similar group of patients having ocular hypertension. The most significant differences appear to be in the results of ophthalmodynamometry, in exercise habits, and cardiovascular disease.[20] At this time, there is no evidence that modifying these features is beneficial in the management of LTG.

Since abnormal blood states may contribute to vascular occlusion, these disorders have been sought as possible etiological factors in the ischemia and necrosis of LTG, as well as being of some predictive value in LTG suspects. However, the available evidence suggests that there is little or no association with these variables.[20,41]

Elevated blood glucose levels and an increase in circulating lipoproteins have been studied in some detail. Winder[94] found that the incidence of blood glucose abnormalities did not exceed that of age- and sex-matched normal population values. This finding may be contrasted with that of Richler and associ-

ates[95] who found that diabetes, together with the male gender and low diastolic blood pressure, were risk factors for the progression of visual field loss in established POAG and LTG patients who were under medical treatment for glaucoma. However, the Winder study[94] showed that as a group, patients with LTG had significantly higher cholesterolemia than normal individuals or people with POAG. These differences were not remarkable and did not apply to all LTG patients, so the effect of hypercholesterolemia does not appear to be distinctive for LTG. It is also of interest that treatment of the hypercholesterolemia did not appear to affect the short-term progress of the disease.

In conclusion, systemic vascular occlusive risk factors appear to play very little part in the pathogenesis of LTG but the benefit of treatment for the maintenance of general health is compelling and may, in addition, confer some benefit in halting the progression of both LTG and POAG.

Table 18–3 summarizes the risk factors believed to be associated with LTG.

Differential Diagnosis
Table 18–1 summarizes the conditions that should be considered in the differential diagnosis of LTG.

Open-Angle Glaucoma. Differentiation between POAG and LTG is not only important from a diagnostic viewpoint but also because the treatment of POAG has a specific goal of IOP reduction to normal levels. However, there is no known universal threshold for IOP-induced damage and there is considerable overlap in the IOP levels found in normal eyes. By definition, the differential diagnosis between POAG and LTG is based on IOP and is, therefore, tied to the level of IOP adopted as the upper limit of normal. A reasonable clinical guide would be that IOP over 21

TABLE 18–3. RISK FACTORS ASSOCIATED WITH LOW-TENSION GLAUCOMA[a]

Family history of glaucoma
Migraine
Carotid artery disease
Myopia
Diabetes or raised blood glucose levels
Hypercholesterolemia

[a] See text for discussion of reliability of these associations.

mm Hg at any assessment would be the determining factor. The reliability of this assessment of IOP over an extended period of time depends on how often the IOP is measured throughout the day and the duration of the investigation.

Despite many studies comparing the clinical features of POAG and LTG, there is a disappointingly small range of signs for the clinician to seek as reliable evidence of one disease rather than the other. Loss of neuroretinal rim tissue may be more localized or shifted inferotemporally in LTG. Scotomas in early LTG may be situated closer to fixation whereas diffuse visual field damage may be more evident in POAG. Careful studies in cases with apparently normal IOP may reveal that the pressure varies more widely than expected, and there may be systemic disorders to suggest a pathological optic nerve change unrelated to IOP. However, many cases of LTG will be clinically indistinguishable from POAG except on the basis of IOP.

Other Glaucomas. Angle closure glaucoma commonly presents in a mild subacute form that is virtually symptomless and has similar disc and field changes to those seen in POAG and LTG. The IOP in these eyes may be within normal levels when the patient is examined and the condition misdiagnosed as LTG. This diagnostic error is unlikely if gonioscopy is performed.

Steroid-Induced Glaucoma. Some 5% of people experience a large increase in IOP on use of topical steroids.[96] Glaucomatous damage may occur in these susceptible individuals during the use of steroids, but IOP usually normalizes and the progression of the disease is halted with discontinuation of the drug. These cases resemble a nonprogressive form of LTG and the differential diagnosis is made through careful history directed towards uncovering a prior use of steroids, particularly topical applications, and after ensuring that progression has truly ceased.

Glaucomatocyclitic Crisis. Glaucomatocyclitic crisis is an acute, often recurrent form of self-limiting glaucoma that occurs in conjunction with a mild anterior uveitis. Recurrence is rare in subjects more than 60 years old, so that the elderly patient with the condition may attract a diagnosis of LTG unless a careful history is taken. Signs of fine keratic precipitates should be sought to confirm this diagnosis.

Glaucoma Secondary to Uveitis. Trabecular damage may occur in severe anterior uveitis and lead to an increase in outflow resistance with increased IOP.

Although this damage is usually permanent, causing chronically raised IOP, it is possible that some recovery of trabecular function may take place leaving a LTG-like clinical presentation. Clinical evidence of postinflammatory changes in the anterior chamber should alert the clinician to the differential diagnosis in these cases.

Pigmentary Glaucoma. Pigmentary glaucoma may be confused with LTG.[97] In pigmentary glaucoma IOP may be normal between attacks of trabecular obstruction by pigment granules while the disc and fields show damage. With time, pigmentary glaucoma tends to "burn out." The iris pigment in the region of the zonules may be totally lost and the iridolenticular contact altered through miosis of the pupil with age, at which time the IOP tends to return to normal as the trabecular clogging by pigment is reduced. However, the signs of pigment dispersion in the anterior segment, the extremely deep anterior chamber, iris transillumination, and the association with myopia should clearly point to prior episodes of elevated IOP in pigment dispersion syndrome. Gonioscopy will reveal a very heavily pigmented trabecular meshwork, even in the burnt-out cases.

Anterior Ischemic Optic Neuropathy. Anterior ischemic optic neuropathy, or occlusion of the short posterior ciliary arteries, is relevant to a discussion of LTG not only because AION must be differentiated from LTG, but also because it has been thought there may be common pathological mechanisms. The acute form of AION is a disease of vascular occlusion, generally being a consequence of systemic hypertension, diabetes, carotid artery insufficiency, or arterial inflammatory disease[98] and thus is subdivided into arteritic and non-arteritic forms. Its clinical features are a sudden onset, symptomatic visual loss associated with "pale" disc edema (often sectoral) and nerve fiber layer hemorrhaging on and close to the disc. Altitudinal visual field defects are a clinical feature of AION, although it has been suggested that some defects so described are in fact simply dense arcuate defects extending beyond the central field.[17] It is also known that optic disc cupping resembling that seen in glaucoma may develop following arteritic AION.[99] The condition is rarely bilateral at initial presentation although the second eye is involved in a later episode in 40% of cases.[100] On the other hand, it is uncommon for AION to recur in the same eye,[100] so that progression of visual loss beyond the initial acute stage is not likely. Figure 18–5 illustrates the acute stage of AION and the late stage optic disc atrophy that mimics glaucoma.

Since LTG is also associated with glaucomatous cupping, frequent disc hemorrhaging, nonprogressive field loss and has various vascular etiological theories, particularly shock and hemodynamic crises, it is tempting to suggest that LTG represents a minor, subacute or chronic form of AION. Indeed, some cases of sectoral AION have resulted in nerve fiber bundle defects with more than passing similarity to LTG.[73] However, there are some important distinctions both in clinical and histological findings to clearly show that the underlying mechanisms are different (Table 18–4).

1. Nerve fiber loss in AION is more extensive than in LTG and is generally found in the superior region of the nerve head[74] in contrast to the more localized loss in the inferior portion that is typical of LTG.
2. The patterns of field loss show a clear predilection for the superior optic nerve head and papillomacular bundle in AION whereas the inferotemporal region of the disc is the most frequent target in LTG.[71,73]
3. Optic disc edema is present at the onset of AION, whereas even local disc edema associated with disc hemorrhage has not been reported in LTG.

4. Generalized or sectoral optic atrophy without excavation is the rule following AION,[21,73] despite occasional reports of optic disc cupping.
5. Visual acuity and symptomatic field loss are occasionally seen in LTG but frequently occur in AION.[101]

It seems unlikely that LTG and AION share common etiologies. If they had the same mechanism, cases of LTG in one eye and AION in the other would be expected. Instead, it has been postulated that, for anatomical reasons yet to be determined, the superior regions of the optic nerve are susceptible to acute ischemia, while the inferotemporal regions of the disc are sensitive to chronic ischemia.[73] Whether or not chronic ischemia is the result of raised IOP or another factor, the vascular theory of LTG is still consistent with this hypothesis.

Although the differences in clinical presentation are usually clearcut in early cases of AION and LTG, there are also similarities and overlap of the spectrum of signs. It is tempting to suggest that some cases of LTG may represent a minor degree of AION caused by only partial occlusion of major vessels, or occlusion of minor vessels supplying the disc.

LTG is commonly, although not necessarily, bilateral at presentation. AION is rarely bilateral at pre-

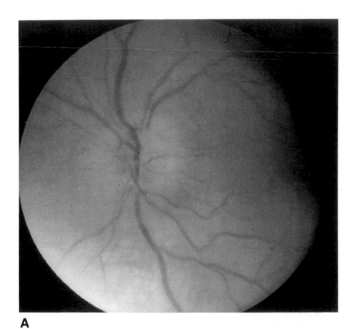

A

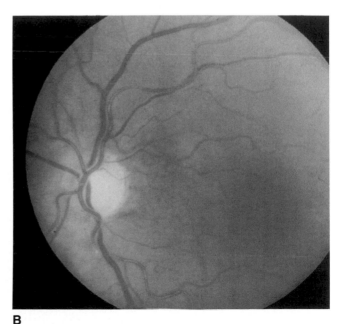

B

Figure 18–5. A. Anterior ischemic optic atrophy (AION) presents acutely as a pale, swollen optic disc, which may be localized to the area representing the watershed of one or more occluded short posterior ciliary arteries. **B.** Following resolution of the acute phase, the disc may assume the appearance of glaucomatous atrophy. Because IOP is within normal limits, a resolved case of AION may be mistaken for low-tension glaucoma. (*See also* Color Plate 18–5.)

TABLE 18–4. DISTINGUISHING FEATURES OF LOW-TENSION GLAUCOMA AND ANTERIOR ISCHEMIC OPTIC NEUROPATHY (AION)[a]

Feature	Description of Most Common Feature	
	LTG	AION
Onset	Gradual	Acute
Progression	Progressive in true LTG only	Varies, but usually nonprogressive
Central visual loss	None early	Commonly severe
Typical visual field defect	Superior	Inferior altitudinal
Disc hemorrhages	On disc margin and inferior most common	Over disc swelling and adjacent retina
Disc contour (initially)	Notched or cupped	Swollen
Disc cupping (long duration)	Inferotemporal, tilting of cup axis	Superior if any
Color of disc	Gray	Pale
Association with temporal arteritis	None	Common

[a] These features are generalizations and should be applied with care in individual cases.

sentation and, if the second eye is involved, this occurs at a later time. Also, LTG tends to be relatively slow in progression and is associated with cupping or notching rather than a swollen disc. Of course, the disc edema in AION is temporary and is followed by optic atrophy so that some time after the attack, it may be more difficult to separate the conditions. Probably some cases of resolved AION are misdiagnosed as nonprogressive LTG.

Compressive Lesions of the Optic Nerve. Pressure and traction of the optic nerve may be followed by a pale optic disc and various degrees of visual loss in the presence of a normal range of IOP. Duke Elder and Scott[102] list the following causes: previous edema of the disc from any cause, pressure or traction from a sclerosed artery in contact with the nerve, aneurysms, bony deformities, tumors of the optic nerve or adjacent tissues, inflammation, and traction during severe exophthalmos in thyroid disease. In many instances, the additional signs and symptoms, or history typical of these conditions will provide the cues necessary to distinguish them from LTG. There may be a need for neuro-ophthalmological consultation where equivocal signs are present in a case with a provisional diagnosis of LTG.

Optic Nerve Trauma. Trauma to the forehead can cause injury to the optic nerve, which is followed by descending optic atrophy. Although the visual loss from such injuries is usually complete, this is not necessarily the case and paracentral field defects may be the only permanent defect.[102] In conjunction with the pale optic disc following atrophy and normal IOP, this condition could be mistaken for LTG. Careful history taking will help avoid this error.

Congenital Disc Anomalies. A number of congenital ocular anomalies give rise to visual field defects or optic disc appearances that could be mistaken for LTG but are accompanied by IOP that remains in the normal range. These include optic nerve head pits (Fig. 18–6), coloboma of the disc, optic nerve drusen (Fig. 18–7), tilted disc (Fig. 18–8), and situs inversus. In classical presentation and when not accompanied by secondary complications, these anomalies should present no diagnostic difficulties.

The appearance of most of these conditions and any associated visual field loss remains stationary, although exceptions to this general rule are seen in optic nerve pits and optic nerve drusen. Optic nerve pits are associated with arcuate visual field defects and the resulting hiatus of the retinal nerve fiber layer provides a pathway along which liquid vitreous may percolate to the inner retina. The consequent retinal edema may cause an additional loss of vision and could be mistaken for progression of optic nerve pathology. Disc drusen may cause progressive field defects and hemorrhage onto the surface of the disc. Small, glistening cyst-like excrescences on the nerve head and a flat or even raised disc contour with little or no physiological cup should suggest the correct diagnosis. However, progression of drusen formation may cause worsening of vision while also complicating the ophthalmoscopic appearance. These may cause the correct diagnosis to be overlooked and LTG to be considered among the alternatives.

Treatment

There is no doubt that IOP of 40 mm Hg and over causes optic nerve atrophy leading to typical glaucomatous visual field defects and that reduction of this pressure to normal values is beneficial in preserving vision. The extrapolation of this benefit to cases of LTG is unproven[103] and there is some evidence of little correlation between survival of visual field and the lowering of IOP in POAG patients with only modest increases in IOP.[104–106] In a report, perhaps more relevant to LTG, Hitchings[107] studied six patients having LTG who had one eye surgically treated to lower IOP while the other eye remained untreated

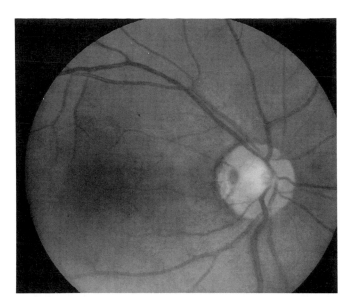

Figure 18–6. Optic nerve head pit. A congenital localized hiatus in the nerve head appears either as a hole or as a plug of glial tissue. This localized absence of axons gives rise to an arcuate scotoma, which could lead to an erroneous diagnosis of low-tension glaucoma in the presence of normal IOP. (*See also* Color Plate 18–6.)

as a control. Follow-up visual field studies suggested no difference in the rate of visual field loss in the operated and unoperated eyes. It is, therefore, difficult to justify treatment of LTG by lowering IOP further, although this is the sole ocular parameter that can be manipulated in this disease. A clinician must find attractive the view, albeit unproven, that lowering the IOP improves the vascular perfusion pressure in the lamina and prelaminar regions of the optic nerve with resulting improved prognosis for the visual field. The objects of treatment are to limit the extent of pathological damage and to help the patient feel that something is being done to this end. At least the latter objective is met by lowering the IOP in LTG.

There are two basic tenets to be satisfied before treatment is undertaken. The first is to ensure that the diagnosis of LTG is correct so that a potentially treatable condition is not overlooked and, the second, to ensure that the disc and field changes are progressing. A full neurological and vascular work-up is advisable when LTG is suspected and, if this proves negative, a carefully managed program of visual field and IOP monitoring should be carried out to determine whether or not the field is stable and to ensure

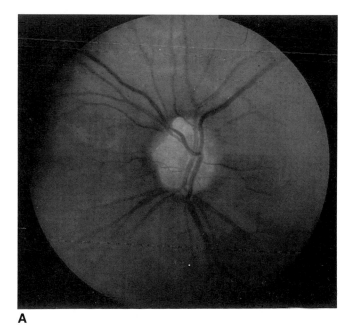

A

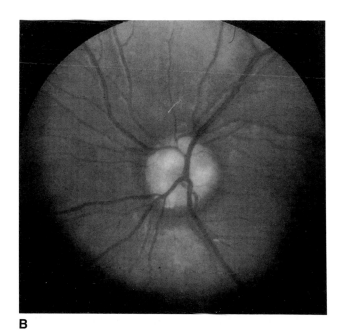

B

Figure 18–7. Optic disc drusen. These deposits within the optic nerve nerve head may be visible as bubble-like excrescences on the surface of the disc **(A.),** or be partly buried and appear as a mildly raised nerve head **(B.).** In some instances the drusen may be totally hidden below the disc surface. Disc drusen are commonly associated with arcuate nerve fiber loss and, because IOP is usually normal, the condition could be mistaken for low-tension glaucoma. (*See also* Color Plate 18–7.)

glaucoma, open angle glaucoma and pigmentary glaucoma with the program Delta of the Octopus perimeter 201. *Doc Ophthalmol Proc Series.* 1987;49:349–363.

79. Anderton S, Coakes RC, Poinooswamy S, Clarke P, Hitchings RA. The nature of visual loss in low tension glaucoma. *Doc Ophthalmol Proc Series.* 1985;42:383–386.

80. Glowazki A, Flammer J. Is there a difference between glaucoma patients with rather localised visual field damage and patients with more diffuse visual field damage? *Doc Ophthalmol Proc Series.* 1987;49:317–320.

81. Hitchings RA, Spaeth GL. Fluorescein angiography in chronic simple glaucoma and low tension glaucoma. *Br J Ophthalmol.* 1977;61:126–132.

82. Krieglstein GK, Langham ME. Influence of body position on the intraocular pressure of normal and glaucomatous eyes. *Ophthalmologica.* 1975;171:132–145.

83. Tsukahara S, Sasaki T. Postural changes in IOP in normal persons and in patients with primary wide open angle glaucoma and low tension glaucoma. *Br J Ophthalmol.* 1984;68:389–392.

84. Brown B, Morris P, Muller C, Brady A, Swann P. Fluctuations in intraocular pressure with sleep. *Ophthal Physiol Optics.* 1988;8:246–248.

85. Kitazawa Y, Horie T. Diurnal variation of intraocular pressure in primary open angle glaucoma. *Am J Ophthalmol.* 1975;79:557–566.

86. Perkins ES, Phelps CD. Ocular pulse amplitudes in low-tension glaucoma. *Klin Monatsbl Augenheilkd.* 1984;184:303–304.

87. Perkins ES, Phelps CD. Open angle glaucoma, ocular hypertension, low tension glaucoma and refraction. *Arch Ophthalmol.* 1982;100:1464–1467.

88. Cennamo G, Reccia R, Pignalosa B, Vassallo P. Low-tension glaucoma: Our clinical experience. *Ophthalmologica.* 1981;183:77–80.

89. Jampol LM, Miller NR. Carotid artery disease and glaucoma. *Br J Ophthalmol.* 1978;62:324–326.

90. Cockburn DM. Signs and symptoms of stroke and impending stroke in a series of optometric patients. *Am J Optom Physiol Opt.* 1983;60:947–953.

91. Christy NP. The anterior pituitary. In: Beeson PB, McDermott W, eds. *Textbook of Medicine.* 14th ed. Philadelphia: W.B. Saunders, 1975:1691.

92. Jordan RM, Kendall JW, Kerber CW. The primary empty sella syndrome. *Am J Med.* 1977;62:569–579.

93. Yamabayashi S, Yamamoto T, Sasaki T, Tsukahara S. A case of "low tension glaucoma" with primary empty sella. *Br J Ophthalmol.* 1988;72:852–855.

94. Winder AI. Circulatory lipoprotein and blood glucose levels in association with low-tension and chronic simple glaucoma. *Br J Ophthalmol.* 1977;61:641–645.

95. Richler M, Werner EB, Thomas D. Risk factors for the progression of visual field defects in medically treated patients with glaucoma. *Can J Ophthalmol.* 1982;17:245–248.

96. Armaly MF. Effect of corticosteroids on intraocular pressure and fluid dynamics. *Arch Ophthalmol.* 1963;70:482–491.

97. Ritch R. Non-progressive low tension glaucoma with pigmentary glaucoma. *Am J Ophthalmol.* 1982;94:190–196.

98. Hayreh SS. *Anterior Ischemic Optic Neuropathy.* Heidelberg: Springer Verlag; 1975:23.

99. Sebag J, Thomas JY, Epstein DL, Grant WM. Optic disc cupping in arteritic anterior ischemic optic neuropathy resembles glaucomatous cupping. *Ophthalmology.* 1986;93:357–361.

100. Boghen DR, Glaser JS. Ischemic optic neuropathy. The clinical profile and natural history. *Brain.* 1975;98:689–708.

101. Beck RW, Savino PJ, Smith CH, Sergott R. Anterior ischemic optic neuropathy: Recurrent episodes in the same eye. *Br J Ophthalmol.* 1983;67:705–709.

102. Duke Elder S, Scott GI. Neuro-ophthalmology. *System of Ophthalmology.* Vol 12. London: Henry Kimpton; 1971:222.

103. Holmin C, Thorburn W, Krakau CET. Treatment versus no treatment in chronic open angle glaucoma. *Acta Ophthalmol.* 1988;66:170–173.

104. Smith RJH. The enigma of primary open angle glaucoma. *Trans Ophthalmol Soc UK.* 1986;105:618–633.

105. Cockburn DM. Does reduction of intraocular pressure prevent visual field loss in glaucoma? *Am J Optom Physiol Optics.* 1983;60:705–711.

106. Schulzer M, Mikelberg FS, Drance SM. Some observations on the relation between intraocular pressure reductions and the progression of glaucomatous field loss. *Br J Ophthalmol.* 1987;71:486–488.

107. Hitchings RA. Low tension glaucoma—Is treatment worthwhile? *Eye.* 1988;2:636–640.

108. Kitazawa Y, Shirai H, Go FJ. The effect of Ca^{2+}-antagonist on visual fields in low-tension glaucoma. *Graefe's Arch Clin Exp Ophthalmol.* 1989;227:408–412.

109. Gillies WE, West RH. Timolol maleate and intra-ocular pressure in low-tension glaucoma. *Aust J Ophthalmol.* 1982;10:183–185.

110. Goldberg I. Argon laser trabeculoplasty and the open angle glaucomas. *Aust NZ J Ophthalmol.* 1985;13:243–248.

111. Epstein DL, ed. *Chandler and Grant's Glaucoma.* 3rd ed. Philadelphia: Lea & Febiger; 1986:421.

112. Pederson JE. Ocular hypotony. *Trans Ophthalmol Soc UK.* 1986;105:220–226.

Chapter 19

ANGLE CLOSURE GLAUCOMA

Thomas Stelmack

Angle closure glaucoma is distinguished from open-angle glaucoma by the location of the aqueous outflow obstruction. A closed angle prevents any aqueous humor from reaching the trabecular meshwork (TM), resulting in an elevation of intraocular pressure (IOP), regardless of the outflow facility of the TM. In contrast, open-angle glaucoma occurs because of an increased resistance to aqueous outflow at the level of the trabeculum, Schlemm's canal, aqueous vein, or episcleral venous plexus. There is no blockage of the flow of aqueous into the anterior chamber angle. The two types of glaucoma, therefore, are quite distinct in their pathophysiology (Fig. 19–1).

Multiple names are applied to this clinical entity. They include general terms such as angle closure glaucoma, closed-angle glaucoma, and narrow angle glaucoma, as well as chronic narrow angle glaucoma, primary angle closure glaucoma, pupillary block glaucoma, creeping angle closure glaucoma, and ciliary block (malignant) glaucoma. Of the generic terms, angle closure glaucoma (ACG) is descriptively more accurate since its scope is sufficient to include closed and previously closed angles, as well as those at risk of closure.

TYPES OF ANGLE CLOSURE GLAUCOMA

Angle closure glaucoma can be initially classified into *primary* or *secondary* forms (Fig. 19–2). *Primary* ACG has a genetic and anatomical basis where *secondary* ACG occurs from some other etiology, i.e., inflammation or cataractogenesis. Each can further be subclassified by whether the block of aqueous flow is occurring primarily at the level of the *ciliary body, pupil,* or *iris*.

Angle closure glaucoma can occur in various stages from prodromal to intermittent (subacute), acute, chronic, and absolute.

RISK FACTORS

Racial and Ethnic Differences

Approximately 2% of the white population will present with narrow anterior chamber angles, although only 5% of these (0.1%) will experience angle closure attacks. Therefore, the examination needs to include a complete battery of tests to identify which

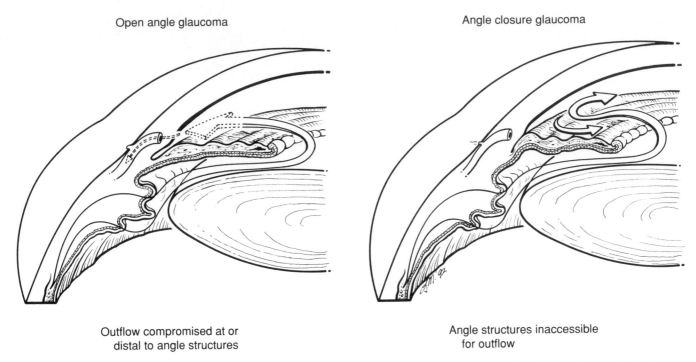

Open angle glaucoma

Angle closure glaucoma

Outflow compromised at or
distal to angle structures

Angle structures inaccessible
for outflow

Figure 19–1. Open-angle glaucoma is characterized by an open inlet with aqueous flowing directly into the angle structures. In ACG, the iris covers the angle structures, not allowing aqueous access to the trabecular meshwork.

narrow angle patients are at greatest risk to develop ACG.[1]

American blacks have a lower incidence of acute ACG than American whites.[1,2] In fact, Central African blacks have no ACG.[3] However, if chronic ACG is included, American blacks and whites have an equal incidence of ACG. This relationship also exists with Asians and other populations with darkly pigmented irides.

Southeast Asians and Japanese are more likely to have angle closure than open-angle glaucoma.[4,5] However, their general incidence is lower than for northern Europeans. South American Amazon Indians[6] have a higher incidence of ACG than American Indians, where it is virtually nonexistent, even though both groups presumably have similar Asian ancestry.[7] Australian aborigines, whose ancestry is Southeast Asian, have no ACG.[8]

With the exception of the Eskimo population of North America, where the incidence is 40 times that

of European descendants living in the same area,[9–13] acute ACG is much less prevalent than open-angle glaucoma. The incidence of angle closure in whites of European descent is 20% of open-angle glaucoma.[14,15]

It should be apparent that when these subpopulations are examined, the genetic and clinical pictures are mixed, and no one definite pattern becomes apparent. This suggests a polygenetic hereditary pattern or one that can be masked.

Environmental factors seem to play a minimal role. Only with the Eskimos of Denmark,[16] where a lower incidence of angle closure exists, can environmental differences be implicated. This assumes that these Eskimos are otherwise genetically similar to those of North America.

Gender, Age, and Histocompatibility

The risk of acute angle closure seems to drop by 50% for each successive generation.[17] Females are affected more frequently except for American blacks where the incidence is equal with men. Most closures occur between the ages of 55 and 65. Of interest, there is no association with HLA typing.[18] Also, a prior history of ACG in a relative offers little prognostic information.

Ocular

When examining biometric characteristics, it becomes apparent that eyes with shorter axial lengths are at

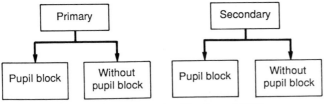

Figure 19–2. The classification of ACG.

greatest risk for developing ACG.[19] As emmetropization attempts to refractively compensate for these potentially hyperopic eyes, smaller radii of curvature for the anterior and posterior corneal surfaces,[20] steeper crystalline lens curvatures, and an anteriorly displaced lens occur. These optical compensatory changes result in a smaller corneal diameter, thicker crystalline lens, and a shallower anterior chamber, physical findings highly correlated with ACG[21] (Table 19–1).

If this correlation were 100%, it would be easy for the clinician to predict which eyes were most at risk for ACG. Whoever met the criteria would receive a prophylactic laser peripheral iridectomy. However, there are non-hyperopic eyes that exhibit these same physical characteristics and also eyes that develop ACG without these anatomical features.

There have been attempts to find either a numerical relationship between specific ocular biometric characteristics that will predict ACG or some other factor that explains why only some eyes with these characteristics go on to develop ACG.[22] Three ratios show the most promise in predicting when an individual with gonioscopically narrow angles may change from the prodromal to an active stage of the disease. Using immersion A-scan ultrasonography, Panek[23] reported that the lens thickness/axial length ratio was the most accurate, and with factoring for age factored in, became even more predictive. Anterior chamber depth/axial length ratio was significant, but less predictive, as was lens thickness at age 20. These ratio studies were done on gonioscopically narrow angles or eyes whose fellow eye had a documented attack of ACG.

The ratios do not resolve the question of accurately describing the phenotype of the ACG patient.[24] Tornquist[22] did find anterior chamber depth to be genetically determined, but this represents only one factor influencing the possibility of an angle closure attack. Theories about close iris-lens apposition[23] and peripheral iris flaccidity[24] as additional contributing factors have not as yet produced good supportive data. The clinician, therefore, should be cognizant of the prevalence of ACG in hyperopic eyes, but as yet still needs clinical observations to judge who is at greatest risk.

MECHANISMS OF ANGLE CLOSURE

Angle closure occurs when all functioning TM is completely blocked from the anterior chamber preventing aqueous outflow. Three basic mechanisms exist that independently or in concert produce this blockage: pupillary block, peripheral iris apposition to the TM/cornea (peripheral anterior synechiae), and anterior displacement of the ciliary body and iris.

Historically, most theories attribute ACG, especially primary ACG, to pupillary block.[25,26] With the exception of Mapstone's controlled landmark studies on pharmacological provocation of angle closure,[27]

TABLE 19–1. MEAN VALUES (WITH STANDARD DEVIATIONS) FOR VARIOUS OCULAR DIMENSIONS OF EYES WITH PRIMARY ACG COMPARED TO NORMAL EYES

Parameter	Normal	ACG	Difference	References
Corneal diameter (mm)	11.76(0.42)	10.85(0.37)	.91	Delmarcelle, et al[19]
	11.05	10.72	.33	Tomlinson, Leighton[21]
Anterior chamber diameter (mm)	12.26(0.54)	11.31(0.67)	.95	Lee, et al[24]
Anterior corneal radius (mm)	7.67(0.24)	7.61(0.29)	.06	Lowe[1]
	7.92(0.29)	7.64(0.25)	.28	Delmarcelle, et al[19]
	7.65	7.55	.10	Tomlinson, Leighton[21]
Posterior corneal radius (mm)	6.46(0.26)	6.23(0.34)	.23	Lowe, Clark[20]
True anterior chamber depth (mm)	2.8(0.36)	1.8(0.25)	1.00	Lowe, Clark[20]
	2.91(0.40)	1 72(0.22)	1.19	Delmarcelle, et al[19]
Lens thickness (mm)	4.50(0.34)	5.09(0.34)	.59	Lowe, Clark[20]
	4.46(0.42)	5.43(0.46)	.97	Delmarcelle, et al[19]
	4.67	5.23	.56	Tomlinson, Leighton[21]
Anterior lens radius (mm)	10.29(1.78)	7.96(0.99)	2.33	Lowe, Clark[20]
Axial length (mm)	23.10(0.82)	22.01(1.06)	1.09	Lowe, Clark[20]
	22.58	22.06	.52	Tomlinson, Leighton[21]
Lens thickness/axial length	1.91(0.44)	2.27(0.29)	.36	Panek, et al[23]
		2.27(0.17)		
Anterior chamber volume (μL)	149.54(35.13)	91.28(24.38)	53.26	Lee, et al[24]

(*Modified from Lowe RF, Lim ASM.* Primary Angle-Closure Glaucoma. *Singapore: PG Publishing; 1989:20.*)

Hence, it is important to aggressively break synechiae with a mydriatic/cycloplegic combination before they become recalcitrant to pharmacological disruption. Once formed, adjacent areas of the pupillary margin are more readily affected by recurrent inflammation, and may lead to enough synechiae formation to cause a pupillary block.

Pupil block may also occur from noninflammatory mechanisms. When the crystalline lens becomes significantly hydrated or the nucleus enlarges during cataractogenesis, phacomorphic ACG results. Following cataract extraction, the vitreous can prolapse anteriorly and block the pupil. Intracapsular cataract extractions may include a prophylactic peripheral iridectomy (PI) or sector iridectomy to reduce the possibility of pupillary block from anterior displacement of the vitreous face. The PI allows aqueous to pass into the anterior chamber if the pupil is blocked. There have been instances where the vitreous is blocking not only the pupil but also a PI site as well, causing angle closure.

Most posterior chamber IOLs are implanted without a PI, since it is felt that the posterior capsule and lens will prevent anterior vitreous displacement. If zonular detachment occurs from blunt or surgical trauma, vitreous can encircle the optic of the posterior chamber IOL and cause a block. This may also occur in cases of blunt trauma where the vitreous extends around the equator of the crystalline lens.

Pupil block may also occur where the offending structure lies anterior to the iris. For example, a crystalline lens may completely dislocate into the anterior chamber and block the flow of aqueous by occluding the anterior surface of the iris. More common are cases of anterior chamber IOLs, which in combination with a small pupil aperture, cause pupil block. A Choyce style anterior chamber IOL, if undersized, can rotate in a propeller-like fashion and block not only the pupil but also the PI. Hence, a double PI separated by a distance greater than the width of the haptic is commonly used. Many of the recent flexible haptic style anterior chamber IOLs do not have this problem due to their narrower haptics.

Anterior lens dislocation from inborn errors of metabolism (homocystinuria), other disorders that weaken zonules (e.g., Marfan's syndrome), and even infectious diseases such as syphilis, can produce pupil block.

Peripheral Iris Apposition

Iris block may occur from a primary anatomical anomaly such as iris plateau configuration or secondarily from inflammation. The primary mechanism of iris plateau configuration is an uncommon laxity that extends from the last iris roll peripherally to the iris root (Fig. 19–4). On pupil dilation, this area of iris will be "bunched" and forced against the TM. Pupil dilation, whether physiological (adrenergic response or due to a dark environment) or pharmacological, will occlude the angle. Since there is theoretically no pupil block occurring, a PI should be of little value for prophylaxis or treatment. In some cases, however, a PI allows the angle to remain open on dilation in a patient with iris plateau configuration. If this treatment mode is not effective, the term iris plateau syndrome is applied.

Secondary mechanisms of peripheral iris apposition can occur from inflammation, repeated angle closure attacks that may be due to pupil block, angle fibrosis, or excessive secretion of Descemet's membrane. In these cases, the angle slowly becomes occluded and the term "creeping" is often applied. Some clinicians distinguish between chronic and creeping angle closure but they represent similar mechanisms. Adhesions form in the anterior chamber angle as the peripheral iris root "creeps" toward the TM or cornea. When a sufficient degree of the angle is compromised, chronic ACG occurs.

Chronic inflammation, such as in sarcoidosis, can cause deposition of inflammatory material that is "sticky" and can result in the formation of peripheral anterior synechiae (PAS). Initial elevation of IOP may occur from an open-angle mechanism, however, when fibrotic tissue invades the angle, a tenacious attachment occurs. With contraction of the fibrin, occlusion of the angle occurs. Eventually all 360° of the angle may be affected.

There are three syndromes where the corneal endothelial cells oversecrete leading to Descemet's membrane extending over the TM. As this membrane contracts, PAS develops with subsequent increase in IOP. These syndromes include essential iris atrophy, Chandler's syndrome, and iris nevus (Cogan-Reese) syndrome.

Intermittent angle closure attacks occurring over time can cause increasing areas of adhesion of the iris to the TM or cornea. Even when the block is broken spontaneously or medically, often some clinical evidence of apposition is present. Areas of pigment clumps at the TM or anterior to Schwalbe's line become important clinical markers indicating previous (a)symptomatic attacks that have remitted. This appearance of pigment is different from the pigment of dispersion syndrome where a homogeneous layering of pigment is seen in the angle rather than clumps.

Neovascularization of the iris may begin at the pupillary frill or in the angle. Once present in the angle, however, fibrosis occurs as it does in the retina and vitreous. This fibrotic tissue contains the newly formed vessels and, as it contracts, functions like a zipper and closes the angle. Treatment lies in eliminating the neovascular etiology by panretinal photocoagulation. Ischemic retinal disease, such as proliferative diabetic retinopathy, is a predisposing factor. Ischemic central retinal vein occlusions can be more devastating because of the relatively short (90 days) time course to neovascularization of the iris.

Anterior Uveal Displacement

Ciliary block (malignant) glaucoma is a complex and not well-understood form of ACG. Hence, its definition has been revised several times. The current criteria include previous acute or chronic ACG, a shallow anterior chamber, an anterior displaced lens, lens- or vitreous-induced pupil block, zonular weakness, thickened anterior hyaloid membrane, anterior rotation or at least thickening of the ciliary body, and posterior aqueous displacement with expansion of the vitreous.[30]

The most common characteristic, however, is the anterior displacement of a geometric plane that includes the ciliary body and iris. The mechanism for this displacement is either anterior rotation/swelling of the ciliary body or anterior vitreous displacement. Another mechanism for anterior uveal displacement is a tumor. A ring melanoma of the ciliary body, as it increases in size, will move the ciliary body and iris significantly forward.

Combined Mechanism

It is possible for a patient with open-angle glaucoma to develop ACG. Chronic miotic therapy will narrow an otherwise open angle.[31] Two theories account for this narrowing, anterior rotation or shifting of the ciliary body, and anterior displacement of a flaccid peripheral iris. The treatment of the glaucoma will be difficult without addressing both components of the glaucoma.

The converse, ACG with an open-angle component, can also occur, especially if there was an inflammatory component to the ACG or the TM was compromised from iris apposition or damaged due to intermittent IOP elevation.

CLINICAL PRESENTATION

Angle closure glaucoma can present clinically through a variety of signs and symptoms that are summarized in Table 19–2. The disease often progresses in four stages: prodromal, intermittent (subacute), acute, and chronic. A fifth stage, absolute

TABLE 19–2. SIGNS AND SYMPTOMS OF ACUTE ANGLE CLOSURE GLAUCOMA

Signs	Symptoms
Conjunctival and ciliary injection	Red eye
Cells and flare	Photophobic
Elevated IOP	Halos/blurred vision
Mid-dilated pupil	Nausea/emesis
Segmental iris atrophy	
Corneal edema	
Glaukomfleken or cataract	
Optic disc congestion	
Central retinal artery	
Pulsation/occlusion	

glaucoma, may occur if the disease becomes recalcitrant to treatment or is left untreated. Figure 19–5 shows how these stages interrelate.

The most common presentation of primary ACG is a series of intermittent or subacute episodes that eventually lead to a lasting acute attack or the slow closing of the angle (chronic angle closure). Chronic angle closure occurs when a sufficient degree of the anterior chamber angle has been closed by PAS.

During the *prodromal stage,* the anterior chamber angle has biometric characteristics making it capable of closure and will often respond positively to provocative testing. Individuals with anatomically narrow angles may progress to the next stage, *intermittent closure,* during which either the entire angle (360°) or part of the angle (incomplete) will close and spon-

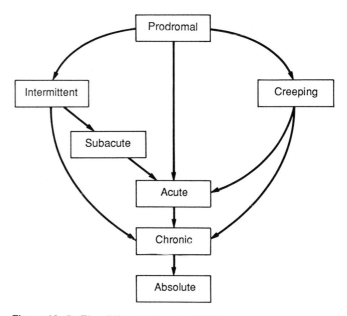

Figure 19–5. The different stages of ACG and how they interrelate.

taneously reopen. *Subacute* attacks may occur with increasing frequency over time, producing greater damage to the optic nerve.

The prodromal and intermittent stages represent the greatest challenge for the clinician. The patient may be asymptomatic or have symptoms that are vague, since the episode will remit spontaneously. A careful history along with gonioscopic and biomicroscopic evidence of closure or risk of closure are helpful.

During the intermittent or subacute stage, symptoms may vary significantly, especially by race. The IOP level, how rapidly the IOP elevated, the patient's threshold of pain, and his or her level of awareness all influence the patient's reaction to ACG. A blue-eyed white with an IOP that has rapidly elevated to greater than 40 mm Hg will often be symptomatic. In contrast, a black or Asian patient with darkly pigmented irides will tend to have less symptoms and may be entirely asymptomatic. The difference may be due to the fact that a black or Asian patient having a subacute attack of ACG is unlikely to have iris ischemia because the iris stroma is thicker and less compromised by elevated IOP. The black or Asian patient may, however, become symptomatic at a higher level of IOP.

The patient's "description" of symptoms during the intermittent stage of ACG will also vary. The classically described symptom of seeing a diffraction gradient in the form of a ring or "halo" around a point source of light (e.g., light bulb) results from corneal edema produced when aqueous is forced through the corneal endothelium into the stroma forming cystic areas of fluid. These cysts produce a prismatic effect similar to what occurs when a rainbow is seen in a waterfall or rainstorm. However, not all corneal edema will be cystic; hence, some patients will complain of having "steamy," "blurred," or "foggy" vision.

To elicit whether these symptoms may have occurred at some time in the past, suggesting a previous intermittent attack, the clinician can present to the patient the analogy of emerging from a heavily chlorinated swimming pool, when on viewing a light bulb, rings of light are seen, or the surrounding area appears as if in a fog. The clinician should keep in mind that nuclear sclerotic cataracts as well as corneal edema from other etiologies may also produce halos.

During a subacute attack, an aching pain is usually felt in the globe and radiates to the temporal area of the head following the innervation pattern of the ophthalmic branch of the trigeminal nerve (CN V1). It results from iris ischemia and inflammation following a rapid rise in IOP. On the other hand, the pain may also be dull, not acutely perceived and there-

fore be ignored. Its absence on history should not exclude the fact that it may have previously occurred. As already stated, blacks and Asians tend to have less pain with intermittent ACG. Sinusitis asthenopia, trauma, and temporal (giant) cell arteritis among others can also produce a similar type of pain.

Conjunctival and ciliary injection may occur in response to iris ischemia and uveitis. Although a red eye has potentially multiple etiologies, this sign in concert with others mentioned can provide helpful diagnostic information. The presence of ciliary injection (flush) as well as a mid-dilated and fixed pupil are corroborative physical findings that support ACG as the diagnosis. Photophobia results from the uveitis, corneal edema, or attempted constriction of an ischemic iris sphincter muscle. This symptom is usually easier to elicit.

Nausea and vomiting can occur from histamine release, changes in parasympathetic tone, or patient apprehension. These symptoms are more common in acute ACG when IOP elevates rapidly in a more sensitive eye, e.g., a blue irides white.

Either prodromal or intermittent ACG can progress to chronic or acute angle closure. In *chronic* ACG, PAS develops throughout the angle usually as a result of previous intermittent attacks of angle closure. Darkly pigmented irides of the black and Asian populations are more susceptible to creeping than intermittent ACG and often progress to chronic rather than acute ACG.

As opposed to the immediate and severe visual loss that occurs in acute ACG, intermittent, chronic, and creeping ACG produce visual field loss similar that seen in primary open-angle glaucoma, often with central vision remaining intact until the late stages of the disease.

Patients with *acute* ACG on the other hand are more likely to be symptomatic (Table 19–2), often arriving in the emergency room or doctor's office presenting with many of the associated signs and symptoms previously described for intermittent angle closure. However, with acute ACG the pain is more intense, and blurred vision from corneal cystic edema is worse, often resulting in a significant loss of visual acuity to a level of 20/80 to finger counting. The gonioscopic view of anterior chamber structures through the cornea is difficult, often requiring the use of a topical hyperosmotic agent, i.e., glycerin (Ophthalgan). Also, the conjunctival and circumlimbal vasculature is injected and the pupil is often mid-dilated and fixed (Fig. 19–6).

Vision loss from acute ACG occurs from both corneal edema and vascular compromise of the anterior optic nerve. Compression of the arterial vascula-

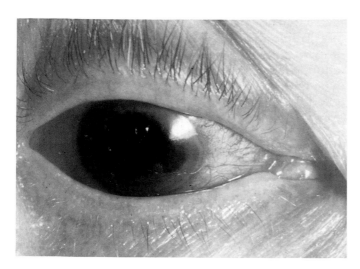

Figure 19–6. An angle closure attack typically presents with a red eye, cloudy cornea, and a mid-dilated pupil. (*See also* Color Plate 19–6.)

ture produces ischemia that may cause disc edema. As IOP continues to elevate, infarction of these vessels can occur. If the IOP approaches the ophthalmic artery diastolic pressure, collapse of the central retinal artery can be seen in the form of pulsation, which makes management of the attack more immediate since central retinal artery occlusion is eminent. The ophthalmic artery pressure is dependent on the status of the internal carotid artery. If perfusion of the internal carotid artery is low, there is a greater chance of occlusion of the central retinal artery during an attack of ACG. Central vision may, therefore, be affected very early during an acute attack. Also, peripheral vision loss is more complete and immediate if left untreated. In contrast, vision loss that results from corneal edema is usually reversible as is that which occurs from optic nerve ischemia if IOP is aggressively lowered.

If there have been previous significant angle closure attacks, segmental iris atrophy may be present from iris ischemia. Also, the lens epithelium may have been damaged, producing subcapsular white flecks called "glaukomfleken" that over time, as new lens fibers are formed, lie deeper in the cortex. In addition, the pupil may be misshapen. Other than documenting previous occurrence, these findings have limited clinical significance.

The initial diagnosis of *ciliary block glaucoma* is difficult, but there are certain features that should immediately alert the clinician to the possibility of this disease. These include previous glaucoma, previous cataract surgery, the presence of vitreal pro-

lapse from surgery or blunt trauma, choroidal detachment (effusion), and cyclodialysis. Ciliary block glaucoma should also be considered when pharmacological management of acute ACG is unsuccessful. Symptoms, however, may not be different from that of acute or chronic ACG.

CLINICAL EVALUATION

Clinical evaluation of ACG is initiated with the assumption that any one of the stages of ACG may be present. This may range from the asymptomatic patient who is at risk because of an anatomically narrow angle to the patient in acute ACG. Either the patient's history, routine slit-lamp examination findings, or the IOP may prompt the clinician to pursue a gonioscopic examination. A patient with acute ACG may need topical glycerin to clear the cornea before an evaluation is possible.

Biomicroscopic evaluation of the anterior chamber angle was first described and correlated to gonioscopy by Von Herrick and Shaeffer.[14] Using the criteria that an angle is possibly occluded at 20° or less, they developed a slit-lamp screening system. An angle of grade 2 or less indicates either possible, probable, or frank occlusion and represents an indication for further evaluation by gonioscopy.

As an alternate screening method when slit-lamp angle estimation is not possible or a bedside examination is required, a penlight-shadowing technique is useful. A penlight is positioned temporally such that it shines across the plane of the iris toward the nasal limbus. If the iris is flat, it will not obstruct the light beam, hence, the nasal limbus will glow. If the iris does obstruct the beam, the limbus will either dimly glow or remain dark depending on the amount of obstruction.

Gonioscopy is done either indirectly with a mirrored system or directly with a prism (Fig. 19–7) (*see* Chapter 8). The most common and easiest goniolens to use are the single- and 3-mirror Goldmann style, which provide an indirect view of the angle. There is no standard system for gonioscopic evaluation and notation. In fact, there are many systems that have been published in the ophthalmic literature, none of which has gained uniform acceptance. However, there is good correlation between various grading systems when experienced observers clinically assess whether an angle is probably occludable.[32] Gonioscopic examination entails assessing what is termed the "approach" to the AC angle, visible angle structures, the shape of the iris, and the amount of angle pigmentation. The angle width (in degrees) is determined by the approach as well as the position of the

CASE 5

This patient is currently an asthmatic taking Atrovent and Theo-Dur. She also has hypertension and diabetes and is using Aldomet, HCTZ, and insulin. She presented with a hemicentral retinal vein occlusion and IOPs of 32 mm Hg OD and 28 mm HgOS. Visual acuities were 20/20 OD and 20/50 OS. A retinal consult was requested and photocoagulation was applied. She was lost to follow-up at that point. On return approximately 2 years later, she had acuities of 20/20 OD and 20/200 OS and IOPs of 18 mm Hg OD and 20 mm Hg OS. Because of her history, she was followed in 1 month with IOPs of 26 mm Hg OD and 25 mm Hg OS. Gonioscopy revealed open angles. The visual field of the right eye revealed suspicious nasal depression while a visual field was not per-

formed on the left eye because of reduced acuity. Both optic nerve heads showed suspicious temporal excavation of the neuroretinal rims. CD ratios were judged to be approximately 0.75 OU.

The decision was made to treat at relatively low pressures and with a reasonable visual field OD because the patient is one-eyed and has a severely compromised systemic status. Treatment was initiated with Betoptic 0.5% bid because of the asthma and has lowered the IOP to 13 mm Hg OU at the last visit. Unfortunately, the patient's blood pressure is out of control with readings from 148/98 to 170/108 and a drop in the pulse rate from 96 to 68. Stabilization of the cardiovascular status by her primary care physician in concert with our treatment is necessary.

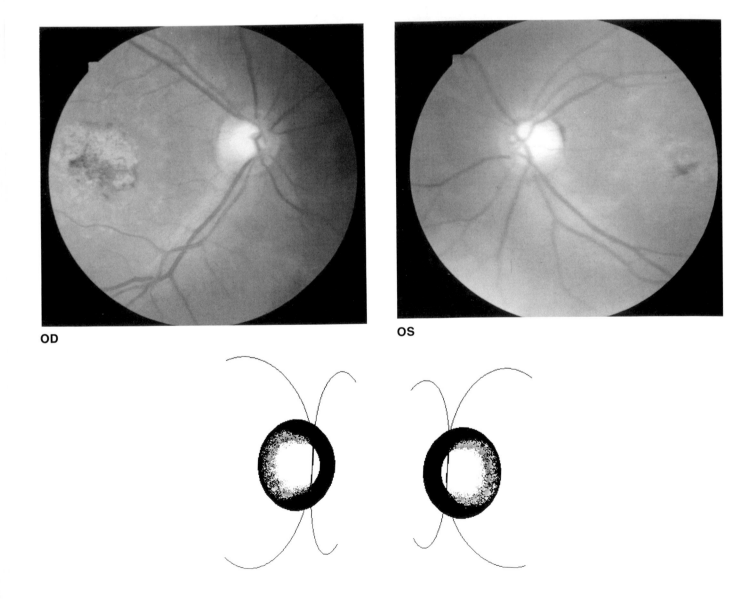

OD   OS

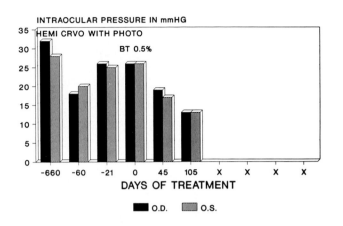

INTRAOCULAR PRESSURE IN mmHG

HEMI CRVO WITH PHOTO

BT 0.5%

DAYS OF TREATMENT

■ O.D.   ▨ O.S.

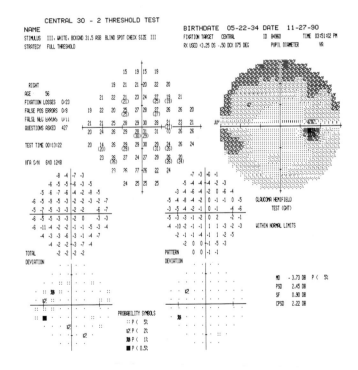

CENTRAL 30 - 2 THRESHOLD TEST

NAME

STIMULUS III, WHITE, BKGRND 31.5 ASB BLIND SPOT CHECK SIZE III

STRATEGY FULL THRESHOLD

BIRTHDATE 05-22-34 DATE 11-27-90

FIXATION TARGET CENTRAL   ID 84960   TIME 03:51:02 PM

RX USED +3.25 DS -.50 DCX 075 DEG   PUPIL DIAMETER   VA

RIGHT

AGE   56

FIXATION LOSSES   0/23

FALSE POS ERRORS   0/8

FALSE NEG ERRORS   0/11

QUESTIONS ASKED   427

TEST TIME 00:13:22

HFA S/N 640 1248

GLAUCOMA HEMIFIELD

TEST (GHT)

WITHIN NORMAL LIMITS

TOTAL DEVIATION

PATTERN DEVIATION

MD   - 3.73 DB   P < 5%

PSD   2.45 DB

SF   0.90 DB

CPSD   2.22 DB

PROBABILITY SYMBOLS

:: P < 5%

▨ P < 2%

▩ P < 1%

■ P < 0.5%

CASE 6   **53-YEAR-OLD BLACK FEMALE**

This patient is taking Premarin, Motrin, and Feldene. She entered our office with the diagnosis of glaucoma taking Betoptic 0.5% bid. At that point, her IOPs were 20/22 mm Hg and 22/18 mm Hg on follow-up. She was then lost to follow-up for 2 years. On return, she presented with IOPs of 20 mm Hg OD and 21 mm Hg OS. Gonioscopy revealed open angles OU. Visual fields showed significant overall depression OD that has progressed over the course of the management with less depression OS initially that has progressed to be similar to OD. The optic nerve heads demonstrate erosion of the rim to the nasal aspect of the disc and a significant notch OD with erosion of the rim

inferior and superior OS. In addition, OS showed an undercutting of the rim. The CD ratio was larger OD than OS and corresponding visual field asymmetry was noted. A significant nerve fiber layer defect can be seen in the right eye as indicated by the two arrows on the photo.

The patient was switched to Betagan 0.5% bid plus pilocarpine 1% qid with a subsequent lowering of IOP that went back up the next visit. Target pressures were in the 16–17 mm Hg range. This patient presents the problems of severe visual field loss, eroded optic nerve heads, and a history of noncompliance. She is scheduled for ALT.

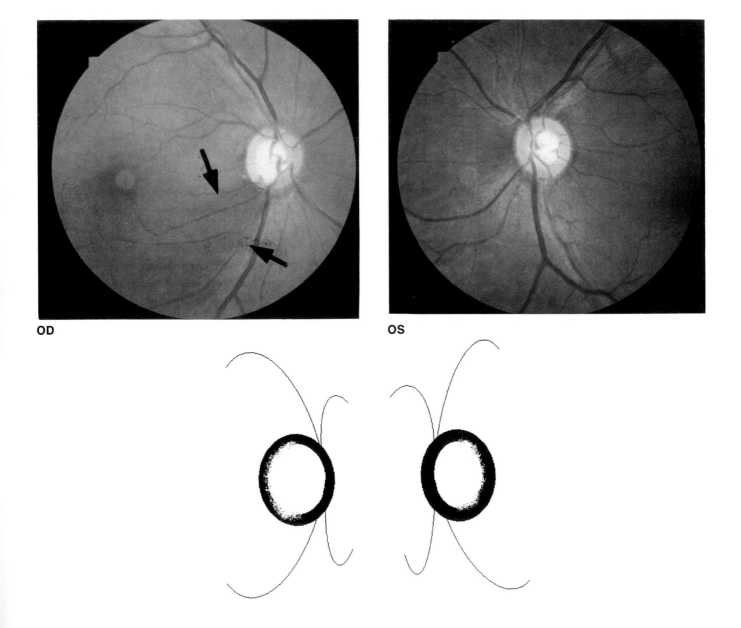

OD   OS

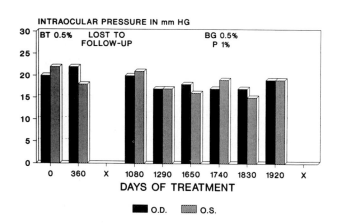

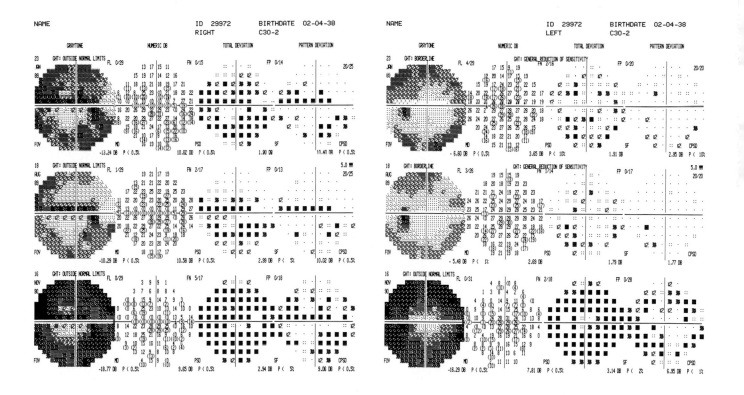

CASE 7   **44-YEAR-OLD BLACK FEMALE**

This patient is currently taking no systemic medication nor does she have any allergies. She presented initially with IOPs of 20 mm Hg OD and 27 mm Hg OS. Visual acuities have remained 20/20 over the course of management. Gonioscopy revealed open angles OU. Initial visual fields showed a generalized depression in the total deviation pattern with mean deviation of 8.68 OD and 11.05 OS. The optic nerve heads were both excavated temporally, which is consistent with the generalized depression of the fields. CD ratios were difficult to judge because of the shape of the discs.

Treatment was initiated at IOPs of 28 mm Hg OD and 33 mm Hg OS with Betagan 0.5% bid. The pressures dropped to 21/25 mm Hg and pilocarpine 1% qid was added. The pressures actually rose to 23/26 mm Hg and the pilocarpine was switched to 2%. Pressures stayed at 22/26 mm Hg so pilocarpine 4% was tried. Pressures hovered around 20 mm Hg for a few months until they finally rose to 26 mm Hg and 28 mm Hg at which time ALT was scheduled for OS. Finally, ALT was performed 180° OD and 360° OS with pressures now at 14 mm Hg OU with continued use of Betagan 0.5% bid and pilocarpine 2% qid. Medical therapy may be modified depending on the behavior of the IOPs. Both blood pressure and pulse have remained steady over the course of treatment.

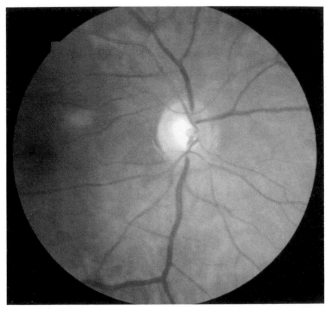

OD

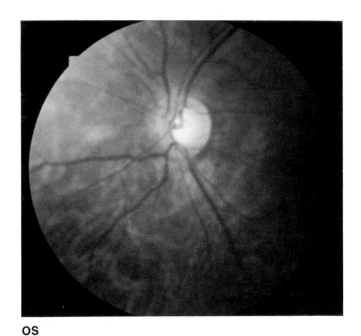

OS

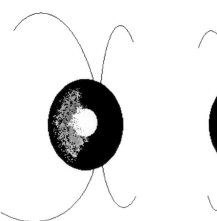
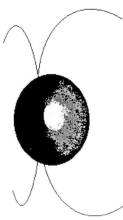

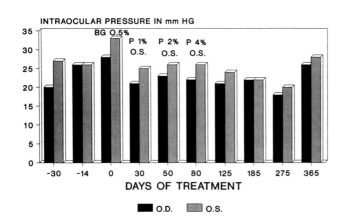

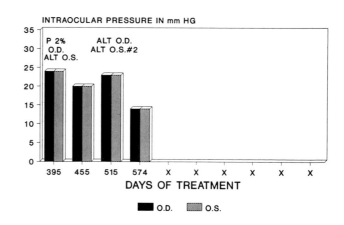

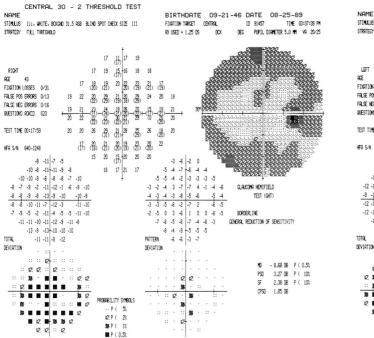

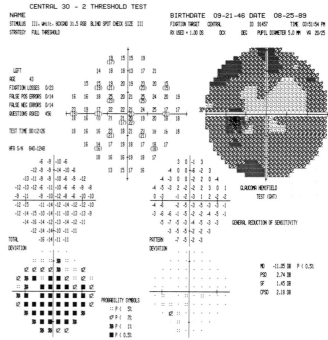

CASE 9   **70-YEAR-OLD BLACK MALE**

This patient is an insulin-dependent diabetic on 20 units of NPH in the AM. He presented with IOPs of 28 mm Hg OD and 30 mm Hg OS. Over the course of management, the patient has had visual acuities in the 20/20 to 20/40 range with mild nuclear sclerotic cataracts. Gonioscopy revealed angles open in all quadrants that have remained that way. Initial visual fields demonstrate severe glaucomatous defects with only limited central vision. The optic nerve heads have severe glaucomatous optic atrophy with severe saucerization. CD ratios were 0.95 OU. The discs and visual fields indicate the necessity to lower the IOPs as far as possible.

Treatment was initiated with Timoptic 0.5% bid with BP RAS at 175/80 with a pulse of 84. The BP RAS has stayed between 135/82 and 156/92 with the pulse at a low of 72 during the entire course of treatment. Timoptic alone did not control the IOP so Propine 0.1% bid was added. This combination did not bring the IOP below 20 mm Hg so ALT was advised first 180° OD then 180° OS. After the initial post-laser IOP rise OU the pressure is running in the 18 to 19 mm Hg range with the use of both Timoptic and Propine. Continued attempts at compliance are necessary. Unfortunately, further ALT may be necessary to get the pressure below the 16 mm Hg range.

A filtering procedure may be indicated soon in this case because of the advanced nature of the glaucomatous damage.

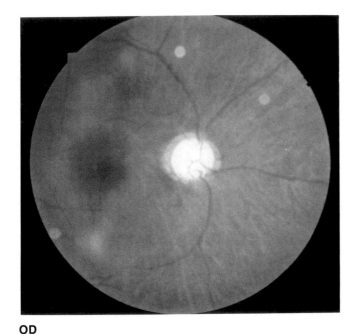

OD

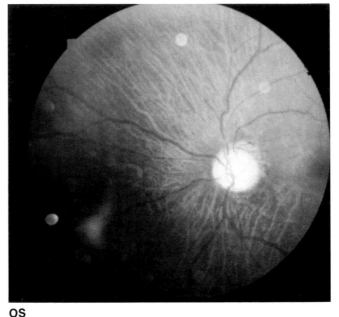

OS

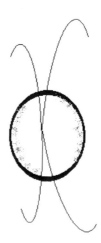

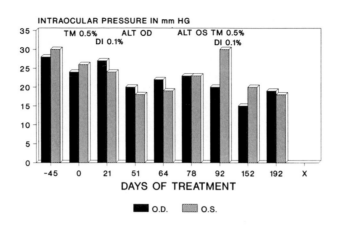

INTRAOCULAR PRESSURE IN mm HG

DAYS OF TREATMENT

■ O.D. ▨ O.S.

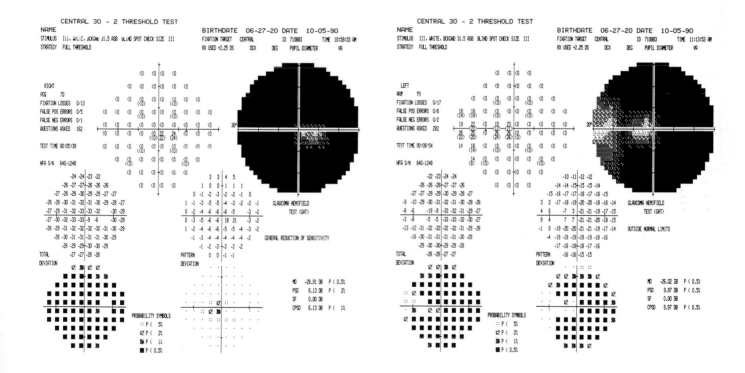

duty to test for
tients than for
dard of care ex
not differentiate
this rather dema
decision of a mu
in the state of V

The case wa
who, at 22 years
lenses by an opl
on numerous o
vision that the
lenses. After aln
ogist performed
tion, determinir
that had reduce
profound impai
physician had l
tonometry durir
his care. He ans
pected of ophtl
testing for glauc
bracket since th
was extremely l
pert witnesses t
at the trial also
below the stand
try was not a t
below 40 years
the ophthalmolc
favor.

The case wa
by the plaintiff,
gist's conduct v
injury, and, in a
tional method c
court reversed tl
The defendant |
theory of "liabil

Although th
of the plain
this alone s
claim. Whe
simple, we
results of tl
ease can be
tion and wh
tected over
should be
though they
within the |

This decisic
among legal and
the case involve

Chapter 21

MEDICOLEGAL ASPECTS OF GLAUCOMA

John G. Classé

Glaucoma has become the subject of considerable legal inquiry, generally acknowledged as the leading cause of large malpractice claims against optometrists[1] and as one of the most frequent causes of claims against ophthalmologists.[2,3] There are several reasons for glaucoma's popularity as a source of litigation: the diagnostic techniques necessary to detect the disease are neither invasive nor time consuming, the medical and surgical management used to control the disease are generally effective, and there are grave consequences for vision if the disease goes undiagnosed and untreated. These factors, combined with the prevalence of the disease, have elevated glaucoma to its position as a leading cause of litigation involving eyecare practitioners.

The majority of legal claims involving glaucoma allege failures of diagnosis, but errors in management have also been the subject of litigation. Before specific clinical and legal issues can be discussed, however, it is necessary to describe the legal basis on which liability can be imposed, the tort of negligence.

NEGLIGENCE

Negligence may be defined as "conduct which falls below a standard established by the law for the protection of others against an unreasonable risk of harm."[4] Proof of negligence in a malpractice case requires the plaintiff (the one filing the claim) to establish, by a preponderance of the evidence, the following four elements[5]:

1. A duty, such as that existing between doctor and patient, that obligates the doctor to conform to a certain standard of care in order to minimize the risk of injury to the patient
2. A breach of this standard of care by the defendant doctor
3. Actual, physical injury to the patient
4. Proximate cause, which is the legal link between what the doctor did (or did not do), and the injury suffered by the patient

Each of these elements must be proven in order for the plaintiff to state a case for which damages may be awarded. Expert testimony must be used to prove elements two, three, and four and, although any of these elements may become the focus of attention at a trial, the most common source of contention in a malpractice case is proof of the breach of the standard of care by the defendant doctor.

A doctor is expected to possess that degree of skill and learning that is commonly found among like

practitioners an(
diagnosis and n
tion.[6] To detern
formed to these
hypothetical ide
son," endowing
fendant with "r
question: "Wha
done under the
the conduct of th
lishes the standa
case, and much
is directed towa
permitted to tesi
would be expect

Because th
through the testi
witnesses are pe
to the exact star
can (and do) var
ing, and viewpc
itself can evolve
peutic skills pro{
of defining the l
a particular case

The evolvin
be illustrated by
occurred in 193{
who was experie
work respondec
offered by a loc;
ined and fitted v
ployed by the
quently to the st
the optometrist
spectacles but, 6
the optometrist
was "completel\
cian, who diagi
tachment secon
woman sued the
that he should l
ferred her for tre
ination. After a
she appealed t
Court. The cour
of the optometr;
to establish tha
pected to diag
course of an ord

In a case k
setts,[8] a patient
with spectacles
his optometrist,
vision. The optc

This case once again illustrates the need to perform tonometry on a routine basis. Other diagnostic tests are also essential, particularly ophthalmoscopy, which often enables an astute clinician to make the diagnosis on the basis of optic nerve changes. Open-angle glaucoma typically progresses more rapidly in one eye than its fellow eye, and differences between the two eyes in cupping of the optic nerve head are often the signal that disease may be present. Such an observation will be greatly facilitated by the use of mydriasis and the enjoyment of stereopsis, which may be achieved through the use of fundus biomicroscopy with a 60-, 78-, or 90-diopter lens. The use of ophthalmoscopy is often of critical importance in suspecting the presence of low-tension glaucoma (see Chapter 18), because this form of the disease does not produce tonometry readings that would alert the clinician to the possibility of optic nerve injury. Assymmetry associated with focal excavation of the cup and field loss that is close to the point of fixation are the diagnostic clues that reveal the possibility of this enigmatic disease.[17]

Likewise, pigmentary glaucoma can pose a significant diagnostic challenge, for the disease is often encountered in patients in their 30s or even 20s. Discovery of pigmentary dispersion syndrome, i.e., Krukenberg's spindle, iris transillumination, and pigment in the anterior chamber angle, should alert the clinician to the likelihood of glaucoma. If suspicious findings are encountered, testing should be performed to rule out the possibility of disease.

In an example case, an optometrist was fitting a myopic young woman in her 20s with contact lenses when he noticed a vertical line of pigment on the endothelium while observing a trial lens through a slit-lamp. He recognized the need to investigate this finding, but the patient had been placed in a time slot for a contact lens fitting and the optometrist decided to dispense the contact lens out of stock, have the patient return the next day for follow-up, and then perform further diagnostic testing. The patient did not keep the appointment, however, and in fact did not return until almost a year had elapsed. At this examination, the optometrist, noting the finding of endothelial pigment, performed ophthalmoscopy, which revealed the patient's cup-to-disc ratio had changed from .2 to .4, and tonometry, which revealed intraocular pressures (IOPs) of 26 and 39 mm Hg. The optometrist referred the patient for treatment, but he was subsequently sued for negligence, with the patient averring that she had not been told of a finding that indicated the possibility of disease, and that the optometrist's failure to communicate the significance of this finding to her prevented her from

seeking care to rule out the presence of pigmentary glaucoma.[18]

To make a definitive diagnosis of pigmentary glaucoma, gonioscopy will be required, as will, of course, ophthalmoscopy and a visual field assessment (see Chapter 17).

In most cases, testing of the visual field is necessary to make the diagnosis of open-angle glaucoma, and it is wise to employ the most sensitive means available, perimetry performed at threshold, when attempting to advise the patient as to the presence of disease.[19] Sensitive visual field testing is also necessary when monitoring glaucoma suspects (discussed later). Routine testing of the visual field, however, is usually limited to screening tests such as confrontation or the tangent screen. Practitioners should not assume that negative screening tests rule out the presence of disease, since patients with open-angle glaucoma often do not evidence a field defect unless perimetry is performed.

Because open-angle glaucoma exists in many different forms, it is appropriate for clinicians to use the full panoply of diagnostic tests available to them, even when examining routine patients, and wise clinicians will employ tonometry, ophthalmoscopy, and visual field testing to rule out the presence of disease. Failure to diagnose open-angle glaucoma, in any form, due to the omission of these tests, will be difficult to defend if litigation should result.

Angle Closure Glaucoma

There are three forms of angle closure (see Chapter 19): (1) the *acute form*, a dramatic, violent attack caused by closure of the entire anterior chamber angle; (2) the *subacute form*, which is of shorter duration and involves closure of the angle for intermittent periods of time; and (3) the *chronic form*, which is a silent, gradual closure of the angle that often mimics open-angle glaucoma. Because of the markedly elevated IOP and potential for significant injury to the optic nerve found in acute angle closure, it is this form of the disease that most often results in litigation.

Misdiagnosis of an angle closure can incur sizable damages. In a representative case, a woman complaining of extreme eye pain, blurred vision, nausea, and vomiting was examined by an intern at a hospital emergency room. Her cornea was so edematous that the intern could not see the fundus. Feeling that a consultation was necessary, the intern contacted an ophthalmological resident by telephone and described the woman's symptoms. The resident diagnosed the condition as conjunctivitis, prescribed a topical antibiotic, and recommended that the intern release the patient without further examination. Consequently, the woman was not seen by an ophthalmologist until 2 weeks had passed, at which time the diagnosis of acute angle closure glaucoma was made and treatment was initiated. Despite undergoing nine surgeries, the woman lost vision in both eyes, and the prednisolone that was administered to relieve her symptoms caused her to develop diabetes. She sued for damages, alleging negligence for failing to make the diagnosis on a timely basis.[20]

Eyecare practitioners may precipitate an iatrogenic angle closure following mydriasis used for the purpose of conducting a dilated fundus examination. Arguments have been proposed, both pro and con, as to the advisability of dilating a pupil where the risk of angle closure is significant.[21] The prevalence of angles susceptible to closure in the general population has been estimated to be 2 to 6%.[22] For these patients, it is the duty of the eyecare practitioner to advise them of the risk of angle closure and to describe for them the benefits to be derived from dilation, so that they may either consent to have the procedure performed or reject it. The legal basis for this obligation to warn on the part of the practitioner is the doctrine of informed consent and, as long as the practitioner has complied with this duty, he or she will not be liable, even if an angle closure occurs.[23] When communicating with patients, practitioners should be certain to comply with specific consent requirements, which vary from state to state (described later).[24] Appropriate documentation should also be employed, either by the use of handwritten entries (Fig. 21–1) or by employing printed forms that are signed by the patient (Fig. 21–2).

If an angle closure does occur secondary to dilation, it will most likely be due to pupillary block,[25] which causes iris bombe′ and the sequelae of closure,

elevation of IOP, and symptoms of pain, nausea, and blurred vision. In these cases, there will be no signs or symptoms until 2 to 4 hours after the patient has left the office. Practitioners must be prepared to respond to complaints from patients who have received dilation and who describe symptoms suggestive of an angle closure. Failure to do so may result in liability. In an example case,[26] the patient of a physician called him several hours after receiving a dilated fundus examination, complaining of headache and discomfort. The physician suggested that the patient take an analgesic and get some rest, but he did not recommend an examination. Because the symptoms persisted, the patient consulted another physician the next morning, who found that the patient had suffered an acute angle closure that required immediate treatment. The patient sued the physician who had failed to examine her.

Discovering the risk of angle closure is not the only situation in which the doctrine of informed consent must be considered. It may also be applicable when a clinician encounters suspicious findings, such as those indicating a patient is a glaucoma suspect.

DUTY TO DISCLOSE SUSPICIOUS FINDINGS

Should a practitioner discover, during the course of an examination, a suspicious finding that indicates the possibility of disease, the practitioner is under a legal duty to make the patient aware of this finding and, if the patient consents, to undertake such additional testing as will be necessary to rule out the presence of disease.[27] This duty is applicable to a finding of elevated IOP.

Patient was informed of the need for a dilated fundus examination because of the 5-year period since her last eye examination, but she declined to have the procedure performed. She was advised of the need to return to clinic without delay if adverse symptoms occur. Otherwise, she is to return for another examination in 1 year.

A

The patient was warned of the need for dilation due to her symptoms of acute onset symptomatic posterior vitreous detachment. She was advised that the only risks of a dilated fundus examination were photophobia and blurred vision of 4 to 6 hours' duration. Despite my recommendation that a dilated fundus examination be performed, she declined the procedure. The symptoms of retinal detachment were described to her and she was advised to return to clinic immediately if they occurred.

B

Figure 21-1. A. Example record entry to document informed consent for a patient who refuses pupillary dilation and has no adverse symptoms. **B.** Example record entry to document informed consent when a symptomatic patient refuses pupillary dilation.

Informed Consent for Dilation of the Pupil

Dilation of the pupil is a common diagnostic procedure used by optometrists to better examine the interior of the eye. It allows a more thorough examination by making the field of view wider and by permitting the doctor to see more of the inside of the eye. Being able to examine the inside of the eye is essential to determining that your eye is healthy.

To dilate the pupil, eye drops must be administered. They require roughly half an hour to take effect. Once your pupils are dilated, it is common to be sensitive to light, a symptom that is usually alleviated by sunglasses. If you do not have any sunglasses, a disposable pair will be provided for you. Another common symptom is blurred vision, especially at near. It will require about 4 to 6 hours for your vision to return to normal. During this time you must exercise caution when walking down steps, driving a vehicle, operating dangerous machinery, or performing other tasks that may present a risk of injury. If you have any special transportation needs, please let us know so that they can be arranged prior to dilation.

In about 2% of people, there is a possible complication of dilation of the pupil; it has been determined that you fall into this category. You must understand this complication before you give your consent to have this procedure performed.

The doctor's examination has revealed that there is a possibility of elevating the pressure inside your eye when dilation is performed. The medical term for this eventuality is "angle closure glaucoma." Because of this possibility, once your eye is dilated and the interior of the eye has been examined, the pressure will be checked again. Should it become elevated, it will be necessary to lower the pressure by administering eyedrops and oral medication. Afterwards, it may be necessary to refer you to an eye surgeon for treatment with a laser to prevent further occurrences of this kind.

Because of the structure of your eyes, it is possible for an angle closure to occur at some other time, when the symptoms may not be recognized and treatment may not be immediately provided. Such an eventuality could seriously affect your vision. Therefore, there is a benefit to you in having dilation performed today and in allowing this complication, if it occurs, to be diagnosed and treated immediately.

The decision to undergo dilation is yours. You may choose not to have dilation performed, but because of your history, symptoms, or examination findings, the doctor recommends that dilation of the pupil be used today to examine your eye for disease. If you have any questions concerning the procedure, please ask them so that we may answer them. Then please sign your name in the appropriate place below to signify your decision.

☐ I understand the risks and benefits of pupillary dilation and I consent to have the procedure performed.

☐ The risks and benefits of pupillary dilation have been adequately explained to me and I understand them, but I do not wish to undergo the procedure.

_____   _____

Date   Signature of Patient

© 1990 John G. Classe

Figure 21–2. Example informed consent document for dilation of the pupil when a patient has a narrow anterior chamber angle.

The law applicable to suspicious tonometry findings was established by a 1979 case brought in the state of Washington.[28] A 54-year-old "severely myopic" woman who was a contact lens wearer consulted an ophthalmologist about problems with her vision, which she characterized as "blurred," with "poor focus," and "gaps" in her visual field. The ophthalmologist performed an examination, during the course of which he performed tonometry, determining that the patient's IOPs were 23.8 mm Hg by Schiotz. Despite this finding, he did not perform a dilated fundus examination or an assessment of her visual field. He attributed her visual problems to her contact lenses and, when asked by the patient if he had checked her for glaucoma, he assured her that she did not have the disease. The patient was seen a dozen times over the course of the next 2 years by the ophthalmologist or his partner, but it was not until the end of this period that she was diagnosed as having open-angle glaucoma "with probable ischemic optic neuropathy superimposed due to increased blood pressure." Despite medical and surgical attempts at management, the patient ultimately ended up with 20/200 acuity and a significant loss of visual field that left her functionally blind.

She sued the physicians for negligence and for a breach of the doctrine of informed consent, and they defended the claim by asserting that the primary cause of the vision loss was a series of strokes that had reduced blood flow to the optic nerve and caused permanent injury. The physicians prevailed at trial and she appealed, but the Washington Court of Appeals affirmed the decision. She appealed again, to the state supreme court, which held in her favor, ruling that the ophthalmologists had failed to conform to the requirements of informed consent. In the written opinion of the case, the court described its rationale for imposing liability.

> The basis for this duty is that the patient has a right to know the material facts concerning the condition of his or her body, and any risks presented by that condition, so that an informed choice may be made regarding the course which the patient's medical care will take. The patient's right to know is not confined to the choice of treatment once a disease is present and has been conclusively diagnosed. Important decisions must frequently be made in many non-treatment situations in which medical care is given, including procedures leading to a diagnosis, as in this case. These decisions must all be taken with the full knowledge and participation of the patient. The physician's duty is to tell the patient what he or she needs to know in order to make them. The existence of an abnormal condition in one's body, the presence of a high risk of disease, and the existence of alternative diagnostic procedures to conclusively determine the presence or absence of that disease are all facts which a patient must know in order to make an informed decision on the course which future medical care will take.[29]

This case drew its share of commentary,[30] because it had obvious implications for the management of glaucoma suspects. Since eyecare practitioners may encounter patients who have elevated IOPs

and no measurable visual field loss, the duty to warn takes on several facets.

First, the clinician must make the patient aware of the significance of the finding and of the diagnostic tests that may be employed to rule out the presence of disease. Since measurement of the visual field is a necessary aspect of this testing, the choice of method by which the visual field will be measured is itself subject to the demands of informed consent. Screening tests, such as confrontation or the tangent screen, are not as sensitive as perimetry performed at threshold, and, if a clinician intends to use these less sensitive tests to assess the patient's condition, the patient must be appraised of this decision and must give an informed consent to have these techniques employed. Otherwise, the clinician is duty bound to refer the patient to another provider who can perform the more sensitive testing. The practitioner's duty is to explain the distinctions between alternative techniques so that the patient understands them. If the patient consents to less sensitive methods (that may be more readily available), the practitioner has fulfilled his duty under the law and may proceed.

Second, the management of glaucoma suspects is itself a matter requiring careful dialogue between practitioners and patients. Within the medical profession, there is a division of opinion as to how glaucoma suspects, i.e., individuals with elevated IOPs and no discernible visual field loss, may best be managed. Some favor continued observation and testing until field loss is measured,[31] while others recommend placing the patient on medical therapy immediately[32] (see Chapter 14). Practitioners must explain these alternatives to affected patients so that they can share in the decision-making process to determine which alternative is preferable for them. Failure to do so can result in a breach of the doctrine of informed consent.

Third, the practitioner who chooses to manage patients and monitor their condition when it is decided that medical treatment is not appropriate, must ensure that patients understand the necessity for periodic testing and must offer a program that is in keeping with the standard of care. Glaucoma suspects must be regularly tested since between 5 and 15% actually develop visual field loss due to the presence of disease.[33] Should glaucomatous changes be detected, the patient should be promptly referred or placed on the medical therapy necessary to arrest the progress of the disease. A small amount of visual field loss, if detected during the course of periodic evaluations undertaken with the consent of the patient, does not give rise to an action for damages because the patient has agreed to run the risk of this small loss rather than be placed on medical therapy. Thus, the practitioner will not be held liable for this resulting "injury."

Of course, the duty to warn is also applicable if tests other than tonometry indicate the possibility of disease, such as suspicious optic nerve cupping observed during ophthalmoscopy or a visual field loss found by perimetry. In any of these instances, the practitioner must communicate the significance of these findings to the patient and offer further diagnostic testing. Furthermore, the practitioner would be well advised to carefully document these communications in the patient's record, so that the record reflects the agreement reached between the two parties as to the care to be offered. Failure to provide supporting documentation can be a fatal flaw in the defense of a liability claim.[34]

NEGLIGENCE IN MANAGEMENT

Even though a practitioner makes the correct diagnosis and institutes treatment, there can still be liability if therapy is negligently performed or if necessary therapy is omitted. Claims alleging negligent management of open-angle glaucoma generally fall into three categories: (1) improper therapeutic regimen, (2) failure to monitor IOP on a periodic basis, and (3) inadequate or improper disclosures concerning care. Of course, failure to conform to the standard of care in other areas of management can also lead to liability.[35]

Improper Therapeutic Regimen
A practitioner is expected to select the regimen that is appropriate for the patient's condition. If an unreasonable course of therapy is chosen, the practitioner will be liable for any resultant injury to the patient. When drug therapy is instituted, the practitioner must use the appropriate concentration and dosage and must ensure that there is no unreasonable risk of injury to the patient due to adverse effects. In an example case,[36] a 5-diopter myope who had been on topical drug therapy for open-angle glaucoma was changed to echothiophate iodide. About 3 weeks after he began using the drug, he noticed spots in his field of vision and, 4 days later, he experienced the classical symptoms of a retinal detachment. Because the physicians who treated him were not immediately available, he had to wait a week before receiving an examination, which revealed that the detachment had progressed to involve the macula, greatly reducing his visual acuity. After surgery was unable to restore his vision, he filed suit, alleging that a non-

miotic drug should have been used, since for myopic patients such as himself the risk of retinal detachment was significant.

In another case,[37] a woman whose bilateral glaucoma had been successfully treated for years with acetazolamide and the usual topical antiglaucoma medications developed kidney stones, a known complication of the acetazolamide. After surgery was performed to remove the calculi, she was placed on a regimen of topical drugs only, and her IOPs were well controlled without the acetazolamide. She filed suit, alleging that a systemic drug with known complications such as acetazolamide should not have been used until it had been established that topical drugs could not effectively control her IOP.

Failure to Monitor IOP on a Periodic Basis
Since the control of IOP is an integral aspect of drug therapy, failure to monitor IOP on a periodic basis, if this failure results in injury to the patient, can create liability. In this regard, a practitioner is expected to examine a patient with sufficient frequency to stay abreast of the case, and this issue was the basis for a 1955 lawsuit in the state of Washington.[38] A woman who had suffered recurring subacute angle closures was hospitalized following an automobile accident and, four days after admission, she complained of intense pain in one eye. She was examined by an ophthalmologist, who measured the IOP in the affected eye to be about 50 mm Hg by Schiotz tonometry and prescribed miotics to alleviate the condition. Over the course of the next 2 weeks, the physician took tonometry readings that indicated her IOP had dropped to about 30 mm Hg. Following the last reading, the ophthalmologist was out of town for several days and, during this interval, the woman experienced a loss of vision due to an acute angle closure, with her eye suddenly becoming what she described as "stony hard." She was dismissed from the hospital without further treatment but soon thereafter consulted another practitioner, who performed surgery on the eye. The loss of vision was permanent, however, and she brought suit against the ophthalmologist, alleging that he had breached the standard of care by "failing to attend her in a manner consistent with the demands of her condition."

Practitioners who anticipate being absent while patients require on-going care should provide for a substitute during the period of absence. Patients should receive adequate notice that the substitute is available, and the substitute should be prepared to manage these patients as circumstances dictate.

In another case involving an ophthalmologist,[39] a woman suffering from chronic bilateral iritis was given topical and systemic steroids and atropine, but, after 2 months of use, she began to see flashing lights, wavy lines, and spider webs. She returned for evaluation, receiving an "eye injection" as treatment. Her difficulties persisted, and she began to feel "pressure" in one eye, yet at three examinations over the course of the next month the physician failed to measure her IOPs, choosing instead to increase her medication. Four days after the last examination, she returned again, complaining of intense eye pain, and the diagnosis of acute angle closure glaucoma was made. It was then discovered that the pharmacist who had filled the ophthalmologist's prescription had mistakenly provided the patient with isoptocarpine rather than atropine. The woman filed suit against the pharmacist and the physician, alleging in part that the physician had been negligent in failing to test her IOP and detect the dangerous condition created by the incorrect drug.

At follow-up examinations, clinicians should endeavor to determine if patients have been using their medication in the prescribed manner and with the frequency desired.

Inadequate or Improper Disclosures

Because of the doctrine of informed consent, a practitioner is under a legal duty to disclose to a patient the expected or unexpected risks of a procedure, the alternative methods of treatment that are available, and the conditions that could be reasonably anticipated if the patient fails to give his consent. Whenever medical or surgical management of glaucoma is necessary, practitioners should be certain to communicate these matters to patients (and to document that they have done so).

When describing the risks of treatment, the practitioner does not have to discuss risks that are remote. A case can be used to illustrate the distinction between common and remote risks.[40] A woman with open-angle glaucoma was treated with acetazolamide and developed bruising, which is an early sign of aplastic anemia, an extremely rare side effect of the drug. She allegedly informed the ophthalmologist who had prescribed the acetazolamide of this development, but he had her continue use of the medication. The patient eventually was diagnosed as having aplastic anemia. She sued the ophthalmologist for negligence, alleging that he should have warned her of this remote but serious side effect of acetazolamide. The physician testified that acetazolamide was commonly used for treatment in cases such as hers, that he had warned her of the common side effects of the drug, and that he was not required to advise her of every possible adverse effect since that

could result in poor compliance with medical therapy. He also denied that she had reported the bruising to him. After a trial, the jury found in his favor.

In states that have adopted the "professional community rule,"[a] a practitioner is expected to divulge that same degree of information as would ordinarily be divulged in the professional community by practitioners acting under the same or similar circumstances. Thus, the standard is established by what practitioners customarily do.[41]

In states that have adopted the "reasonable patient rule,"[b] a practitioner must divulge such information as would allow a reasonable patient to make an informed decision as to whether to undergo the course of therapy involved.[42] This standard is determined by the patient's need to know information that is material to his ability to make a decision rather than by what practitioners customarily do.

Practitioners should be aware of the particular rule that is applied in their jurisdiction, for failure to observe it can lead to liability. The worse situation is one in which the practitioner makes misleading statements or uses silence to prevent making disclosures. In such cases, the practitioner's conduct may be construed as fraud. A sample case[43] may be used to illustrate the importance of such a determination.

A man of Dutch extraction went to an ophthalmologist complaining of an ocular foreign body. The physician told him that the pressure in the eye was elevated and performed "simple surgery" to alleviate the condition. Despite these efforts, the patient eventually lost his sight in the eye, a result that the physician attributed to progression of the glaucoma. Seeking a second opinion, the man consulted another ophthalmologist, who concurred with the diagnosis and treatment rendered by the first physician. Eight years later, during the course of an examination by a third ophthalmologist, the patient learned that he did not have glaucoma and that the condition from which he suffered could have been alleviated and his vision

---

[a] As of 1981, jurisdictions following the "professional community rule" are: Alabama, Arizona, Arkansas, Colorado, Delaware, Florida, Georgia, Hawaii, Idaho, Illinois, Indiana, Kansas, Massachusetts, Michigan, Mississippi, Missouri, Montana, Nebraska, New Hampshire, New Jersey, New York, North Carolina, North Dakota, Oregon, Tennessee, Texas, Utah, Vermont, Virginia, and Wyoming. (*See* Rosoff AJ. *Informed Consent: A Guide for Health Care Practitioners.* Rockville, MD: Aspen; 1981.)

[b] As of 1981, jurisdictions following the "reasonable patient" rule are: Alaska, California, District of Columbia, Kentucky, Louisiana, Maryland, Minnesota, New Mexico, Ohio, Oklahoma, Pennsylvania, Rhode Island, Washington, and Wisconsin. (*See* Rosoff AJ. *Informed consent: A Guide for Health Care Practitioners.* Rockville, MD: Aspen; 1981.)

spared if the appropriate diagnosis and treatment had been received earlier. He brought a lawsuit against the two ophthalmologists, alleging that they had been negligent, and they defended the claim on the basis of the statute of limitations. After the case was dismissed on this basis by the trial court, the man appealed, arguing that the ophthalmologists had made misrepresentations that had prevented him from determining their culpability. The appellate court reinstated the case, even though the lawsuit was filed 10 years after the physicians had examined the patient, holding that their affirmative misrepresentations had tolled, i.e., stopped, the running of the statute of limitations.

One important disclosure that should not be neglected is the risk of incurring open-angle glaucoma secondary to the use of certain drugs applied for therapeutic purposes.

DUTY TO WARN OF THE ADVERSE EFFECTS OF DRUG THERAPY

Open-angle glaucoma is a known complication of various kinds of drug therapy (*see* Chapter 17). Once again, the doctrine of informed consent obligates practitioners to make the appropriate disclosures to patients, and the standard of care requires practitioners to examine patients with sufficient frequency to detect these complications before serious injury occurs.

In a typical case,[44] a hairdresser who was allergic to some of the dyes used at work consulted an ophthalmologist, seeking relief from the watering, redness, and itching of the allergy. The physician prescribed topical steroids, and their use considerably diminished the patient's symptoms, to the extent that she continued to use the steroids for a period of almost 2 years, at the conclusion of which time it was found that she had developed bilateral cataracts and

bilateral glaucoma. She sued the ophthalmologist, alleging that he had been negligent for allowing her to obtain prescription refills over such a lengthy period of time and that he had breached the doctrine of informed consent by failing to warn her of the potential adverse effects of long-term topical steroid therapy.

In a similar case,[45] a young child who was suffering from conjunctivitis was taken by her mother to a pediatrician, who prescribed an antibiotic-steroid combination to alleviate her symptoms. The mother used the ointment intermittently over the course of the next 2 years to treat the child, refilling the prescription six times. During this period of time, the child was seen by the pediatrician, but at none of the examinations did he assess her IOPs or suggest that the child be seen by an eyecare practitioner for that purpose. The child developed bilateral open-angle glaucoma that severely eroded her field of vision. She sued the pediatrician for failing to monitor the effects of the drug.

Prescriptions for medications with known side effects, such as steroids, should be carefully controlled, particularly with respect to refills. The number of allowable refills should be written on the prescription, as should the statement "Changes in refill instructions are not permitted without the approval of the prescriber." Copies of prescriptions should be retained in patients' records. Warnings should be issued to patients when long-term therapy is anticipated, and these communications should likewise be documented and retained.

RECORDKEEPING

The preceding discussion has identified several clinical steps that, if followed, will diminish the likelihood of a legal claim (Table 21–1).

If litigation should occur, a practitioner's records will be subjected to scrutiny during legal proceed-

---

TABLE 21–1. CLINICAL PROCEDURES THAT MINIMIZE LIABILITY FOR GLAUCOMA

Perform tonometry as a routine procedure.

Use ophthalmoscopy to compare the optic nerveheads. Whenever possible, use fundus biomicroscopy to employ the advantages of stereopsis.

Periodically assess the visual field, even in routine patients.

If suspicious findings are incurred during the course of an examination, discuss them with the patient and perform such follow-up testing as is appropriate to rule out the presence of disease.

Conform to the requirements of the doctrine of informed consent when discussing management options with glau-

coma suspects. If periodic visual field testing is performed, use the most sensitive means available (i.e., perimetry testing at threshold) or refer the patient to another practitioner who can provide this testing.

Follow accepted drug therapies when managing glaucoma patients.

Warn patients of the expected adverse effects of drug therapy and monitor patients with sufficient frequency to detect complications before they cause significant injury.

Document all test results, important communications, and recall and referral appointments in the patient's record.

ings.[46] There are three essential aspects of care that require adequate documentation: (1) examination findings, (2) warnings and instructions, and (3) recalls and referrals. Failure to document these aspects of patient care can seriously impair the defense of a negligence claim.

Examination Findings

When recording examination findings, practitioners should endeavor to use descriptive terminology rather than words or abbrevations that provide no information, such as "normal," "unremarkable," and "WNL" (within normal limits). Since assessment of the optic nerve is an important part of the examination for glaucoma, the written description should include cup-to-disc ratio (".3/.4"), an evaluation of the nervehead rim ("NRRI", which means "neuroretinal rim intact"), color ("no pallor"), and distinctness of the nervehead margins ("margins distinct"). Concentric or focal excavations of the nervehead, asymmetry of cup-to-disc, and other significant findings should be supplemented with drawings, photographs, or word descriptions. Tonometry findings should include the instrument used (if more than one type of instrument is commonly used for testing), the time of measurement, and the actual readings (if more than one reading is taken). Visual fields are highly subjective in nature, and screening fields should contain a notation as to the reliability of the responses ("patient could not appreciate blind spot"). Likewise, difficulties noted during perimetry should be recorded ("patient frequently moved eyes from fixation"). The use of descriptive terminology greatly strengthens a practitioner's defense of a liability claim.[47]

Warnings and Instructions

Because of the doctrine of informed consent, communication with the patient is necessary when suspicious findings are encountered, when alternatives to treatment are available, and when there are common risks of treatment (especially with drug therapy). Practitioners may document informed consent either through handwritten entries or through the use of printed forms, but it is essential that one of these alternatives be chosen whenever elevated IOPs are discovered, patients must be monitored as glaucoma suspects, pupillary dilation is required for patients with extremely narrow angles, medical therapy with common side effects must be used, or other circumstances necessitating disclosures are encountered. Failure to document the patient's consent to proceed with diagnosis or treatment, if an adverse result occurs, greatly handicaps a practitioner's defense.[48]

Recalls and Referrals

If a patient must return for follow-up, the appointment should be scheduled before the patient has left the office, even if the date of the appointment is several months away. The patient's record should contain a notation that a recall appointment has been scheduled and describe the purpose of the appointment ("RTC 6-6-91 for tonometry, fields, and ophthalmoscopy"). The patient should be contacted by telephone or mail shortly before the scheduled date as a reminder of the appointment. If a patient fails to keep a recall appointment, it is not the optometrist's legal duty to contact the patient to schedule another appointment but, in cases in which a patient is suspected of having disease or is being treated for disease, it is wise to do so.[49] The second appointment should be duly recorded and, if the patient again fails to appear, further effort on the part of the optometrist will depend on the circumstances. In extraordinary cases, it may be necessary to send the patient a letter, describing the necessity for examination and informing the patient that loss of vision may occur unless follow-up care is provided. If a patient must be referred to another practitioner, the optometrist and patient should determine the specific practitioner and an appointment should be made for a specific date and time. The identity of the practitioner and the date of the examination should be documented in the patient's record. If a patient fails to see the practitioner, again the optometrist has no further legal responsibility but, if the circumstances warrant, may choose to contact the patient to schedule another appointment. In rare cases, a letter admonishing the patient to keep a referral appointment may be appropriate.

It is advisable to use the problem-oriented recordkeeping system[50] since it is well accepted by both the legal and the medical professions, is efficient, and lends itself to episodic care such as is found in the follow-up of glaucoma suspects or of patients receiving medical therapy. Although recordkeeping can become burdensome at times, its importance should not be underestimated by practitioners. Adequate recordkeeping will often be a defendant practitioner's shield, while inadequate records will prove to be his Achille's heel. The importance of adequate recordkeeping cannot be overemphasized.

REFERENCES

1. Classé JG. Standards of care when diagnosing or treating the glaucomas. *Optom Clin.* 1991;1(1):192–204.
2. Bettman JW. A review of 412 claims in ophthalmology. *Int Ophthalmol Clin.* 1980;20:133.

3. Bettman JW. Seven hundred medicolegal cases in ophthalmology. *Ophthalmology*. 1990;97:1379–1384.

4. *Black's Law Dictionary*. 4th ed. St. Paul, Minn: West;1968.

5. Prosser WL. *Law of Torts*. 4th ed. St. Paul, Minn: West;1971:31.

6. Prosser WL. *Law of Torts*. 4th ed. St. Paul, Minn: West;1971:149–150.

7. *Hampton v Brackin's Jewelry and Optical Co., Inc.*, 237 Ala. 212, 186 So. 173 (1939).

8. *McMahon v Glixman*, 393 N.E.2d 875 (1979).

9. Duke-Elder S, Jay B. Diseases of the lens and vitreous. In: *System of Ophthalmology*. St. Louis: C.V. Mosby; 1969:392–398.

10. National Society to Prevent Blindness. *Vision Problems in the United States*. New York: National Society to Prevent Blindness; 1980.

11. *Helling v Carey*, 83 Wash.2d 514, 519 P.2d 981 (1974).

12. 519 P.2d at 981.

13. Wechsler S, Classé JG. *Helling v Carey*: Caveat medicus (Let the doctor beware). *J Am Optom Assoc*. 1977;48:1526–1529.

14. Godio L, Ruskiewicz J, Chao W. The impact of a court decision on the actual practice of eye care. *Am J Optom Physiol Optics*. 1982;59:267–270.

15. Classé JG. *Helling* revisited: How the "tale" wagged the dog. *J Am Optom Assoc*. 1987;58:343–345.

16. *Whitt v Columbus Cooperative Enterprises, Inc.*, 64 Ohio St.2d 355, 415 N.E.2d 985 (1980).

17. Alexander LJ, Fingeret M, Jennings BJ, Thimons JJ. Grand rounds: Low tension glaucoma. *Optom Clin*. 1991;1(1):255–265.

18. Classé JG. A review of 50 malpractice claims. *J Am Optom Assoc*. 1989;60:694–706.

19. Classé JG. Legal aspects of visual field assessment. *J Am Optom Assoc*. 1989;60:936–938.

20. *Kim v New York Hospital*, 25 ATLA Law Rep 328 (1982).

21. Bartlett JD. Dilation of the pupil. In: Bartlett JD, Jaanus SD, eds. *Clinical Ocular Pharmacology*. 2nd ed. Boston: Butterworths; 1989:400–407.

22. Cockburn DM. Prevalence and significance of narrow anterior chamber angles in optometric practice. *Am J Optom Physiol Optics*. 1981;58:171–175.

23. Classé JG. *Legal Aspects of Optometry*. Boston: Butterworths; 1989:300–301.

24. Rosoff AJ. *Informed Consent: A Guide for Health Care Providers*. Rockville, Md: Aspen; 1981;75–185.

25. Fingeret M, Kowal D. Acute glaucomas: Diagnosis and treatment. *Optom Clin*. 1991;1(1):165–191.

26. Bettman JW. A review of 412 claims in ophthalmology. *Int Ophthalmol Clin*.1980;20:132.

27. Ravzi E. Informed consent in Washington: Expanded scope of material facts that the physician must disclose to his patients. *Washington Law Rev*. 1980;55:655.

28. *Gates v Jensen*, 92 Wash.2d 246, 595 P.2d 919 (1979), reversing 20 Wash. App. 81, 579 P.2d 374 (1978).

29. *Gates v Jensen*, 92 Wash.2d 246, 595 P.2d 922–923 (1979), reversing 20 Wash. App. 81, 579 P.2d 374 (1978).

30. Thal L. *Gates v Jensen*: Another precedent for glaucoma testing. *J Am Optom Assoc*. 1981;52:349–353.

31. Chandler PA, Grant WM. Ocular hypertension versus open-angle glaucoma. *Arch Ophthalmol*. 1977;95:585–586.

32. Phelps CD. Ocular hypertension: To treat or not to treat? *Arch Ophthalmol*. 1977;95:588.

33. Eskridge JB. Ocular hypertension or early undetected glaucoma? *J Am Optom Assoc*. 1987;58:747–766.

34. Louisell DW, Williams H. *Medical Malpractice*. New York: Matthew Bender; 1978:185.

35. Bettman JW. A review of 412 claims in ophthalmology. *Int Ophthalmol Clin*. 1980;20:132.

36. *Weaver v Grace*, 21 ATLA Law Rep 64 (1978).

37. Bettman JW. A review of twenty-two medicolegal claims. How they might have been avoided. *Surv Ophthalmol*. 1983;28:54.

38. *Hurspool v Ralston*, 290 P.2d 981 (1955).

39. *Harris v Groth*, 99 Wash.2d 438, 663 P.2d 113 (1983).

40. *Tarter v Linn*, 578 A.2d 453 (Pa. Super 1990).

41. Rosoff AJ. *Informed Consent: A Guide for Health Care Providers*. Rockville, Md: Aspen; 1981;33–38.

42. Rosoff AJ. *Informed Consent: A Guide for Health Care Providers*. Rockville, Md: Aspen; 1981;38–41.

43. *van Bronckhorst v Taube*, 341 N.E.2d 791 (Ind. App. 1976).

44. Bettman JW. A review of 412 claims in ophthalmology. *Int Ophthalmol Clin*. 1980;20:59.

45. *Aetna Casualty and Surety Co. of Illinois v. Medical Protective Co. of Ft. Wayne, Ind.*, 575 F.Supp. 901 (Ill. 1983).

46. Classé JG. *Legal Aspects of Optometry*. Boston: Butterworths; 1989:215–233.

47. Classé JG. A review of 50 malpractice cases. *J Am Optom Assoc*. 1989;60:697.

48. Classé JG. *Legal Aspects of Optometry*. Boston: Butterworths; 1989:295–301.

49. Classé JG. *Legal Aspects of Optometry*. Boston: Butterworths; 1989:194–195.

50. American Optometric Association. *Scope of Practice: Patient Care and Management Manual*. St. Louis: American Optometric Association; 1986.

Index

Page numbers followed by *f* refer to figures and by *t* to tables.

Page numbers followed by f refer to figures and by t to tables.

Page numbers followed by *f* refer to figures and by *t* to tables.

Page numbers followed by *f* refer to figures and by *t* to tables.

Page numbers followed by *f* refer to figures and by *t* to tables.

Page numbers followed by *f* refer to figures and by *t* to tables.

Page numbers followed by *f* refer to figures and by *t* to tables.